LESLIE BECK'S NUTRITION GUIDE TO MENOPAUSE

Leslie Beck, a registered dietitian, is a leading nutritionist who has helped over 2000 individuals achieve their nutrition and health goals. She is the bestselling author of *Managing Menopause with Diet, Vitamins and Herbs, Leslie Beck's Nutrition Guide for Women, Leslie Beck's Nutrition Encyclopedia,* and *Leslie Beck's 10 Steps to Healthy Eating* and is a contributing author in *Rose Reisman's Sensationally Light Pasta & Grains.* Leslie writes nutrition articles for national magazines, is the nutrition expert for CTV's *Canada AM*, and is host of the Discovery Channel's *Foodstuff,* a daily nutrition program aired nationally.

Leslie has worked with many of Canada's leading businesses and international food companies. She regularly delivers nutrition workshops to corporate groups in Toronto and Vancouver. Having a strong interest in sports nutrition, Leslie acts as nutrition consultant to the Toronto Raptors and has worked with the Canadian International Marathon (1995–1997.) She often holds nutrition workshops for Toronto's marathon and running clinics. Leslie keeps fit herself by running, cycling, and weight training.

Born and raised in Vancouver, B.C., Leslie obtained her bachelor of science (dietetics) from the University of British Columbia and proceeded to complete the dietetic internship program at St. Michael's Hospital in Toronto. She is a member of the Dietitians of Canada, the College of Dietitians of Ontario, and the Consulting Dietitians of Ontario. She lives in Toronto.

Visit Leslie Beck's website at **www.lesliebeck.com**.

Also by Leslie Beck

Leslie Beck's 10 Steps to Healthy Eating

Leslie Beck's Nutrition Guide for Women

Leslie Beck's Nutrition Encyclopedia

Leslie Beck's
Nutrition Guide to Menopause

Natural Strategies with Diet, Vitamins and Herbs

Leslie Beck, RD

VIKING
CANADA

VIKING CANADA
Published by the Penguin Group
Penguin Books, a division of Pearson Canada, 10 Alcorn Avenue, Toronto, Ontario, Canada M4V 3B2
Penguin Books Ltd, 80 Strand, London WC2R 0RL, England
Penguin Putnam Inc., 375 Hudson Street, New York, New York 10014, U.S.A.
Penguin Books Australia Ltd, 250 Camberwell Road, Camberwell, Victoria 3124, Australia
Penguin Books India (P) Ltd, 11, Community Centre, Panchsheel Park, New Delhi – 110 017, India
Penguin Books (NZ) Ltd, cnr Rosedale and Airborne Roads, Albany, Auckland 1310, New Zealand
Penguin Books (South Africa) (Pty) Ltd, 24 Sturdee Avenue, Rosebank 2196, South Africa

Penguin Books Ltd, Registered Offices: 80 Strand, London WC2R 0RL, England

First published 2003

10 9 8 7 6 5 4 3 2   1

Manufactured in Canada.

NATIONAL LIBRARY OF CANADA CATALOGUING IN PUBLICATION

Beck, Leslie (Leslie C.)
   Leslie Beck's nutrition guide to menopause : natural strategies with diet, vitamins and herbs / Leslie Beck.

Title of previous edition: Managing menopause with diet, vitamins and herbs.
Includes bibliographical references and index.

ISBN 0-670-04386-9

1. Menopause—Complications—Alternative treatment.
2. Menopause—Nutritional aspects. I. Title.

RG186.B424 2003   618.1'75   C2003-900415-5

Visit Penguin Books' website at **www.penguin.ca**

To my mother and my female clients.

Your questions, your openness and your trust in me

made writing this book possible.

Contents

Introduction

If you are a woman in your 40s, 50s, 60s, or 70s, this book is a must have. Perhaps you are experiencing changes in your monthly menstrual cycle, or uncomfortable physical symptoms such as hot flashes. Or maybe you are a woman in your postmenopausal years and you're concerned about protecting your bones and your heart. Whether you are perimenopausal or postmenopausal, whether you are taking hormones or not, this book will help you make smart changes to your diet, add the right vitamin and mineral supplements to your daily routine, and choose the safest and most effective herbal remedies to ease your symptoms. In short, this book will help you stay healthy and feel better the natural way, before, during, and after menopause.

As a professional nutritionist (registered dietitian), I have been giving women of all ages advice on diet and supplements for the past 15 years. When I see a client, I assess her diet, supplement routine, medical history, risk factors, exercise habits, and other lifestyle factors. Armed with this information, I then develop a customized nutrition plan that will help each woman achieve her health and fitness goals.

My private practice is located in the heart of downtown Toronto's financial district. As a result, many of my clients are aging baby boomers—women and men who are taking charge of their health care. They want to eat smart, take the right supplements, and exercise more to stay healthy and full of energy into their later years. And, many of my clients want to avoid taking medications.

Over the past 10 years, I have seen an increasing number of women who want nutrition advice for managing menopause. If a woman comes to see me because she wants to lose weight or lower her cholesterol level, she invariably also asks me what she can do for her hot flashes, or what supplements she should be taking in light of her most recent bone density test, or what food she should eat to help reduce her risk of breast cancer. And in light of recent news about the risks of HRT, many women have consulted me for nutrition advice after stopping their medication. Now that they are no longer taking estrogen, what should they do to ease their hot flashes? To protect their heart and bones? Weight gain, mood swings, hot flashes, and memory problems are common concerns among my female clientele—not to mention the risks of heart disease, osteoporosis, and breast cancer.

My clients are not alone with their health concerns. Today in Canada almost 3.5 million women are between the ages of 40 and 54, the phase of life when levels of certain hormones are changing and dwindling. As baby boomers get older, the number of women in this situation will only increase. What's more, the number of women entering the postmenopausal years is expected to increase by 50 percent over the next decade. The demand for advice on menopausal health issues will continue to grow.

I realized there was a real need for this book back in the mid-1990s. Many women I met were frustrated by the lack of information available to them. Books on diet and nutrition were few and far between. My clients complained that their doctors were unable to answer their questions because they lacked training in nutrition and alternative therapies. And let's face it, most busy doctors don't have the time to assess your diet and develop a nutrition plan for you. If you want sound advice that's tailored to your lifestyle, a visit to a qualified nutritionist is in order. Registered dietitians are university-educated experts who are trained in how nutrition affects both health and disease.

New scientific information about menopause

A lot has changed since I wrote the first edition of this book, *Managing Menopause with Diet, Vitamins and Herbs* (Prentice Hall Canada, 2000). Back in 1999, I could not find one book on menopause that covered diet, nutrition, and herbal remedies in depth. Sure, there were plenty of books on menopause, but most didn't mention nutrition and only skimmed the surface when it came to vitamin or herbal supplements. Since then there has been an explosion of consumer information on natural alternatives for menopause—alternatives that include diet, supplements, and exercise. A large and growing interest among women has created a demand for credible and practical information. Today if you browse the women's health section of your local bookstore, you will be able to find a few more books on nutrition and menopause, and a whole lot more on menopause in general.

But our interest in the topic of so-called natural solutions to menopause is not the only reason for this revised edition; there is more accessible information today. There has also been an increase in the amount of scientific information about menopause. More studies are investigating menopausal health issues and, as a result, more findings are being published in scientific journals. Over the past three years, we have learned more about soy and breast cancer, isoflavones and bone health, and the safety of herbal remedies. Even the recommended dietary allowances for some vitamins and minerals have been revised since the first edition of this book was published. My head spins when I think about how fast science evolves.

One of the most important changes that took place since I wrote the first edition of this book is our understanding of hormone replacement therapy (HRT). In July 2002, findings from the Women's Health Initiative Hormone Study provided greater insight into the health risks associated with HRT. These findings led to new guidelines for doctors about the use of HRT for their patients.

Revised and updated strategies for managing menopause

Now you can understand why I had to update this book—there's so much more to say! This book gives you all the latest information on how certain foods, supplements, and herbs can help you feel better and stay healthy. All my recommendations are based on scientific evidence. Throughout the book, I translate the scientific findings into information you can put into practice. And, of course, I offer plenty of tips, as well as a meal plan that shows you how to incorporate natural strategies into your daily life.

What's new and different about *Leslie Beck's Nutrition Guide to Menopause*? If you have a copy of the first edition, you'll be pleased to know this revised edition offers more than ever. In addition to including findings from the most recent scientific studies from 2000 to 2002 throughout the book, you'll also find:

- A new section devoted entirely to women and hormones—how hormones affect your health and how they change during menopause.
- A menopause rating scale. Are you perimenopausal? Take this quiz to find out. Once you change your diet or incorporate a natural remedy, use the scale to assess improvement in your symptoms.
- The latest findings on hormone replacement therapy (HRT)—the risks and benefits.

- A guide to natural HRT—information about bio-identical hormones and how they might help manage your symptoms with fewer side effects and health risks than conventional HRT.
- An updated appendix on vitamins and minerals—how much you need and what foods you'll find them in.

How this book can help you

Leslie Beck's Nutrition Guide to Menopause is an essential read for any woman who wants to:
- Ease the symptoms of perimenopause, including hot flashes, insomnia, mood swings, menstrual irregularities, and sexual changes.
- Lose weight or prevent weight gain associated with lifestyle habits, advancing age, or HRT.
- Reduce her risk of breast cancer, heart disease, and osteoporosis—health problems most often experienced in the postmenopausal years.

If you are currently taking a medication to manage your symptoms or prevent disease, you'll learn that there are a number of things that you can and should be doing at the same time to stay healthy:
- Incorporating certain foods and supplements to give you more protection from osteoporosis and heart disease than that offered by drugs alone.
- Making dietary changes to help prevent the weight gain often associated with short-term hormone use.
- Eating right to increase your feeling of energy and well-being.

How this book is organized

The book is divided into three parts. Part One: Menopause and Hormones offers a primer on the terminology of menopause and on HRT (both synthetic and natural). Part Two: Managing Your Symptoms focuses on how to relieve symptoms such as hot flashes and night sweats, insomnia, mood swings, forgetfulness and fuzzy thinking, vaginal and bladder changes, and menstrual cycle changes. This is then followed by Part Three: Protecting Your Long-Term Health, which shows you how to prevent weight gain and how to reduce your risk of osteoporosis, heart disease, and breast cancer. Read what's most important to you, depending on what stage of menopause you're in and how it's affecting you.

In Parts Two and Three, I list my recommendations in three categories: dietary strategies, vitamins and minerals, and herbal remedies. For a quick summary of my recommendations, you can skip ahead to the end of these chapters for The Bottom Line sections. At the back of the book, you'll find Leslie's Total Nutrition Plan for the Menopausal Years, with modifications for weight loss, along with other valuable appendices. And all along the way, you'll find quotes from my clients, friends, and relatives, addressing their experiences of perimenopause and menopause. Their words are proof that you're not alone.

I hope you enjoy this book and find it a useful guide to lifelong good nutrition.

Leslie Beck, RD
Toronto, January 2003

Part one

Menopause and hormones

"Human females are unique from all other females on at least two counts: we menstruate, and we cease to be reproductively available after we've lived only half of our life span."

—Susun S. Weed, *Menopausal Years,*

The Wise Woman Way

What is menopause?

"I am 48 years old. I feel great but I haven't had a period for six months. Does this mean I'm menopausal?"

Every woman will experience menopause in her own unique way. Scores of women will complain of hot flashes, restless nights, and unwanted weight gain, but no two women experience the symptoms of menopause in the exact same way. Nor do the health risks associated with menopause affect all women. While hot flashes plague some women during the day, other women experience them during their sleep, and still others don't suffer a single hot flash. And while some women are concerned about their creeping blood cholesterol levels at menopause, others with normal cholesterol readings are more concerned about their bone density test results. For some women, the arrival at menopause means embracing a new stage of life. Indeed, many women report a new-found sense of freedom, self-confidence, and vitality.

Menopause is a natural event—it is not an illness. Menopause and its associated changes begin naturally as your ovaries produce fewer sex hormones. The signs and symptoms associated with the beginning of menopause occur over a period of time, called *perimenopause*. This word means "around menopause." Perimenopause can begin anywhere from 3 to 10 years before menopause, when hormonal changes start to occur. During perimenopause, women will begin to experience symptoms while they are still having their period. For many women, the first sign of perimenopause is an erratic menstrual cycle—skipped, lighter, or shorter periods.

The hallmark of this countdown to menopause is fluctuating levels of the female hormones estrogen and progesterone. Estrogen highs can bring on PMS-like symptoms, including mood swings, fluid retention, and headaches, whereas estrogen lows promise hot flashes, vaginal dryness, and forgetfulness. While perimenopause can start in your late thirties, most women begin noticing symptoms in their 40s.

You're considered to have reached *menopause* when 12 months have passed since your last period. The average age at which a Canadian woman reaches menopause naturally is 51. At menopause, a woman's ovaries no longer produce significant amounts of estrogen and progesterone, and they don't release eggs. It's at this time that women enter the *postmenopause,* the phase of life in which the risk of developing heart disease, osteoporosis, and breast cancer increases.

If you haven't hit menopause yet, you might be wondering when you will. For a clue, ask your mother or older sister when she experienced menopause. Genetics does affect the age menopause occurs; women often enter menopause around the same age as their mothers and sisters. Research also suggests that if you are underweight you might reach menopause earlier than the average Canadian woman. Conversely, if you're overweight, natural menopause could come later. And if you are a current or past smoker, menopause could come one or two years earlier.

Sometimes women enter *premature menopause.* This occurs when the ovaries stop producing estrogen and progesterone before the age of 40. Premature menopause can be brought on by genetics, an autoimmune disorder, or medical treatments such as complete hysterectomy (removal of both the uterus and ovaries), radiation, or chemotherapy. When medical procedures cause menopause, it is often referred to as *induced* menopause. Like natural menopause, premature menopause increases a woman's risk of osteoporosis and heart disease.

The female sex hormones

Hormones are chemicals that are formed in the glands and move to the blood, where they carry messages from one organ to another or to tissues in the body. The female sex hormones, estrogen and progesterone, work closely together to make your menstrual cycle function normally. These sex hormones also play an important role in keeping you healthy.

Estrogen is the main sex hormone that guides your body through the reproductive cycle. Estrogen is actually an umbrella term that encompasses three distinct hormones: estradiol, estrone, and estriol. Each type of estrogen plays a unique role in the body. Later, when I discuss natural hormone replacement therapy (natural HRT) in Chapter

3, I will discuss the significance of these different estrogens. Estrogen not only maintains the health of your reproductive tissues, it also keeps your breasts, bones, skin, and brain healthy. Excessive estrogen levels can cause fluid retention, weight gain, and migraines. Too much estrogen can also overstimulate cells in the breast and uterus, leading to cancer. A deficiency of estrogen can lead to hot flashes, vaginal dryness, skin aging, bone loss, urinary problems, and possibly dementia. Experts generally agree that by-products of estrogen metabolism can lead to breast cancer.

Progesterone balances the amount of estrogen in the body. It enhances estrogen's beneficial effects while preventing problems linked to estrogen dominance. As you'll read below, progesterone is responsible for preparing your body for pregnancy. When your periods start to become erratic during perimenopause, fluctuations in progesterone levels may be the culprit.

Androgens, such as testosterone and dehydroepiandrosterone (DHEA), are most often thought of as male sex hormones, yet every woman produces them in small quantities. After menopause, androgen production can drop by as much as 50 percent. Androgens play a role in maintaining energy, muscle mass, bone density, and sex drive. Both natural and conventional HRT regimens may add testosterone to help combat side effects such as low energy and loss of interest in sex.

Hormones and your menstrual cycle

To understand what's happening to your body during menopause, it helps to know how your hormones normally act during the childbearing years. Your menstrual cycle consists of three phases: the follicular phase (day 1 through 14), ovulation (day 14), and the luteal phase (day 14 to 28). The first day of your period is considered day 1. If your menstrual cycle is longer than 28 days, ovulation will occur later and the follicular phase will be longer. Likewise, if your cycle is shorter than 28 days, ovulation will occur before day 14 and the follicular phase will be shorter.

During the follicular phase of your monthly cycle, your ovaries produce enough estrogen to mature the egg inside your follicle. At the beginning of your cycle, your estrogen levels are low. Your brain responds to a low estrogen level by telling your pituitary gland to release follicle stimulating hormone (FSH). This hormone causes egg follicles to develop and release estrogen. By the end of your follicular phase—just before ovulation—your ovaries are also producing higher levels of male sex hormones,

THE FEMALE MENSTRUAL CYCLE

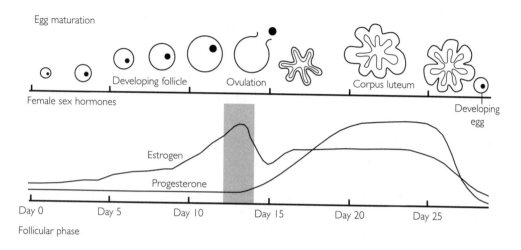

Egg maturation

Developing follicle

Ovulation

Corpus luteum

Developing egg

Female sex hormones

Estrogen

Progesterone

Day 0 Day 5 Day 10 Day 15 Day 20 Day 25

Follicular phase

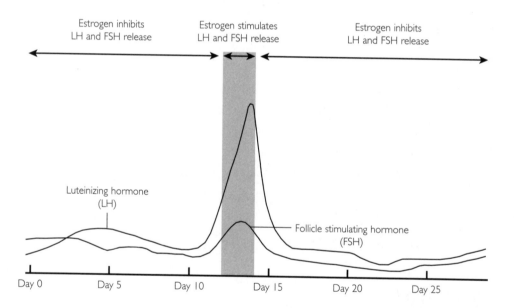

Estrogen inhibits LH and FSH release

Estrogen stimulates LH and FSH release

Estrogen inhibits LH and FSH release

Luteinizing hormone (LH)

Follicle stimulating hormone (FSH)

Day 0 Day 5 Day 10 Day 15 Day 20 Day 25

including testosterone. This may be the reason why many women report feeling more energetic at this time of the month.

When circulating estrogen rises to a critical level, the pituitary gland releases a surge of luteinizing hormone (LH). This influx of LH causes your ovaries to convert cholesterol into progesterone. Together, progesterone, LH, and FSH cause ovulation by telling the follicle to release a mature egg. The empty egg follicle turns into something called the *corpus luteum*, a gland that produces progesterone after ovulation. During the last 14 days of your menstrual cycle, progesterone prepares your body for pregnancy by thickening the lining of your uterus. If conception does not occur, the corpus luteum becomes smaller, estrogen and progesterone levels fall, and your uterine lining is shed, resulting in your period. Lower levels of estrogen and progesterone signal your pituitary gland to release FSH and LH, and the cycle begins anew.

Hormonal changes during perimenopause

As you get older, your supply of eggs and follicles dwindles. When there are fewer follicles, your ovaries produce less estrogen. Lower levels of estrogen tell your pituitary gland that it's time to release FSH and then LH. But now your ovaries are unable to respond to FSH and LH. They can't produce much estrogen and release an egg, and as a result, your brain keeps on telling your pituitary gland to make your ovaries ovulate. So your pituitary gland releases more and more FSH. Perimenopausal women who do not ovulate remain in the follicular phase, building up more and more estrogen. This hormone imbalance can cause breast tenderness, bloating, headache, mood swings, and cramps. You'll read in Chapter 4 how this constant production of FSH can also trigger hot flashes.

If no egg is released from your ovary, there's no corpus luteum and, consequently, no progesterone secretion. Without progesterone your body won't shed its uterine lining, and you'll miss a period. With overall lower levels of hormones, your periods will also become shorter, and eventually they will cease.

How to determine if you are perimenopausal

BLOOD TESTS

It's easy to determine if you are at menopause: either 12 months have passed since your last period or a blood test comes back in the menopausal range. Most of these blood tests measure the amount of FSH and LH in the blood. At menopause and afterward, FSH and LH levels are at their highest. Unfortunately, these blood tests are unreliable indicators of *perimenopause*. That's because during perimenopause, FSH and LH levels fluctuate considerably, depending on the state of your follicles. A blood test might show normal hormone levels even if you are in the midst of the transition. The same test, taken the following month, could reveal a high FSH level if you don't release an egg.

Some blood tests measure the total amount of estrogen, progesterone, and testosterone, but these too are unreliable because they measure bound, or inactive, hormones. When the sex hormones manufactured by the glands in your body are released into the bloodstream, they are bound to carrier proteins. Only a small fraction of a given amount of sex hormone breaks loose from the carrier protein in the bloodstream and is free to enter tissues, where it acts. This free or unbound hormone is active, or bioavailable, to your body's tissues. A more reliable method, although less commonly used, is to measure unbound (free) estrogen, progesterone, and testosterone levels. Keep in mind, however, that free hormone levels can fluctuate throughout the day. This means that where you stand compared with the normal range may be affected by when your blood test is done.

SALIVA TESTS

A growing number of physicians are measuring levels of free estrogen, progesterone, and testosterone from saliva samples. Scientists have found that the levels of unbound sex hormones in saliva are comparable to levels present in the bloodstream and bioavailable to tissues in the body. The advantage to saliva testing is that it is quick and painless—all you have to do is spit into special containers provided by your doctor, at specific times during the day. While this method is becoming more popular, it may be still unfamiliar to many doctors, so it is worth asking about.

CHART YOUR SYMPTOMS

Clearly, one of the best ways to assess whether you are in perimenopause is to track your symptoms. Keeping a menopause diary will help you determine what symptoms, if any, are bothersome and to what degree they are affecting your life. This information can help you and your health care provider decide what course of action is best to take—nutritional and herbal, natural HRT, or conventional HRT. Of course, nutritional remedies such as diet, vitamins, and minerals should form the baseline health plan for all women, regardless of what approach to menopause they take.

Keeping a menopause diary is also a useful way to assess improvement in symptoms once you begin on a course of treatment. The most reliable menopause symptom index used by doctors and researchers today is called the menopause rating scale (MRS).[1] It was developed in 1994 by an expert group of German, Austrian, and Swiss scientists as a replacement for the outdated Kupperman menopause index. The MRS registers every menopause symptom recognized today. (In contrast, the Kupperman index overlooked important symptoms and underscored the importance of others.) Take a moment to complete the menopause rating scale below.

MENOPAUSE RATING SCALE (MRS II)[2]

Which of the following symptoms do you have at the moment? For each symptom you are experiencing, place a tick in the box that best describes the intensity of that symptom. If you don't have the symptom, place a tick in the box "none."

		None 0	Mild 1	Moderate 2	Severe 3	Very Severe 4
1	HOT FLASHES Ascending feeling of heat, outbreaks of sweating	☐	☐	☐	☐	☐
2	HEART COMPLAINTS Palpitations, racing heart, galloping heart, feeling of being stifled	☐	☐	☐	☐	☐
3	SLEEP DISORDERS Difficulty falling asleep, difficulty staying asleep, waking up too early	☐	☐	☐	☐	☐
4	DEPRESSIVE MOODS Despondency, sadness, weepiness, lack of drive, mood swings	☐	☐	☐	☐	☐
5	IRRITABILITY Nervousness, inner tension, aggressiveness	☐	☐	☐	☐	☐

	None 0	Mild 1	Moderate 2	Severe 3	Very Severe 4
6 ANXIETY Inner restlessness, panic	☐	☐	☐	☐	☐
7 GENERAL DECREASE IN VITALITY; MEMORY IMPAIRMENT Physical and mental fatigue, difficulty concentrating, forgetfulness	☐	☐	☐	☐	☐
8 SEXUALITY Decrease in sexual desire, sexual activity, and satisfaction	☐	☐	☐	☐	☐
9 URINARY TRACT DISORDERS Pain on urination, frequent urge to urinate, involuntary passing of urine	☐	☐	☐	☐	☐
10 VAGINAL DRYNESS Feeling of dryness of the vagina, difficulties with sexual intercourse	☐	☐	☐	☐	☐
11 JOINT AND MUSCLE PAINS Pain mainly in the finger joints, arthritis-like pains, tingling	☐	☐	☐	☐	☐

Interpreting your results

The MRS is used in scientific research studies. This means it is designed to compare the effect of a treatment on symptoms in *groups* of women. Although its use is not intended for an individual woman, I do think it is nevertheless a useful tool to help you determine which symptoms are troubling you the most. Once you pinpoint those symptoms, you and your health care provider can implement an appropriate treatment plan. For instance, upon reviewing the eleven symptoms, you may find that you rated hot flashes as mild and sleep disturbances as moderate. This may lead you to decide that you can live with the occasional hot flash, but finding a natural solution to your insomnia is a priority. If you find that many of your symptoms are moderate or severe, discuss solutions for them all with your physician.

Once you start on a course of therapy, be it a herbal remedy, dietary modification, physical activity, or medication, you can use the MRS again to assess your symptom improvement. You can also add up the scores for all eleven symptoms to get your total menopause score. The total possible score is 44. While this score has little use on its own, it might be interesting to see by how much your score decreases after treatment.

The hormone replacement therapy (HRT) dilemma

"For years I was told that estrogen would keep my heart and bones in good shape as I got older. That's why I took HRT for the past 11 years. The latest news about HRT really scared me. I literally put down the newspaper and picked up the phone to call my doctor."

2

Ever since the introduction of Premarin (a synthetic estrogen derived from the urine of pregnant mares) to North America in the 1940s, physicians have viewed estrogen replacement therapy (ERT) as the logical solution to the consequences of natural estrogen loss. In the 1950s, Ayerst Laboratories, manufacturers of Premarin, launched a massive education program for doctors that focused on menopause, menopausal symptoms, and the health risks of estrogen deficiency.

In its earliest days, ERT was used to treat hot flashes. It was also thought to keep women looking youthful. In the 1960s, the use of estrogen was heavily promoted in *Feminine Forever*, a book written by New York gynecologist Dr. Robert Wilson and supported financially by Ayerst Laboratories. Dr. Wilson presented menopause as a "deficiency disease" and urged women to save their femininity, prolonging their attractiveness to men. As you might expect, ERT use soared and, by 1966, Premarin was the most frequently dispensed drug in the United States.

At first, women were prescribed Premarin alone. In 1977, however, American researchers reported that women taking Premarin had a much higher rate of endometrial cancer than nonusers. It was then discovered that adding a progestin to estrogen could prevent the increased endometrial cancer risk. ("Progestin" is a general term for a substance that causes some or all of the biologic effects of progesterone; the term is often used to specifically refer to the synthetic derivatives of progesterone in oral contraceptives and hormone replacement therapy.) By the mid-1980s, progestins were routinely added to ERT for women who had not undergone a hysterectomy (that is, they still had an intact uterus). The combination of estrogen and progestin is known as combined hormone replacement therapy (HRT).

Over the next two decades, researchers reported that women on such hormone regimens had a lower risk of bone loss and heart disease compared with nonusers. In fact, more than 30 studies suggested that estrogen was an important strategy for not only preventing heart disease in healthy women, but also reducing the risk of a recurrent heart attack in women with the disease. Because of these studies, there was a shift from prescribing ERT and HRT for short-term symptom relief to prescribing it for long-term use for disease prevention. This meant that these hormones were prescribed for a therapy regimen of five or more years. Soon, however, studies began to indicate that taking estrogen for longer than five years increased the risk of breast cancer. And findings from clinical trials emerged that did not agree with earlier findings about the benefits of ERT and HRT.

HRT: More harm than good

Before 1998, ERT and HRT were considered the gold standard treatment in the prevention of heart disease and osteoporosis. Doctors across the country routinely prescribed HRT to their patients approaching menopause. Hormone replacement seemed to protect a woman's future health, and it was also effective in alleviating perimenopausal hot flashes, mood swings, and sleep disturbances. But today, hormone replacement is no longer considered the first line of approach in managing menopause.

Recently, there has been a lot of confusion about hormone therapy in light of research findings indicating that the risks of taking HRT (estrogen plus progestin) outweighed the benefits. In July 2002, the Women's Health Initiative (WHI) study arm investigating combined HRT was abruptly halted after five years. Sponsored by the National Institutes of Health, the WHI followed more than 27,000 healthy women, aged 50 to 79, taking either HRT or estrogen only. The goal was to determine whether HRT protected from heart disease and osteoporosis, as well as increased the risk of cancer and blood clots.

After a little more than five years of study, the results revealed that women taking

HRT were at increased risk of heart disease, blood clots, stroke, and breast cancer. Although the risks were small, it was enough to stop the investigation of combined HRT. The hormone regimen was found to protect from hip fracture and colon cancer, but more women suffered a serious health problem than a positive one. The data indicate that if 10,000 women take HRT for one year, as compared with 10,000 women not taking HRT, eight more will get breast cancer, seven more will have a heart attack, eight more will have blood clots in the lungs, and eight more will have a stroke. The increased risk of breast cancer did not appear until after four years of taking HRT, and the longer a woman remained on the hormone combination, the greater her risk. The risk of blood clots was highest during the first two years of HRT use.[1]

RISKS AND BENEFITS OF HRT

Increases the risks of:	Reduces the risks of:
Coronary heart disease	Colon cancer
Blood clots	Dementia
Breast cancer	Depression
Gallbladder disease	Osteoporotic bone fracture
Stroke	Urinary tract infection
	Relieves menopausal symptoms

Women in the study taking estrogen only (women who had undergone a hysterectomy) were told to continue taking their study pills as before, since neither a favourable or unfavourable risk-benefit profile could be detected. Some data suggest that the risk of breast cancer may be higher on combined HRT than on unopposed estrogen. The actual breast cancer risk in the ongoing ERT arm of the WHI may not be available until 2005, when the study is scheduled to conclude.

The WHI is not the only study to turn up disappointing results regarding heart disease. The Heart and Estrogen/Progestin Replacement Study (HERS) studied 2763 American postmenopausal women with established heart disease. The women were randomly assigned to take combined HRT or a placebo pill. The initial study ended after four years when the results indicated that the risk of heart attack was higher after the first year on HRT, but reduced after the third year of use. With this information, women were asked to consider staying on their assigned treatment after consultation with their physician. In all, 93 percent of women continued treatment for an additional three years. After almost seven years of follow-up, the researchers concluded that combined HRT did *not* reduce the risk of heart attack or death from heart disease.[2]

Two points are noteworthy about the WHI and HERS trials. First, both studies used oral estrogen plus oral progesterone therapy (0.625 milligrams conjugated estrogen daily plus 2.5 milligrams of medroxyprogesterone acetate daily). The same findings may not apply to different hormone doses and different routes of administration. Second, most of the women in these studies began their assigned treatment (HRT or placebo) at least 10 years after menopause. Neither trial investigated perimenopausal women, women with early menopause, or women with premature menopause. Therefore, we don't know if the same risks (and benefits) observed in this group of women apply to younger women.

Where does HRT stand today?

While many questions remained unanswered, this new knowledge about HRT has led the Society of Obstetricians and Gynecologists of Canada and the North American Menopause Society to revise guidelines on the appropriate use of combined HRT. Here's the lowdown on the appropriate use of HRT, given recent scientific findings:

- The primary use of combined HRT is to treat menopausal symptoms such as hot flashes, night sweats, and mood swings in women with a uterus. Short-term use of HRT is still considered a reasonable option for most women, with the exception of those with a history of breast cancer, heart disease, blood clots, or stroke. In otherwise healthy women, the risk of suffering a health problem is extremely low. Experts consider short-term therapy to be anywhere from six months to four or five years. HRT should be tapered off and eventually stopped after using it for the planned treatment period, unless there is some compelling reason to continue.

- The use of either combined HRT or estrogen-only therapy should be used for the shortest duration possible and at lower-than-standard doses. Currently, it is unknown whether patches and creams are any safer than pills.

- Combined HRT should *not* be used as a treatment for heart disease; ask your doctor to discuss other options with you.

- Because of the risks associated with HRT, you should discuss with your doctor alternative therapies for the prevention of postmenopausal osteoporosis, along with the risks and benefits of each.

- Women who have been on HRT for five years or longer should talk with their doctor about whether to continue on it.

After reading this unsettling news about HRT, you might be wondering if this therapy is right for you. If you are considering starting on HRT, review with your doctor why you want to start the regimen, the health benefits to you with HRT use, and your increased health risks with HRT use. An individual risk profile is essential to guide you and your doctor in making the decision to use any HRT or ERT regimen.

Discontinuing your HRT

If you are an HRT user and now wondering if you should stop your medication, consult your doctor. As when considering starting HRT, you need to understand the reasons you started the therapy, your benefits and risks using it, and what the alternatives are. If you decide to discontinue HRT, ask your doctor the best way to do so. If you have a history of severe menopausal symptoms, you may be better to taper off HRT rather than quitting cold turkey. Stopping your medication abruptly can bring on hot flashes, often severe ones. Slowly decreasing your pills over 6 to 12 weeks will help prevent the recurrence of hot flashes. Your doctor will determine an appropriate tapering-off regimen for you.

Natural hormone replacement therapy

"I am very fortunate to have an open-minded doctor. At my request, she researched the topic and finally wrote me a prescription for natural HRT. It took a few tries before we got a formulation that works best for me. I feel so much better—my sleep is improved and my hot flashes are virtually gone."

3

If you are suffering from hot flashes, insomnia, or mood swings, you may decide that short-term use of conventional HRT is not right for you. One option then to consider is natural HRT. A number of my clients have chosen this therapy, with positive results. The term "natural" is slightly misleading when it comes to hormones; "natural HRT" is in fact a misnomer. The correct term to use is bio-identical hormone replacement therapy. Bio-identical hormones have an identical chemical structure to the ones produced in your body. Here's a look at the estrogens produced in the body:

Estradiol (accounts for 10–20 percent of estrogen produced) is produced mainly by the ovaries and is the major estrogen in premenopausal women. It is also the form of estrogen used in estrogen patches. Estradiol is considered a potent estrogen and may increase the risk of breast cancer.

Estrone (10–20 percent) is the main estrogen in postmenopausal women. It is made primarily in the liver from other hormones. Like estradiol, estrone is also potent in action and may promote breast cancer.

Estriol (60–80 percent) is a weak form of estrogen and is not associated with cancer-promoting activity. It is created from the metabolism of estone and estradiol. Estriol is at its highest level during pregnancy. When given as bio-identical HRT, this estrogen is effective at relieving hot flashes and vaginal dryness and does not seem to produce unwanted side effects such as breakthrough bleeding, breast tenderness, and headache. However, because estriol is weak in action, it does not provide the bone protection that the other, potent, estrogens do.

Now consider Premarin, the commonly prescribed estrogen preparation derived from the urine of pregnant mares. Premarin consists of mostly estrone and some estradiol; the rest is equilines (horse estrogens). Although this estrone and estradiol are bio-identical to the human body, they are extremely potent and may be linked to breast cancer. Equilines are natural to horses but foreign to humans, and we lack the enzymes needed to metabolize equilines at a safe rate. It's also known that the metabolic breakdown products of Premarin are biologically stronger than those of bio-identical hormones and therefore more likely to cause side effects. Provera, synthetic progestins, is associated with side effects such as mood swings and weight gain. Provera uses natural progesterone as its base but is then altered to form a non-identical hormone. So synthetic hormones such as Premarin and Provera are not bio-identical—they do not exactly replicate the structure of your body's own hormones. Slight differences in chemical configuration means that synthetic hormones act differently in your body and produce different effects. Premarin is often associated with side effects such as bloating, weight gain, and headache, causing many women to discontinue therapy. Because the body metabolizes equilines more slowly, they hang around longer, possibly increasing the risk of breast cancer. The side effects associated with synthetic progestins are not seen with bio-identical progesterone.

Bio-identical hormones come from a variety of sources, including plants (soy, wild yams) and animals (pigs, horses). They can also be produced synthetically in a laboratory. And even hormones extracted from soy or wild yam must undergo several processing steps before a bio-identical hormone is obtained. So, bio-identical hormones are not really natural in the strictest sense of the word. What we mean by "natural" when it comes to hormone replacement is that the preparation contains hormones identical in molecular structure to those made by the human body. Because bio-identical hormones match those hormones our bodies have evolved to utilize, their effects are more natural to the body. That means there is less chance for the side effects that are often associated with hormones foreign to the human body.

Proponents of bio-identical hormone replacement cite the following benefits over synthetic hormones:

- If used at the proper dosage, bio-identical hormones don't have the side effects associated with conventional HRT.
- Bio-identical hormones aren't associated with long-term health risks. The body metabolizes, or breaks down, bio-identical hormones more quickly than synthetic hormones and, as a result, they don't pose the same health risk. In fact, the breakdown products of bio-identical hormones have a much weaker effect in the body, so their effects don't last as long as synthetic hormone metabolites.
- Bio-identical hormone replacement can be individualized to meet a woman's needs. Natural HRT has no "one size fits all." Your doctor can prescribe a preparation based on your hormone test results and symptoms. Unlike conventional HRT, bio-identical hormones can be customized to suit your personal hormonal profile.
- Bio-identical progesterone does not diminish the beneficial effect of estrogen on lowering cholesterol as synthetic progestin does.
- Bio-identical progesterone may protect against osteoporosis and breast cancer.

By now you may be wondering why your doctor hasn't suggested this hormone regimen to ease your menopausal symptoms. Unfortunately, most doctors are unaware of bio-identical hormones. Large-scale clinical trials using these hormones are sorely lacking, and doctors receive little information about natural hormones. And, because little research has been conducted in women using natural HRT, many doctors are hesitant to prescribe it. Bio-identical hormones cannot be patented because they are found in nature: in order for a drug to be patented, it must have a unique structure not found in nature or a unique extraction process, such as that used in the manufacture of Premarin. However, drug companies have no financial incentives to research and develop products that cannot be patented, and, in North America, physicians are educated about prescribing patented drugs. Not only is valid information about bio-identical hormones difficult to find, but it takes time to search out current information, to review it, and then to incorporate it into clinical practice—time many busy doctors don't have.

Compounding pharmacists

Bio-identical hormones are readily available, with a doctor's prescription, from a compounding pharmacist. The practice of compounding medicine dates back to the origins of pharmacy, when pharmacists actually *made* medications, tailoring them to an individual's needs. This practice has declined over the past 50 years. With the advent of drug manufacturing, the role of the pharmacist has changed from a maker of medicine to a dispenser of manufactured pills and potions. Today, with more doctors and patients realizing the benefits of individualized medication, more pharmacists are assuming their traditional role.

When a pharmacist compounds a prescription, he or she takes the raw form of a medication, often a powder, and prepares it to meet the patient's needs. The compounding pharmacist decides on the best delivery route for the medication, be it tablet, capsule, cream, gel, or suppository, and works closely with the prescribing physician to arrive at the best possible dosage for the patient.

If your doctor is unfamiliar with bio-identical hormones and you want to try natural HRT, you might try consulting a compounding pharmacist (see Appendix 5 for a list of compounding pharmacies across Canada), as many have referral lists of doctors who are prescribing bio-identical hormones. It might be simpler to consult a doctor who is already prescribing natural HRT than one who is not familiar with the preparations.

COMPOUNDED HORMONE REPLACEMENT PREPARATIONS

Generic Name	Strength	Source
Triple Estrogen (80% estriol, 10% estrone, 10% estradiol)	Customized	Soy
Bi-estrogen (estradiol, estriol)	Customized	Soy
Estriol	Customized	Soy
Progesterone	Customized	Soy or yams
Testosterone	Customized	Soy

Over-the-counter "natural progesterone" creams

As more women seek natural alternatives to conventional hormone replacement therapy, the use of so-called progesterone creams is on the rise. You've already read that bio-identical progesterone is considered safer and more effective than prescription progestins, and it's relatively inexpensive. While a compounding pharmacist should be your first stop for a high-quality preparation, it might be tempting to save time getting a prescription from your doctor and head straight to the health food store to buy a cream made from wild yam.

Many wild yam products are promoted as "natural progesterone." However, wild yam creams are *not* progesterone, nor do they contain progesterone. Wild yam root contains natural compounds called diosgenins, which are converted to progesterone *in the laboratory*. But this conversion does not occur in the human body. This means you don't get any progesterone by applying a wild yam cream to your body.

Despite that these products do not contain progesterone, a number of my clients have reported improvement in vaginal dryness, mood, and even libido after using them. No scientific studies have investigated the effect of wild yam on menopausal symptoms, so it's hard to say whether these women were merely experiencing a "placebo effect." It is possible that wild yam has some hormonal properties. There's evidence from the lab that diosgenins in wild yam can bind to estrogen receptors in the body. Because wild yam may have estrogenic properties, women with hormone sensitive conditions—breast cancer, endometriosis, and uterine fibroids—should avoid using wild yam products.

It is illegal to sell progesterone over the counter (OTC) in Canada. Progesterone is considered a prescription drug and regulated as such by Health Canada. However, this is not the case in the United States, where progesterone creams may be marketed as cosmetics and sold over the counter. This means you may find a US-manufactured progesterone cream in your local supplement store. And certainly you'll find these products easy to purchase over the Internet. But think twice before you open your wallet! When it comes to American OTC progesterone creams, it's buyer beware, since quality can vary greatly. OTC progesterone products may not contain progesterone concentrations as labelled. According to a British report, 2-ounce jars of Progest cream used in a clinical trial contained 100 milligrams progesterone per ounce rather than the 465 milligrams claimed by the manufacturer. Topical progesterone products marketed as cosmetics require no FDA approval prior to marketing. There is currently no limit on the amount of progesterone allowed in cosmetic products. The bottom line: Don't waste your money. If you want a high-quality and effective product, one from your compounding pharmacist is your best bet.

Here's what you need to know when using a *progesterone* cream or gel:

- Apply to the areas of skin that are thin: your palms, face, neck, upper chest, or inner arms and thighs. This will maximize absorption.
- Use anywhere from 1/8 to 1/2 teaspoon of cream each day. Products will vary according to the amount of progesterone, so follow your pharmacist's instructions.
- To avoid saturating one particular area, alternate the areas to which you apply the cream.
- Progesterone cream, gel, capsules, or drops may be used with prescription estrogens; however, consult your doctor before self-medicating.

I mentioned earlier that every woman experiences menopause differently. Because each woman's menopause is unique, no treatment plan fits all women. But no matter how you experience menopause, this time of life presents you with an opportunity—an opportunity to enhance your quality of life by improving your health habits. It is now time to start down the path to improved nutrition. Healthy eating and physical activity are not optional; both are essential to the health and well-being of all women. Even if you opt for HRT—natural or conventional—you still must implement the nutrition essentials for a healthy menopause. The following chapters will help you incorporate the right foods, vitamins, and minerals in the right amounts into your daily diet. You'll also learn how to safely use herbal remedies to combat hot flashes, insomnia, or mood swings. Enjoy your journey!

Part two

Managing your symptoms

"It's been a bit of a rollercoaster ride—first came the hot flashes, which really disrupted my sleep. Luckily, I now have those under control by making a few simple lifestyle changes. It's the mood swings that I'm trying to cope with now."

Hot flashes and night sweats

"I suddenly have a hot flash. I know that I am beet red from the neck up and the perspiration is starting to run down my forehead. Someone suggests, 'It's very warm in here today,' and I am truly mortified. I have just broadcast to my younger male colleagues that I am menopausal!"

4

Hot flashes are, without a doubt, the most commonly reported symptom of menopause—indeed, for many women, hot flashes are often the first sign that menopause is approaching. Between 60 and 85 percent of North American women experience hot flashes at some point during the perimenopausal or postmenopausal years. Ten to 15 percent of these women experience hot flashes so severe that they interfere with daily life. On average, hot flashes persist for two to three years, but in 50 percent of women who experience this symptom, they last for up to five years before tapering off. A small group of women get hot flashes for periods of 15 years or longer, sometimes experiencing them into their 70s and 80s. Almost all women have severe hot flashes immediately after a hysterectomy (induced menopause).

Anatomy of a hot flash

Hot flashes vary considerably among women in terms of frequency, intensity, and duration. A warning signal often precedes a hot flash. This signal may take the form of an "aura," similar to that experienced by migraine sufferers. The aura may manifest as pressure in the head, a headache, or a wave of nausea. A sensation of heat then starts in the head and neck and spreads to the torso, arms, and then the entire body. Sweating follows and is most intense in the upper body. The perspiration can be drenching, particularly if the hot flashes are nocturnal, occurring during sleep. Some women experience heart palpitations, dizziness, or feelings of tension and anxiety with their hot flashes. Nocturnal hot flashes, or "night sweats," can be severe enough to disrupt sleep, causing insomnia, fatigue, and irritability. (Chapters 5 and 6 cover natural treatment of these symptoms.)

Hot flashes, as I explain in more detail below, actually cool the body, and chills or shakes may follow the flash as a result of the drop in body temperature it has caused. The entire event can last anywhere from a few seconds to several minutes; it can then take up to an hour for the resultant chills to subside. I have some clients who experience hot flashes as often as one every hour, while others report as few as several per week. Hot flashes may disappear for months, only to return when you least expect them. Many women report that stressful events or warm temperatures or warm rooms aggravate hot flashes. Consuming caffeine and alcohol, or even eating a spicy meal, can trigger hot flashes in some women.

Fortunately, hot flashes usually resolve with age and as your body adjusts to the changes of the menopausal years. To understand hot flashes better, let's take a closer look at the hormones involved. If you have already read Chapter 1, this will serve as a quick review.

HORMONES AND HOT FLASHES

Estrogen

The word "estrogen" is a generic term for a group of female sex hormones, including estradiol, estriol, and estrone. Estrogens form in your ovaries, brain, and fatty tissues. At puberty, estrogen stimulates breast development and other female characteristics. Estrogen also stimulates the uterine lining (endometrium) to grow during the preovulatory phase of the menstrual cycle, to prepare you for possible pregnancy.

Follicle stimulating hormone (FSH)

This hormone is produced by your pituitary gland, which is inside your brain. For the first 14 days of your menstrual cycle, FSH stimulates the follicles in your ovaries to produce estrogen. When estrogen levels have risen adequately, the pituitary gland turns off FSH production. After menopause, when your ovaries no longer respond to FSH, your blood levels of FSH stay high. During the perimenopausal years, your FSH levels can fluctuate widely.

Luteinizing hormone (LH)

This hormone is also produced in your pituitary gland, and, like FSH, it acts on your ovaries. LH is released once your estrogen levels rise and FSH is turned off. When your level of LH is at its highest, your ovarian follicle releases an egg (ovulation).

Progesterone

Once you ovulate, your follicle (now called a *corpus luteum*) produces progesterone in addition to estrogen. Progesterone acts to build up the uterine lining. When progesterone and estrogen levels drop, your body sheds its uterine lining through bleeding—a period—and your pituitary gland knows that it's time to start releasing FSH once more.

WHAT CAUSES HOT FLASHES?

Researchers are still trying to understand exactly what occurs in the body that causes a hot flash. Hot flashes begin in the hypothalamus, the region of the brain housing the body's temperature control centre. This "thermostat" decides that you are too hot—even though your body temperature is normal—and attempts to cool you down by increasing your heartbeat and sending more blood to your skin, especially the skin of your head and neck. As a result, the blood vessels in your skin dilate, your skin flushes, and you sweat. The overall effect is that heat escapes from your body. It's ironic that hot flashes are actually your body's way of cooling down (even though you don't need to!).

What might cause the hypothalamus to become confused about your temperature and trigger a hot flash? In a nutshell, hormonal changes are responsible. As you enter the menopausal years, estrogen production drops and ovulation becomes irregular, before stopping altogether. Without enough estrogen, your body can't thicken the lining of your uterus. You'll get irregular periods and, eventually, your periods will cease. Without ovulation, progesterone levels fall. But remember, low estrogen and progesterone levels tell your brain that it's time to release FSH and then LH. But now your ovaries are no longer able to respond to FSH and LH. They can't produce much estrogen or release an egg, so your hypothalamus keeps telling your pituitary gland to make your ovaries ovulate. As a result, your pituitary gland releases more and more FSH (that's why FSH levels are high during menopause). Your hypothalamus is so busy constantly signalling your pituitary gland, its temperature control centre can malfunction, setting off a hot flash even though a temperature adjustment isn't needed. Experts also believe that a drop in estrogen levels may trigger your hypothalamus and, as a result, your body's temperature control system malfunctions.

COPING WITH HOT FLASHES

It is interesting to note that hot flashes don't exist in some cultures. Indeed, in the Japanese language, there is no word for "hot flash." Women in Asian cultures generally make the transition into the menopausal years experiencing very few, if any, of the distressing symptoms suffered by women in our Western culture. In fact, studies show that, compared with women living in Western countries, only 20 percent of Asian women living in China experience hot flashes.[1] Women in these cultures tend to view menopause as a healthy, natural part of aging, rather than as an unwanted medical condition. And researchers have learned that there is definitely a link between a society's attitude toward menopause and the symptoms commonly experienced by women in that society. With today's focus on beauty, sexiness, and thinness, many Western women find themselves at odds with menopause. They are afraid that menopause means becoming old and useless. I vividly remember listening to one client as she described her anxieties about menopause as a fear of "becoming old," "becoming fat," and "knitting all day long." It seems common for women to be afraid that they won't be valued by society after they pass through menopause.

So how does all this relate to my original question: What can we do about hot flashes? We can start by learning from women in Eastern cultures and adopting a more accepting and respecting attitude toward our bodies' natural life cycle changes. And we can pick up other hints from them as well. Japanese women eat plenty of soy foods and fish and very few high-fat animal foods. Their diet certainly contrasts with our North American fare of meat, potatoes, and processed food. The Japanese woman's lifestyle demonstrates that clearing up menopausal symptoms generally requires more than just a shift in attitude—but often less than a prescription for hormones. Over the years, many of my clients, the ones who have been unable to deal with hot flashes simply through minor lifestyle adjustments, have asked me if there is something they can take or eat to alleviate this troublesome symptom. A vitamin or herb perhaps? Specific foods? The answer is yes. Making changes to your diet and your surroundings can definitely help you feel better. Below, I describe the natural approaches for treating hot flashes that I often recommend to the women I see in my private practice. Not only do my clients report improvement, but scientific studies also support the ability of these remedies to ease hot flashes.

Dietary approaches

SOY FOODS AND ISOFLAVONES

Foods made from soybeans are certainly getting plenty of attention these days. (You can find a list of these foods on the following pages). Scientists are learning that soy foods can help ease menopausal hot flashes (along with offering possible protection from osteoporosis, heart disease, and breast cancer, as we'll see in Part Three.) A 12-week Italian study looked at the effects of soy protein on hot flashes in 104 women aged 48 to 61 years. The study found that, compared with the group taking placebo, or dummy pills, the women who consumed 60 grams of soy protein powder daily reported a 26 percent reduction in the average number of hot flashes they experienced by their third week on this regimen, and a 33 percent reduction by the fourth week. At the end of the three-month study, the soy group had a 45 percent decrease in the number of hot flashes experienced daily. In comparison, the placebo group experienced only a 30 percent reduction.[2] Another study carried out by American researchers in North Carolina found that women whose daily diet included a total of 20 grams of soy protein reported significant improvement of hot flashes as well as of other menopausal symptoms.[3]

But I don't want you to think that soy is the magic cure for hot flashes. It's true that a daily intake of soy has helped a number of my clients ease their hot flashes. But, overall, studies don't find it to be a stupendously effective remedy. While it does tend to decrease both the frequency and severity of hot flashes, the effects are generally modest or mild. And all the studies find that participating women who receive the placebo also experience some improvement. If a study finds that women who eat soy every day have 20 percent fewer hot flashes than women taking the dummy treatment, some experts might question the clinical relevance of the finding. Will a 20 percent improvement mean that much to your symptoms? Will it mean moving from 11 hot flashes a day down to nine? I am a fan of soy foods, but I don't want to overstate the effect soy has on hot flashes. On the other hand, I meet many women in my practice who tell me that any improvement is welcome.

What makes soybeans so special? Soybeans contain isoflavones, naturally occurring compounds that are a type of phytoestrogen (plant estrogen). Genistein and daidzein are the most active soy isoflavones and have been the focus of much research. Isoflavones have a molecular structure similar to that of the human estrogen hormones and, as a result, have a weak estrogenic effect in the body. Even though soy isoflavones are about 50 times less potent than human estrogens, they are able to offer women a source of usable estrogen and, along with that, some of estrogen's protective effects. If a woman's estrogen levels are low enough to cause hot flashes during the peri-menopausal or postmenopausal periods, a regular intake of isoflavones from foods such as roasted soy nuts, soy beverages, and tofu may help alleviate the situation. These foods can be incorporated into your favourite recipes and still be as beneficial—the phytoestrogens in soy don't break down when heated.

Types of soy foods

Here's a quick introduction to what these foods are, where you can get them, and how they're used in the kitchen.

Soybeans   You can buy these dried or already cooked (in cans). Dried soybeans need to be soaked in water overnight before cooking. Add cooked soybeans to soups, casseroles, chilies, and curries, or add them mashed to burgers. For a real treat, order *edamame* (green soybeans) as an appetizer the next time you dine in a Japanese restaurant. (Watch out though; it tends to be loaded with salt, so you might want to ask for it without.)

Miso   A traditional Asian flavouring, this paste is made of a fermented mixture of soybeans and grain. Miso is excellent added to soups at the end of cooking, or to marinades and sauces. For soup, use 1/4 cup (50 ml) miso for every quart (or litre) of water.

Soy flour   Soybeans are defatted and finely ground to make a flour, sold in health food stores and some grocery stores. Because soy flour contains no gluten, the wheat protein that adds structure to baked goods, it should be mixed with other flours when baking. Substitute soy flour for up to one-half of the wheat flour in recipes for breads, muffins, loaves, cakes, cookies, and scones.

Soy beverages   These are made from either the juice of ground soybeans or from isolated soy protein. You'll find many brands and flavours in grocery and health food stores. You may need to try a few brands before finding one with a taste you like, but be sure to buy a brand fortified with calcium and vitamin D. Use soy beverages just as you would milk—on cereal, and in smoothies, coffee, lattes, soups, and cooking and baking. And if you're cutting down on sugar, choose an unflavoured beverage.

Soy "meats"   These ready-to-eat soy foods resemble—in appearance, texture, and protein content—burgers, hot dogs, deli cold cuts, and ground meat. You'll find them in the freezer, deli, or produce section of grocery stores. Soy burgers and dogs are already cooked; all they need is reheating. Overcooking will dry them out and probably discourage you from trying them again. Soy ground round is available plain or seasoned, ready to complement a Mexican or Italian meal.

Soy nuts   Also called roasted soybeans, this snack food is available in plain, barbecue, and garlic flavours. Of all the soy foods, soy nuts have the highest amount of isoflavones per serving—2 tablespoons pack roughly 42 milligrams! The good news for those of you who tend to like salty snack foods is that these munchies have less salt, less fat, and more fibre than actual nuts, yet they're tasty and satisfying. However, if you have high blood pressure or are susceptible to retaining fluid, buy unsalted soy nuts.

Tempeh   You'll find this traditional Asian soy food, shaped in small bars, in the refrigerated or frozen food section of health food stores. Made of a fermented soybean-grain mixture, tempeh has a delicious nutty flavour. Slice it and add it to casseroles and stir-fries or grill it in kebabs and burgers. Tempeh is tastiest and most digestible if you simmer it in your favourite marinade for 20 minutes before incorporating it into other recipes.

Texturized vegetable protein (TVP)   Made from defatted and dehydrated soy flour, TVP is sold in packages of granules or small chunks. Rehydrate it with an equal amount of water or broth, then use it to replace ground meat in pasta sauces, lasagna, chilies, and tacos.

Tofu   Made by using minerals or lemon juice to coagulate the juice from soaked, ground, and briefly cooked soybeans, tofu readily picks up flavours during cooking. It comes in soft (silken) and firm varieties. Use soft tofu in smoothies, dips, salad dressings, lasagna, and cheesecake recipes. Firm tofu is best for grilling and stir-frying, or add cubes of it to soups for a protein boost.

How much soy should you eat?

Based on the studies done to date, it appears that a daily intake of 40 to 80 milligrams of soy is needed to reduce hot flashes. As you will notice in the table below, the isoflavone content of soy foods can vary considerably. Depending on the growing conditions and the type of bean, soybeans contain 2 to 4 milligrams of isoflavones per gram of protein. When it comes to food products made with soy protein, such as protein powders and energy bars, the isoflavone content will vary depending on how the isoflavones were removed from the protein in the soybean. Dehulling, flaking, and defatting results in a protein low in isoflavones. Food processing also affects the final isoflavone content of a soy food. For instance, soy hot dogs and soy yogurts may contain only one-tenth of the isoflavone content in the soybeans used to manufacture the food. Texturized vegetable protein and soy flour contain approximately 5 milligrams of isoflavones per gram of protein. Soy beverages and tofu contain about 2 milligrams of isoflavones per gram of protein. Soy sauce, soybean oil, and soy margarines contain no isoflavones. The chart on page 32 will help you plan your soy food consumption so that you get at least 40 milligrams of isoflavones per day.

Soy isoflavones appear to be most effective if they're taken in divided doses throughout the day. Depending on what type of soy food you eat, the isoflavones reach their highest concentration in your bloodstream four to eight hours after eating. Isoflavones are then excreted from the body, usually within 24 hours of consuming the soy food. Scientists have learned that in order to maintain a constant blood level of soy isoflavones, you need to eat soy foods daily, and at regular intervals. Studies have revealed that consuming soy in two or three doses over the course of the day can maximize the effectiveness of soy isoflavones. Based on this information, it makes sense to get 20 to 40 milligrams of isoflavones two times daily to keep your blood levels of isoflavones up. Sounds easy enough—a soy smoothie for breakfast and soy nuts for an afternoon snack!

Cooking with soy foods

I can understand that if you've never tried soy foods before, you might be hesitant to cook with them. Tofu, especially, seems to have a bad reputation—many of my clients aren't used to eating soy foods, and when I mention tofu, I usually see noses turn up. You'd have thought I had just recommended eating Brussel sprouts (though I happen to love them!). Then again, let's face it, a cake of soybean curd doesn't look that appealing and it's definitely a hard food to sneak into the family dinner. It might help to look at this as an opportunity to be adventurous. To assist you, here's a list of 10 ways to enjoy more soy. You can also try one of the recipes in Appendix 3; they all come highly recommended by my clients.

ISOFLAVONE CONTENT OF SOY FOODS

Soy food	Serving size	Isoflavone content (milligrams)
Roasted soy nuts	1/4 cup (50 ml)	40–60
Soybeans, cooked or canned	1/2 cup (125 ml)	14
Soy flour	1/4 cup (50 ml)	28
Soy beverage, most brands	1 cup (250 ml)	20–25
Soy beverage, So Nice	1 cup (250 ml)	60
Soy hot dog	1	15
Soy protein isolate powder	1 oz. (28 g)	30
Tempeh, cooked	3 oz. (90 g)	48
Texturized vegetable protein, dry	1/2 cup (125 ml)	30–120
Tofu, firm	3 oz. (90 g)	22
Tofu, soft	3 oz. (90 g)	28

Source: USDA-Iowa State University Database on the Isoflavone Content of Foods. U.S. Department of Agriculture, Agricultural Research Service, 1999.

10 ways to enjoy more soy

1 Use a calcium-enriched (fortified) soy beverage on cereal or in a breakfast smoothie (see Appendix 3 for recipe).

2 Use a fortified soy beverage in cooking and baking; for instance in soups, casseroles, muffins, and pancakes.

3 Cube firm tofu and add it to soups. A favourite meal of mine is adding chopped tofu to hot and sour soup.

4 Grill firm tofu on the barbecue. First marinate tofu in balsamic vinegar or brush with hoisin sauce, then make tofu kebabs with vegetables.

5 Substitute soft or firm tofu for ricotta cheese in lasagna and cheesecake recipes.

6 Use silken tofu in creamy salad dressing or dip recipes.

7 Replace one-quarter of the all-purpose flour in a recipe with soy flour.

8 Snack on roasted soy nuts—they come in plain, barbecue, garlic, or onion flavours.

9 Replace ground meat with TVP (texturized vegetable protein) or ready-to-use soy ground round in chili, pasta sauce, and tacos.

10 Try veggie burgers (with soy protein) and veggie dogs cooked on the grill. When

buying veggie burgers, make sure you see "soy protein" listed as one of the first few ingredients on the label. And remember, they take only a few minutes to re-heat. Overcooking veggie burgers and veggies dogs will dry them out.

Soy protein powders

If you've tried my recipe ideas and are still not convinced that soy foods are welcome in your daily diet, consider using a high-quality soy protein powder. It's easy to add a tablespoon or two of soy protein powder into a homemade breakfast smoothie or a glass of orange juice. I have many clients who use these powders to ensure they get their daily dose of soy isoflavones.

Before you rush off to the health food store, however, keep in mind that soy pro-tein powders vary in quality. Depending on how the manufacturer extracts the protein from the soybean, you can end up with a little or a lot of isoflavones. Look for prod-ucts made with *isolated* soy protein. Soy protein isolates offer the purest form of soy protein available—the protein is completely separated, or isolated, from the carbohy-drate and fat portions of the soybean. Most soy protein isolates are made using a water extraction process, which preserves the naturally occurring isoflavones. I don't recom-mend buying soy protein concentrates. Many of these are made using alcohol to extract the protein from the bean. Alcohol extraction causes a loss of naturally occurring isoflavones. If you're uncertain how the soy protein you're considering buying is made, call the manufacturer. The chart on page 34 shows how the two protein extraction methods compare.

My advice is to buy a product made with Supro brand soy protein. You'll have to read the ingredient list to find this information. Manufactured by Protein Technologies International using an isoflavone-friendly process, Supro soy protein isolate contains plenty of isoflavones. It's also the soy protein isolate used in most scientific studies. Products that use Supro include Genisoy Protein Powder, Twinlab Vege Fuel, GNC Challenge Soy Protein 95, GNC Challenge Soy Solution, Nutrel Soy Serenity and Soy Strategy, Naturade Total Soy, and Interactive SoyOne.

What about an isoflavone supplement?

If you've been to a health food store lately, you may have noticed a number of isoflavone supplements on the shelf. These supplements are made with isoflavones that have been extracted from soybeans or red clover plants (you'll learn more about red

ISOFLAVONE CONTENT OF WATER- AND ALCOHOL-EXTRACTED SOY PROTEIN POWDERS

Type of soy protein	Serving size	Isoflavone content (milligrams)
Soy protein isolate (water extraction)	2 rounded tbsp. (30 g)	29.3
Soy protein concentrate (water extraction)	2 rounded tbsp. (30 g)	30.6
Soy protein concentrate (alcohol extraction)	2 rounded tbsp. (30 g)	3.7

Source: USDA-Iowa State University Database on the Isoflavone Content of Foods. U.S. Department of Agriculture, Agricultural Research Service, 1999. Release 1.1.

clover supplements later in this chapter). For many of you, popping a soy isoflavone pill with your multivitamin probably seems more appealing than eating a plate of stir-fried tofu. But do these supplements relieve hot flashes? As you will read below, the findings are mixed. (Results from the studies using red clover isoflavones are also mixed, as you'll read later on.)

One small study conducted at the Massachusetts Institute of Technology in Cambridge, Massachusetts, found no significant change in the number of hot flashes or night sweats experienced by postmenopausal women who took a soy isoflavone extract each day. However, other study findings have been positive. A study presented at the 1999 annual meeting of the North American Menopause Society found that an isoflavone supplement made from soy helped reduce the severity of hot flashes in postmenopausal women. A total of 177 women entered the trial. The average age of the trial participants was 55, and all were experiencing five or more hot flashes a day before the study. At the end of 12 weeks, women who had taken two 50-milligram isoflavone tablets daily experienced a significant reduction in the severity of hot flashes compared with women who had been given a placebo.[4]

There were also promising results from a double-blind (neither the researchers nor the subjects know who is getting the treatment or placebo), randomized controlled trial from Brazil that followed 80 postmenopausal women for four months. Half the women received a 100-milligram soy supplement; the others took a placebo. By the end of the study, the women taking the isoflavone supplement experienced significant improvement in symptoms. Researchers from France found similar results. They compared the effect of a soy pill containing 70-milligrams of isoflavones with that of a placebo on hot flashes in 75 women. The women taking the soy extract experienced a 38 percent reduction in the number of daily hot flashes after just one month of treatment. After four months, the women taking the soy supplement had a 61 percent reduction in hot flashes, compared with 34 percent in the placebo group.[5]

So what should you do? Eat isoflavone-rich food or pop a pill? To date, most experts agree that not enough research has been conducted to give the green light to isoflavone supplements. Most studies have been of short duration, so we don't know if it is safe to take these products over the long term. Isoflavones, in food or pill form, behave like estrogen in the body. For this reason, women with hormone sensitive cancers, endometriosis, or uterine fibroids should avoid supplemental doses of isoflavones. I certainly advise that women at high risk of breast cancer stay away from soy isoflavone pills. (Read Chapter 13 for more information on soy and breast cancer risk.) Until we know more about the safety and effectiveness of isoflavone supplements, I recommend that you incorporate phytoestrogen-containing foods into your diet.

Vitamins and minerals

VITAMIN E

If you're eating for a healthy heart, chances are you're already familiar with this antioxidant vitamin (you'll read how vitamin E helps protect you from heart disease in Chapter 12). It's possible that vitamin E might also help reduce hot flashes. Unfortunately, very little research has been done on this subject, and much of it dates back to the late 1940s. Although these studies were not placebo controlled, they did find the vitamin to be effective in reducing hot flashes. I have managed to find one recent study from the Mayo Clinic and Mayo Foundation in Cleveland. During the first four weeks of the study, the researchers gave 120 women with a history of breast cancer 800 international units (IU) of vitamin E daily. After taking vitamin E for four weeks, the women were given a placebo pill. The women did report fewer hot flashes when taking the vitamin E, but the effect was not dramatic.

Despite the limited amount of research, a survey of 438 American women conducted by researchers at Columbia University in New York revealed that 57 percent who had hot flashes took vitamin E, and 27 percent of these women felt that it helped.[6]

It is not completely understood how the vitamin works to reduce hot flashes. Vitamin E has been reported to prevent excessive production of follicle stimulating hormone (FSH) and luteinizing hormone (LH). As discussed at the beginning of this chapter, the higher the levels of these two hormones in your body, the more your blood vessels dilate. This dilation, in turn, increases blood flow to the skin, causing you to feel hotter.

While there's not a lot of scientific support for vitamin E as a therapy for hot flash relief, I am in favour of adding it to your nutrition regimen. As you'll read later in the book, vitamin E has other important health benefits, and it's impossible to get high amounts in your daily diet. The richest sources of this vitamin are vegetable oils, nuts, seeds, avocado, and wheat germ. Whole grains and leafy green vegetables such as kale and collards are also good sources. The recommended daily allowance for vitamin E is 22 IU, an amount that is possible to achieve from foods. But when you consider that one tablespoon of olive oil gives you a measly 2.6 IU of the vitamin, and 2 tablespoons of toasted wheat germ gives you only 4 IU, you can see why you must rely on a supplement to get 400 or 800 IU—the amounts used in the studies.

If buying a vitamin E supplement, choose one labelled "natural source." Although the body absorbs both synthetic and natural vitamin E equally well, your liver prefers the natural form. It incorporates more natural vitamin E into carrier molecules. Also consider choosing a vitamin E supplement that is labelled "mixed tocopherols." Preliminary research shows that one form of vitamin E, gamma-tocopherol, has potent anti-inflammatory effects in addition to its antioxidant properties. Some researchers think gamma-tocopherol may play a role in cancer prevention. If you're taking a blood-thinning medication such as Coumadin (warfarin), don't take vitamin E without your doctor's approval, since it has slight anticlotting properties.

BIOFLAVONOIDS AND VITAMIN C

Bioflavonoids are natural chemicals (phyto, or plant, chemicals) found in plant foods, and are especially plentiful in the inner peel of citrus fruits. They have been reported to have a very weak estrogen-like effect in the body—they are about 50,000 times less potent than your body's own estrogen. Over the years, bioflavonoids have been used to treat hot flashes, as well as vaginal dryness and fluid retention. They're most often combined in a supplement with vitamin C. It makes sense that the two work best together, since citrus fruits are rich sources of both. Despite that I could not find any published clinical studies supporting their use for hot flash relief, it may be worth trying bioflavonoids and vitamin C. They're both relatively easy to get in the diet, and if taken in appropriate amounts in supplemental form, they pose no risk to otherwise healthy women.

To get more citrus bioflavonoids and vitamin C into your diet, aim to eat at least one citrus fruit, such as an orange or grapefruit, each day. Or drink a glass of unsweetened citrus juice. If you make your own juice, you can also juice the fruit rinds to get plenty of bioflavonoids. If you decide to try this, you may want to use unwaxed, organically grown fruits. And make sure to add freshly grated citrus peel to fruit salsas, green salads, salad dressings, and home-baked muffins or loaves.

To supplement, take a 500-milligram vitamin C supplement once or twice a day. There's little point in swallowing much more, since your body can use only about 200 milligrams at one time. I've recommended 500-milligram supplements because this is the most common dose you'll find on the market. If you prefer to take a larger dose, take 500 milligrams twice daily.

Choose a vitamin C supplement with added bioflavonoids—you'll find this information on the ingredient list. The vitamin C supplement I take contains 50 milligrams of citrus bioflavonoids, though some contain as much as 100 milligrams. If you're looking for the most vitamin C for your money, choose a supplement labelled "Ester-C." This is a patented form of the vitamin that laboratory studies have found to be up to four times more available to the body than regular vitamin C (ascorbic acid or ascorbate). Many supplement manufacturers offer Ester-C.

There is some concern that vitamin C supplements can cause kidney stones, though no studies have shown this. Nevertheless, the body converts high amounts of vitamin C to oxalate, a component of kidney stones, and so I advise clients with a history of kidney stones to restrict their vitamin C intake to 100 milligrams per day.

Herbal remedies

Before I discuss the various herbal remedies, here's a rule to follow when buying almost any of them: Always buy a *standardized* product. When an herbal remedy has been standardized, each pill or capsule is guaranteed to give you a specified amount of the active ingredient or a marker ingredient found in the plant. By choosing a standardized product, you're making sure you get a high-quality product. Unstandardized brands could contain little or no active ingredients.

BLACK COHOSH (CIMICIFUGA RACEMOSA)

Also known as squawroot, bugbane, and snakeroot, black cohosh has long been used by North America's aboriginal peoples for treating menstrual and menopausal symptoms. It's also popular in Europe, especially in Germany, where it has been used for more than 40 years by over 1.5 million women. Both my clinical experience with clients and the findings from controlled scientific studies indicate that black cohosh is the most promising herbal remedy for treating menopausal symptoms.

When it comes to relieving hot flashes, some research suggests that black cohosh is just as effective as estrogen therapy. How the herb works, though, is currently under scientific debate. Experts do agree that naturally occurring active compounds in black cohosh are able to lower levels of luteinizing hormone (LH). As you'll recall, high LH levels can trigger hot flashes. These active compounds are called triterpene glycosides or, more generally, phytoestrogens, and are in the same class of compounds as the isoflavones found in soybeans. Where the experts don't agree is how these triterpene glycosides actually lower LH levels. Many German studies seem to indicate that they work by acting like weak estrogen molecules and binding to estrogen receptors. However, recent research has demonstrated that the herb does not have an estrogenic effect and, instead, may lower blood levels of LH by acting on receptors in the brain (remember, it's the hypothalamus that tells your pituitary gland to make LH).[7] Regardless of how black cohosh works to ease hot flashes, its effectiveness has helped many women through menopause. Take a look at the positive results from these well-controlled studies:

- *2002, Germany.* In this randomized double blind trial, 150 peri- and post-menopausal women were given a daily extract of black cohosh (a product called Remifemin) or a placebo. After six months of treatment, the majority of women reported a 70 percent reduction in physical and emotional symptoms, including hot flashes.
- *1991, Germany.* Researchers compared black cohosh with placebo to determine its ability to affect hormone levels in 110 women with menopausal symptoms.

After six months, there was a significant drop in the levels of luteinizing hormone (LH) in the black cohosh group. Again, Remifemin extract was used.

- *1988, Germany.* This study followed 60 women under 40 years of age who had had a hysterectomy. Women were randomly assigned either one of three estrogen medications or a standardized extract of black cohosh root (Remifemin). After six months, all groups had experienced a significant decline in menopausal symptoms. In this study, the herb was just as effective as estrogen in reducing hot flashes.

- *1987, Germany.* In this randomized trial, 80 perimenopausal women were given black cohosh root (Remifemin), standard estrogen therapy, or placebo. After 12 weeks, only the black cohosh extract had significantly improved hot flashes (as well as vaginal dryness and mood changes).[8]

The major advantage black cohosh offers in treating hot flashes is that it doesn't have the side effects associated with hormone therapy. Black cohosh should be your first treatment of choice if estrogen therapy is not an option because of uncomfortable side effects or because you have a higher than average risk of developing breast cancer. Of course, those of you who have had estrogen-positive breast cancer will likely have an important question to pose here. If black cohosh does act like estrogen, will it increase your risk of getting breast cancer again? The answer is no. A recent study found that black cohosh does not cause estrogen-positive breast cancer cells to grow. Furthermore, the researchers showed that the herb was able to inhibit, rather than promote, the growth of cancer cells.[9] The only side effects that have been reported in a small number of women is mild stomach upset and headache.

Earlier in the book, I told you that cancer treatments often trigger early menopause. Indeed, many breast cancer survivors experience hot flashes. Unfortunately, there isn't much research to support the use of black cohosh in this group of women. A recent American study gave breast cancer patients either black cohosh or a placebo pill. After two months of study, the women taking the herbal remedy didn't fare any better than those taking the placebo. Bottom line: Black cohosh didn't make a significant impact on the number or intensity of hot flashes experienced by these women.[10]

As stated above, I often recommend buying the herbal product used in the scientific studies, which, in the case of black cohosh, is Remifemin. This product is available in supplement stores, health food stores, and some pharmacies. Many other brands, however, also use a top-quality extract and offer an effective product. When buying black cohosh, look for the words "triterpene glycosides." High-quality brands state on the label that each tablet or capsule provides 40 milligrams of black cohosh standardized to contain 2.5 percent triterpene glycosides.

Almost all the studies investigating black cohosh and hot flashes used a dose of either 40 milligrams twice daily or 80 milligrams twice daily. This is why many products are sold as 40-milligram tablets or capsules. Remifemin is sold as a 20-milligram tablet, based on a recent study showing that a lower dose of this product is equally effective. If you buy a different brand, I recommend that you start with 40 milligrams twice a day. Don't be impatient. You will likely notice improvement four to eight weeks after you start taking the herb. If you don't notice any change in your hot flashes after six weeks, increase your dosage to 80 milligrams twice daily, but keep in mind that as you increase your dose, you may experience mild stomach upset or, possibly, headache. Black cohosh should not be used if you're taking hormone replacement therapy or medications to treat high blood pressure.

Many menopause supplements sold in pharmacies and health food stores combine black cohosh with a number of other herbs known to ease menopausal symptoms. Such products include Estro-Logic (Quest Vitamins), Menopause Formula (Natural Factors), Meno+ (ehn), and Life Menopause Formula (Shopper's Drug Mart). The herbal formula for Estro-Logic was developed by an American gynecologist, Dr. Kathleen Fry, and a medical herbalist, Claudia Wingo. The product is being studied in a trial of 100 menopausal women. Preliminary findings look promising—the combination appears to be effective at easing a number of common menopausal complaints, including hot flashes. You might consider trying one of these products rather than taking black cohosh alone.

RED CLOVER

Red clover flower tops contain four naturally occurring isoflavones: biochanin, formononetin, genistein, and daidzein. (You'll recall that genistein and daidzein are the same two isoflavones found in soybeans.) When it comes to determining if isoflavone supplements from red clover ease hot flashes, the findings are mixed. Two Australian studies found that red clover supplements had no effect on hot flashes. In one of these studies, 37 postmenopausal women were divided into three groups and given either a placebo or 40 or 160 milligrams daily of isoflavone extract derived from red clover (Promensil). In the second study, 51 postmenopausal women took 40 milligrams of Promensil daily for three months. In both studies, the women reported no difference in menopausal symptoms.[11]

While the studies mentioned above found no difference in the number of hot flashes among postmenopausal women taking a red clover supplement or a placebo pill, researchers from the Netherlands recently observed a 44 percent reduction after three months of supplementation. The study also used the branded red clover extract Promensil. A small US study investigated the effect of Promensil on hot flashes and found similar results. After eight weeks of treatment, women experienced significantly fewer and less intense hot flashes.[12]

Red clover might also help prevent osteoporosis. A 12-month study conducted among 107 women aged 50 to 64 years revealed that red clover (Promensil) slowed down bone loss in the spine among pre- and perimenopausal women. An Australian study found that postmenopausal women taking a different extract of red clover isoflavones, called Rimostil, experienced an increase in bone mass over a six-month period.[13]

The recommended dose of red clover is one tablet daily of Promensil (peri-menopausal women) or Rimostil (postmenopausal women). While both products are made from red clover, each contains a slightly different mix of the four different red clover isoflavones. Promensil seems to be more effective in easing hot flashes, whereas Rimostil may be more effective for bone health.

As with any herbal remedy, there are potential side effects. Red clover may cause skin rash. Women with hormone-sensitive cancers, endometriosis, or uterine fibroids should not use generic brands of red clover. Published data on Promensil indicate that it does not stimulate cell growth in the endometrium, nor does it increase breast density. However, do not assume that other red clover products have been tested for their effect on breast cells. Because red clover isoflavones have an estrogen-like action in the body, it's safer to avoid using them if you have a hormone-sensitive condition.

THE bottom LINE...

Leslie's recommendations for relieving hot flashes

1   Avoid foods that can trigger hot flashes or make them worse. Foods and beverages that contain caffeine are prime culprits. Avoid alcohol altogether if you're experiencing hot flashes or if you're under stress. Finally, stay away from spicy foods.

2   Add one serving of soy food to your daily diet.

3   Gradually increase your soy intake to ensure you're eating 40 to 80 milligrams of isoflavones each day.

4   If you're having trouble eating enough soy to give you 40 milligrams of isoflavones daily, consider adding 1 to 2 tablespoons (15 to 25 ml) of a soy protein powder (made from soy protein isolate) to milk, juice, or a homemade fruit smoothie daily.

5   Start taking 800 IU of vitamin E each day. Buy natural source vitamin E. Vitamin E is fat soluble, so take it with a meal that contains a little fat to help its absorption. Don't take vitamin E if you're on blood-thinning medication. Check with your physician first.

6   To get more bioflavonoids and vitamin C, add one citrus fruit to your diet each day. Add citrus zest to recipes where appropriate.

7   Take a 500-milligram supplement of Ester-C (a patented form of vitamin C) with added bioflavonoids once or twice daily. Or, buy a separate bioflavonoid supplement of 250 to 500 milligrams and take once or twice daily.

8   Consider taking a standardized extract of black cohosh. Start with 40 milligrams of the herb, twice daily, morning and evening (40 milligrams is usually the amount found in one tablet or capsule). If you don't find the herb effective after six weeks, take two 40-milligram tablets twice daily.

9   If black cohosh causes side effects such as stomach upset or headache, consider using red clover, a supplement containing isoflavones. Take one tablet of Promensil daily.

Restless nights and insomnia

"I started waking up to find my body soaking wet and cold and the bed sheets literally drenched. I found myself in a constant state of exhaustion. I had to find a cure for these night sweats if I was going to be able to perform properly during the workday."

5

How many of you have woken up feeling hot and bothered, your bed sheets soaking wet? Night sweats cause disrupted sleep in a good number of women in their peri- and postmenopausal years. While many women have no difficulty falling back to sleep, some simply cannot. Night after night of little sleep leaves them feeling exhausted, and that's when many other menopausal symptoms can emerge. Fatigue can lead to irritability, depression, and forgetfulness. But don't get me wrong—I'm not saying that insomnia is the only reason for these symptoms. Hormonal fluctuations that accompany the perimenopausal years can be responsible too. You'll learn more about these fluctuations and their overall potential impact in Chapters 6 and 7.

When your sleep habits are disturbed regularly for more than three weeks, you are considered to be suffering from *chronic insomnia*. While in some cases insomnia may be the result of nocturnal hot flashes, some experts believe that something else, something unrelated to hot flashes, interrupts sleep in many peri- and postmenopausal women. Insomnia usually results from a combination of factors and is often a symptom of some other physical or mental condition. As well, certain medications may trigger insomnia, so consult your pharmacist about possible side effects of any medications you are taking.

Keep in mind that our sleep patterns change as we age. Research indicates that sleep efficiency decreases from a high of 95 percent in adolescence to less than 80 percent in old age. Consequently, older women have more difficulty falling asleep or staying asleep, and they often find that sleep is not as refreshing as it once was. But there are also many lifestyle and environmental factors that can lead to chronic insomnia. Whatever is causing your sleepless nights—be it hot flashes, stress, or a side effect of a medication—you can take action without resorting to prescribed sleeping aids (or a glass of wine!) before tucking in for the night.

Dietary approaches

CUT DOWN ON CAFFEINE

No doubt you've heard this before: Eat and drink fewer caffeine-containing foods and beverages and you'll sleep better. Still, it's advice that bears repeating. Caffeine stimulates the central nervous system. While one or two cups of coffee in the morning may give you that gentle lift you were hoping for, the fourth or fifth cup can overstimulate your system and cause insomnia (not to mention irritability). My first recommendation to clients wanting to cut down on caffeine is to avoid it in the afternoon. Replace caffeine-containing beverages with caffeine-free or decaffeinated beverages such as herbal tea, mineral water, unsweetened fruit or vegetable juice, and decaffeinated coffee.

How much caffeine is too much?

Health Canada says that a daily consumption of 400 to 450 milligrams of caffeine does not pose any risks for healthy people.[1] However, Health Canada's recommendation is based on studies that have investigated the effect of caffeine on blood pressure and other health conditions, not on your ability to sleep soundly. While Health Canada's upper limit of 450 milligrams won't harm your health, it may keep you up at night—and that may harm your health! Studies have shown that as little as one or two cups of coffee in the morning will affect the quality of your sleep that night. Other studies have found that as little as 100 milligrams of caffeine (the amount found in 4 ounces [125 ml] of coffee) can delay sleep when taken before bedtime, especially in people who don't usually consume caffeine.[2] Caffeine blocks the action of adenosine, a natural brain chemical that slows down the body. If you're having trouble getting to sleep or if you're waking up during the night, aim to consume no more than 200 milligrams per day, and preferably none at all. Use the following chart to find out how much caffeine you're consuming. (And remember that the "grande" size of cup at Starbucks contains a lot more than 8 ounces!)

CAFFEINE CONTENT OF COMMON FOODS AND BEVERAGES (MILLIGRAMS)

Coffee, filter drip, 8 oz. (235 ml)	110–180
Coffee, instant, 8 oz. (235 ml)	80–120
Coffee, decaffeinated, 8 oz. (235 ml)	4
Espresso, 2 oz. (60 ml)	90–100
Tea, black, 8 oz. (235 ml)	46
Tea, green, 8 oz. (235 ml)	33
Cola, 12 oz. (375 ml)	35
Dark chocolate, 1 oz. (30 g)	20–30
Milk chocolate, 1 oz. (30 g)	6
Chocolate cake, 1 slice	20–30
Excedrin, 2 tablets	130
Anacin or Midol, 2 tablets	64

ELIMINATE ALCOHOL

Unfortunately, there are no two ways about it—the effects of alcohol are detrimental to sleep, and consuming alcohol will worsen insomnia. Even if you're not suffering from sleep problems, a few drinks still certainly can affect the quality of your sleep. Swiss researchers have found that having a moderate amount of alcohol six hours before bedtime reduces sleep time and increases wakefulness two-fold. I know that if I enjoy a couple of glasses of wine in the evening, I inevitably wake up a few times that night. Or worse, I wake up at four in the morning and can't fall back asleep. Then I'm forced to drag myself through the next day feeling tired and lethargic. Sound familiar? I can remember the good old days when a few drinks wouldn't bother me—I could stay out late and feel great on less than eight hours of sleep. I now save my alcohol for the weekend, when I can grab a few extra hours of sleep each night. For the sake of sound sleep, a healthy body, and a productive mind, I recommend the same to all my clients.

Why does alcohol affect sleep the way it does? Once absorbed into the bloodstream, alcohol is metabolized, or processed, by your liver at a set rate. If you drink more alcohol than your liver can keep up with (about one drink per hour), alcohol arrives in the brain, where it interferes with brain chemicals called neurotransmitters, which are responsible for transferring messages from one nerve cell to another. Neurotransmitters need to be in proper balance for deep, restful sleep to occur. Alcohol has also been reported to impair the rapid eye movement (REM) portion of sleep, a sleep phase very important for physical, emotional, and mental restoration.[3]

At the same time that alcohol robs you of rest, it also tires you further by dehydrating you. Alcohol's dehydrating effect is due to its ability to depress the brain's production of antidiuretic hormone. Without enough antidiuretic hormone, you lose water and minerals through your kidneys. This, in turn, can increase your feeling of fatigue. This is because water makes it possible for you to digest, absorb, and transport nutrients throughout your body. So when you're dehydrated after an evening of drinking alcohol, your cells receive nutrients (and oxygen) less efficiently. You also need water to help regulate your body temperature. If you drink too much alcohol—even just a couple of drinks—your body will have trouble properly regulating its temperature. If you're well hydrated, your body has enough fluid to release heat that builds up from normal metabolism and exercise; every day your body releases heat through your skin in the form of sweat. If you're dehydrated because you're not drinking enough fluids, or you've enjoyed a little too much wine, your body can't release built-up heat as efficiently because it doesn't have enough fluid to produce sweat. As a result, you may also find your hot flashes get worse after imbibing.

How much alcohol is safe to drink?

I recommend that women consume no more than one drink per day or seven drinks per week. This recommendation is based on our current knowledge of cancer prevention. But if you're suffering from insomnia, or you want to be at your peak the next day, eliminate alcohol from your diet altogether. Instead of having a glass of wine, pour yourself sparkling mineral water and spruce it up with a slice of lime. Or try some of the nonalcoholic wines or beers available. If you're wanting a cocktail, how about a virgin Caesar, tomato juice, or a splash of cranberry juice in soda water?

You can also use a few tricks to lessen the effect of alcohol on your sleep:

Drink alcohol with a meal or snack.   If you drink alcohol on an empty stomach, about 20 percent of it is absorbed directly across the walls of your stomach, reaching the brain within a minute. But when the stomach is full of food, alcohol has less chance of touching its walls and passing through them, so the effect on your brain is delayed.

Drink no more than one drink every hour.   Since the liver can't metabolize alcohol any faster than this, drinking slowly will ensure your blood alcohol concentration doesn't rise too quickly. To help you slow your pace, try alternating alcoholic and nonalcoholic drinks. By the way, one drink is equivalent to 5 ounces (150 ml) of wine, 12 ounces (375 ml) of beer, 10 ounces (310 ml) of wine cooler, or 1.5 ounces (45 ml) of liquor. A pint of beer (500 ml) counts as two drinks!

EAT CARBOHYDRATE BEFORE BED

If your mother ever told you to drink a glass of warm milk to help you sleep, she was smart. A snack rich in carbohydrate, like a glass of milk, a small bowl of cereal, or a slice of toast, provides the brain with an amino acid called tryptophan. The brain needs tryptophan to manufacture a neurotransmitter called serotonin. Serotonin has been shown to facilitate sleep, improve mood, diminish pain, and even reduce appetite.

I don't often recommend snacks after dinner, especially for clients trying to lose weight. But if you follow this suggestion in the spirit I've intended (that is, a *small* snack), you won't gain weight. If you want to find out whether carbohydrate helps you fall asleep, eat a small amount of carbohydrate food, or drink a glass of low-fat milk or soy beverage one hour before going to bed. Try this strategy for a week. If your insomnia does not improve, look at other factors that may be disrupting your sleep.

Vitamins and minerals

VITAMIN B12

Many studies have found that vitamin B12 promotes sleep, especially in people with sleep disorders. Researchers in Japan have used 1.5 to 3 milligrams of the vitamin each day to restore normal sleep patterns in patients. When vitamin B12 was withheld for two months, sleep disruptions reappeared. A German study found that sleep quality, ability to concentrate, and "feeling refreshed" were significantly correlated with B12 blood levels in healthy men and women.[4]

It is not completely understood exactly how this B vitamin works to influence sleep. Some researchers believe it interacts with melatonin, a natural hormone in the body. Melatonin is involved in maintaining the body's internal clock, which in turn regulates the secretion of various hormones. In so doing, melatonin is also thought to help control sleep and wakefulness patterns. Melatonin production is stimulated by darkness and suppressed by light. It seems that vitamin B12 directly influences melatonin release and metabolism and may prevent disturbances in melatonin balance.

The recommended dietary allowance (RDA) of vitamin B12 for healthy adults (women and men) is 2.4 micrograms per day. In 1998, the Food and Nutrition Board of the National Academy of Sciences, an organization of American and Canadian scientists who set RDAs for North America, released a new recommendation for vitamin B12. The board recommended that people over the age of 50 get their B12 by eating foods fortified with the vitamin (such foods contain the vitamin in a ready-to-absorb state), or by taking a supplement. The board made this recommendation because, to absorb vitamin B12 from our diet, the body must first use stomach acid to release it from food proteins. However, as we age, we produce less stomach acid. Indeed, up to 30 percent of older adults produce very little or no stomach acid, a condition called achlorhydria.

Are you getting enough vitamin B12? On page 49 you'll find a list of foods high in B12 that will help you boost your intake in no time.

What about a vitamin B12 supplement?

Vitamin B12 is found in all animal foods—meat, poultry, fish, eggs, and dairy products. If you are eating these foods every day, you are likely meeting your B12 needs. Foods fortified with the vitamin include soy beverages, rice beverages, and breakfast cereals (you'll have to check the label to be sure). However, I do recommend you take a B12 supplement if:

- You're over 50 years of age.
- You're taking antacid medication for reflux (heartburn) or a stomach ulcer.
- You're a strict vegetarian who eats no animal foods, and you don't use fortified soy or rice drinks.

Vitamin B12 supplements come in 500- or 1000-microgram sizes. To ensure you're meeting your requirements, I recommend taking 500 micrograms once a day, with a meal. The active form of vitamin B12, called methylcobalamin, is preferred over cyanocobalamin. No adverse effects have been reported in healthy people taking B12 supplements.

VITAMIN B12 CONTENT OF COMMON FOODS (MICROGRAMS)

Beef, flank, cooked, 3 oz. (90 g)	2.8
Chicken breast, cooked, 5 oz. (140 g)	0.3
Chicken leg, cooked, 6 oz. (180 g)	0.2
Pork centre loin, cooked, 3 oz. (90 g)	0.5
Mussels, cooked, 3 oz. (90 g)	20
Salmon, sockeye, cooked, 3 oz. (90 g)	4.9
Tuna, canned and drained, 3 oz. (90 g)	2.5
Egg, 1 whole	0.6
Cheese, cheddar 1 oz. (30 g)	0.2
Cottage cheese, 1%, 1/2 cup (125 ml)	0.7
Milk, 1 cup (250 ml)	0.9
Yogurt, 3/4 cup (175 ml)	0.9
Fortified soy drink, 1 cup (250 ml)	1.0
Fortified rice drink, 1 cup (250 ml)	1.0

Source: *Nutrient Value of Some Common Foods*, Health Canada, 1999. Adapted and reproduced with the permission of the Minister of Public Works and Government Services Canada, 2003.

Herbal remedies

VALERIAN *(VALERIANA OFFICINALIS)*

Native to Europe, this plant has a mild sedative effect on the central nervous system. Valerian root makes getting to sleep easier, and it increases the amount of time you spend in deep sleep. The herb also appears to have antianxiety and mood-enhancing properties. Unlike popular prescribed sleeping pills, valerian does not lead to dependence or addiction. And it usually doesn't cause a morning "hangover." When compared with drugs such as Valium and Xanax, valerian binds very weakly to brain receptors.[5]

Scientists have learned that valerian promotes sleep by increasing the levels of a brain chemical called gamma-aminobutyric acid (GABA). GABA plays a key role in reducing feelings of stress and anxiety. Scientists can actually measure an increased concentration of GABA in the brains of individuals who have taken valerian. It seems that not only is valerian able to increase the amount of GABA secreted by the brain, it also helps prevent the levels from falling too quickly. The net result for someone who takes valerian is that GABA levels stay high for a longer time.

Much of the research on valerian and sleep dates back to the mid-1980s and early 1990s. At least 10 controlled clinical studies have evaluated valerian's effects in both healthy people and patients with sleep disorders. In one double-blind study (neither the researchers nor the subjects knew who was getting valerian or placebo), 89 percent of those taking 400 milligrams of valerian root reported improved sleep; 44 percent of the study participants taking valerian reported perfect sleep. Two other studies conducted with healthy people found that valerian was able to significantly reduce the time it takes to fall asleep and improve the quality of sleep. In both studies, participants used 400 to 450 milligrams of valerian daily.[6]

Although the active ingredients in valerian have not yet been confirmed, many experts attribute the herb's effect to certain essential oils found in the root. For this reason, I recommend that you buy a product standardized to contain at least 0.5 percent essential oils or 0.8 percent valerenic acid. Take 400 to 900 milligrams in capsule or tablet form, from 30 minutes to one hour before bedtime. If you wake up feeling groggy, reduce the dose. Don't expect results overnight. One German study found that the herb worked better for people suffering chronic insomnia when used over a period of time.[7] Valerian has a delayed onset of action; it may take two to four weeks to achieve an improvement in sleep.

This herbal remedy may cause stomach upset and headache. Although most studies find no effect of valerian on morning alertness and concentration, valerian may occasionally cause morning drowsiness. Do not combine valerian with alcohol or sedative medications. Valerian should not be taken during pregnancy and breastfeeding, as reliable information on its use during this time is insufficient.

Other ways to help yourself sleep

Here are some further suggestions for increasing your likelihood of getting a restful night's sleep:

1 *Avoid eating heavy meals and smoking cigarettes in the evening.* Heavy meals and rich foods take longer to digest and may make it difficult to fall asleep. If you smoke cigarettes, avoid doing so before bedtime, as nicotine can stimulate your system and make it difficult to fall asleep.

2   *Don't forget about exercise.* Regular physical activity can bring on a feeling of
     tiredness later in the day. Research shows exercise also helps you rest better by
     increasing your blood level of melatonin, which, as I discussed above, plays an
     important role in regulating sleep-wake cycles. I recommend a minimum of three
     to four cardiovascular exercise sessions each week. Try brisk walking, jogging,
     biking, stair climbing, swimming, cross-country skiing, or aerobics classes. If you
     haven't been exercising at all, consult with your doctor before you begin a
     program. Then start at 20 minutes per session, gradually building up to 30 to 45
     minutes per session. Avoid exercising too close to bedtime (in other words, after
     dinner), as vigorous activity before going to bed may keep you awake a little
     longer.

3   *Get into a nighttime routine that you associate with going to sleep.* Reading a book,
     drinking a cup of chamomile tea, or taking a warm bath can all help slow your
     mind and body, preparing you for sleep. Avoid watching television or doing
     office work within one hour before your bedtime. Instead, do something that
     helps you quiet your mind and relax. Keep your bedroom at a comfortable
     temperature. Sleeping in a room that is too warm or too cold can cause sleep
     disturbances.

4   *Practise relaxation techniques* if worries and tension related to stress are keeping
     you awake. Learn about deep breathing or meditation. I have many clients who
     regularly practice yoga and can't say enough about its relaxing effect. If these
     techniques don't work for you, consider speaking with a stress management
     counsellor.

5   *Visit your family doctor* if you've tried all of the above and you still can't sleep (or
     if you have no energy during the day). Both poor sleep patterns and ongoing
     fatigue may be the symptoms of an underlying health problem. A physical exam
     and blood tests can often help determine the cause.

Sleep disturbances can cause a loss of restorative sleep, the period during which your
body rebuilds its vital forces. Depression, stress, obesity, muscle cramps, restless legs,
and sleep-related breathing disorders such as sleep apnea can all interfere with a good
night's rest. You doctor may refer you to a sleep disorder clinic to help determine the
underlying cause of ongoing sleep disturbances.

THE bottom LINE...

Leslie's recommendations for coping with insomnia

1   Avoid eating dinner close to bedtime. Try to leave a window of at least three hours between eating your evening meal and retiring for the night. And avoid eating heavy meals if insomnia is plaguing you.

2   Cut back your caffeine intake to a daily maximum of 200 milligrams. Remember, though, that it's preferable to avoid as much caffeine as possible.

3   If you drink alcohol and don't want to give it up (which I recommend doing if you're experiencing sleep problems), aim for no more than one drink per day or seven drinks per week. To lessen alcohol's impact on your brain, have your drink with a meal or a snack.

4   Try a light carbohydrate-rich snack 30 to 60 minutes before going to bed to increase the level of sleep-promoting serotonin in your brain. Good choices include a banana, a slice of toast, a glass of milk or calcium-fortified soy beverage, or a small bowl of cereal. Some experts even recommend a baked potato!

5   Make sure you are getting enough B12 in your diet. If you can't get enough B12 through food, or if you don't produce enough stomach acid to absorb it efficiently, take 500 micrograms of vitamin B12 daily in supplement form.

6   For short-term insomnia, consider taking 400 to 900 milligrams of valerian root extract 30 minutes to one hour before bedtime. Buy a product standardized to contain at least 0.5 percent essential oils or 0.8 percent valerenic acid. Use valerian to manage acute bouts of insomnia. Long-term (longer than three months) daily use of valerian may cause headaches and sleepiness in some individuals.

7   Don't forget to investigate other possible causes of chronic sleep problems: a lack of exercise, too much stress, or a possible medical problem.

Mood swings

"One minute I feel fine; the next minute I am irritable, cranky, irrational, and depressed for no particular reason. I am normally a high-energy-type person, but I find that I just can't get myself in gear these days, no matter how well I eat, sleep, or exercise."

6

Most women describe the mood swings of perimenopause as being like those of premenstrual syndrome (PMS). They talk about crying at the drop of a hat, or blowing up at a family member for no good reason. Some women describe day-long bad moods, during which everyone and everything annoys them. If you've ever suffered through these kinds of feelings during the premenstrual stage, you know they're not fun. And that they can be disruptive to your personal and work life.

Not all women experience mood swings during the transition years, however. Studies show that if a woman has had a hysterectomy, she's more likely to become depressed.[1] But mood swings are not an inevitable consequence of menopause. While you might feel mildly depressed, your next-door neighbour might never experience a strong mood shift during her perimenopausal years. It's my clinical observation that women who tend to be irritable and cranky during the premenstrual stage experience the same mood swings, often more intense, at perimenopause. Those mood changes may be minor for some women and major for others.

Mood swings are partly due to hormone fluctuations. Although we don't yet fully understand what happens in the body during a woman's menstrual cycle, we do know that natural chemicals in the brain, called neurotransmitters, respond to hormonal fluctuations that occur during the cycle. Neurotransmitters are responsible for the transfer of messages from one nerve cell to another. These chemicals are released at the end of a nerve cell when a nerve impulse arrives there. Once they are released, neurotransmitters move to the next nerve cell and alter the membrane of that second cell so as to either inhibit or excite it. The neurotransmitters that excite nerve fibres make us more alert, while the ones that inhibit nerve fibres calm us down.

The hormonal ups and downs of perimenopause may also make us more sensitive than usual to our feelings. And certainly for some women, the approach of menopause itself can be upsetting. If you're unhappy or dissatisfied with your life, the signal that one life phase is ending and a new one is beginning can be distressing. Sometimes a feeling of unfulfillment, whether it's a result of boredom at work or an unhappy marriage, can create anxiety about the postmenopausal years. We fear that if we're not happy now, menopause will make matters worse. Other women fear they are leaving behind their youthful, productive years.

Regardless of what is responsible for your mood swings, there are things you can do to calm them down. If they're interfering with your enjoyment of life, it's especially important to take action. Consult your family doctor if my suggestions don't help and your mood changes continue to disrupt your life.

Dietary approaches

For centuries, people have used food to alter their mood. What our ancestors didn't realize was that, by eating certain foods, they were actually influencing their brain chemistry. Modern science, however, now recognizes that the foods we eat can affect our mood by modifying the brain's production and release of neurotransmitters. The brain and nervous system rely on 30 to 40 neurotransmitters to do their work; researchers believe that five or six of these can be affected by food. Nutrients like carbohydrates, proteins, and vitamins are able to cross the "blood-brain barrier"—a physiological mechanism that limits the types of substances that can enter the brain—and be converted into neurotransmitters.

Studies have shown that specific neurotransmitters affect our mood in predictable ways. It's not known for sure, though, whether eating meals designed to increase the level of certain neurotransmitters is an effective way to re-create the moods inspired by that neurotransmitter. Keep in mind that everyone is different and we may not all respond in the same way. What is true, however, is that any drastic change in your normal eating patterns (crash dieting, bingeing on sweets, or skipping meals) can alter neurotransmitter levels and your mood. So the first step to smoothing out your mood is to eat at regular intervals throughout the day. No more meal skipping! And don't wait longer than four to five hours between meals; if you do need to, grab a between-meal snack. The second step? Eliminate caffeine and alcohol, two beverages known to increase anxiety, irritability, and feelings of depression. Your next step? Read on.

CARBOHYDRATE-RICH FOODS

Without a doubt, carbohydrates have been one of the most widely studied nutrients in terms of their effect on mood. High-carbohydrate meals have been associated with a calming, relaxing effect and even drowsiness. A high-carbohydrate meal, such as pasta, increases the brain levels of an amino acid called tryptophan. The brain then uses tryptophan to make the neurotransmitter serotonin. Many studies have linked high serotonin levels with happier moods and low levels with mild depression and irritability. Most of the research in this area has been done with women who have PMS. One study found that meals high in carbohydrates improved mood in young women within 30 minutes of consumption. Another study found that when women with PMS took a high-carbohydrate drink, their mood improved within 90 minutes.[2]

If you're feeling depressed or irritable, try a high-carbohydrate meal that contains very little protein. Protein foods are made up of many different amino acids, so the more protein you eat, whether it's chicken, meat, or fish, the more amino acids that will enter your bloodstream. And that means there will be many other types of amino acids available to compete with tryptophan for entry into the brain. Remember that you want tryptophan levels to rise in your brain so that you can produce more serotonin, which can make you feel calm and relaxed. Try pasta with tomato sauce, toasted whole-grain bread with jam, or a bowl of cereal with low-fat milk.

If your mood needs a boost during the day, reach for a high-carbohydrate beverage (available at health food stores and sports equipment stores). These drinks are used by athletes to help rebuild muscle carbohydrate stores after a hard workout. They're sold as powder mixes and ready-to-drink and come in a variety of flavours.

The next time you're in the United States, drop by a pharmacy to pick up a liquid dietary supplement called PMS Escape. It's a powdered drink mix, available in several flavours, made from a blend of carbohydrates, vitamins, and minerals. It's thought to boost serotonin levels in the brain. The product was developed by Judith Wurtman, a research scientist at the Massachusetts Institute of Technology and a pioneer researcher of the carbohydrate-serotonin connection.

CHOCOLATE

Chocolate is thought by some researchers to have a mood-enhancing ability. They attribute this to a number of its ingredients:

- The sugar in chocolate triggers the release of serotonin in the brain, producing a calm, relaxed feeling. Interestingly, though, one recent study that looked at chocolate addicts found that after they ate chocolate, mood did not improve. In fact, these women felt guilty after eating chocolate. The researchers summarized: "Although chocolate is a food which provides pleasure, for those who consider themselves chocolate addicts, any pleasure experienced is short lived and accompanied by feelings of guilt."[3]
- The caffeine in chocolate stimulates the central nervous system to give you a quick lift. Since milk chocolate contains very little caffeine, dark chocolate is more likely to give you a hit.
- Chocolate contains fat-like compounds that have been shown to target receptors in the brain and produce heightened sensitivity and euphoria.[4]
- Chocolate contains *phenylethylamine*, a chemical that some experts say stimulates feelings that people experience when in love. Its feel-good chemicals have long been associated with feelings of love, safety, and comfort.

Other experts argue that our love of chocolate is purely sensory, and that it's our desire for chocolate's wonderful smell, flavour, and rich texture that keeps us coming back for more. Indeed, at this time, most of the evidence linking chocolate with mood improvement is anecdotal. Still, it's nice to be able to justify that (occasional) chocolate bar. Pass the Godiva, please!

OMEGA-3 FATS FROM FISH

It seems that the type of fat you eat can affect your mood. Scientists have learned that levels of omega-3 fats are lower in people who are depressed.[5] These special polyunsaturated oils are important components of nerve and brain cell membranes and help cells communicate messages effectively. Omega-3 fats may also be crucial for the formation of brain hormones that help stabilize mood.

The best sources of omega-3 oils are cold-water fish. Salmon, trout, mackerel, herring, sardines, and anchovies are all good choices. I recommend that you eat fish three times per week. Fish contains two special omega-3 fats with long, barely pronounceable names: docosahexaenoic acid (DHA) and eicosapentaenoic acid (EPA). It's a lack of DHA that seems to be an important factor in depression. DHA may work to ease depression by altering the structure of cell membranes in the brain, making them more responsive to the effects of serotonin. It's also thought that DHA has anti-inflammatory effects in the brain, which can influence mood.

You might be wondering if fish is safe to eat after hearing reports of mercury contamination. It's true that some species of fish accumulate high levels of mercury, which can cause health problems. These fish include swordfish, shark, tuna steak, and king mackerel. Women in their childbearing years and children under the age of 15 should eat these fish no more than once per month. Other people should limit their consumption to no more than once per week. According to Health Canada, mercury is not an issue with canned tuna, as the tuna used for canning is young and hasn't had time to accumulate mercury. However, recent reports suggest that if you eat canned tuna day after day, you might be getting too much mercury. Some experts say that the amount of canned tuna that is safe to eat each week should be based on your body weight. To be safe, aim for no more than 5 ounces (150 g) each week. You might also want to stick with albacore or chunk light varieties, as they have less mercury than solid white or chunk white types. Fortunately, the fish that contain the most omega-3 fats do not pose a mercury concern. So go ahead and enjoy your salmon steak or sardine sandwich a few times each week. (You'll learn in Chapter 12 that a regular fare of oily fish also wards off heart disease.)

If you don't care to eat fish, there are other ways to get more DHA into your cell membranes.

Fish oil capsules

Unless you are allergic to fish, you can take a fish oil supplement. Research suggests that fish oil supplements improve symptoms in patients with clinical depression. Boston researchers from Harvard University and the Brigham and Women's Hospital studied 30 people with manic depression (also known as bipolar disorder) who were taking medication. The four-month study found that compared with placebo pills, people taking a daily dose of omega-3s from fish oil capsules had significantly longer remission periods from their depression. In fact, those who took the fish oil were three times more likely to maintain stable moods.[6]

If you opt for taking supplements, choose a product that contains both EPA and DHA. While proportions of EPA and DHA can vary among supplements, most brands of fish oil contain 18 percent EPA and 12 percent DHA. Fish oil supplements vary considerably in the amount and ratio of DHA and EPA. As well, look for a supplement that has vitamin E added, which helps prevent the oils from going rancid. And finally, avoid fish *liver* oil capsules. Fish liver oil is a concentrated source of vitamins A and D, which can be toxic when taken in large amounts for long periods. Take a 500-milligram capsule once or twice a day.

The downside? For starters, fish oil supplements can cause belching and cause a fishy taste in the mouth. High doses can cause nausea and diarrhea. Because fish oil "thins" the blood, exercise caution if you are taking other blood-thinning medication, such as aspirin, warfarin (Coumadin), and heparin. If you take these drugs, consult your physician before taking fish oil capsules. If you are being treated for depression, *fish oil supplements should never replace your medication. Always discuss any alternative or complementary treatment with your doctor first.* Also keep in mind that the research cited above involved people with serious depression, serious enough to put them on medication. For most people, following my recommendations for getting enough omega-3 fat into the daily diet is their best bet.

FLAXSEED, WALNUT, AND CANOLA OILS

Our bodies use foods rich in a fat called alpha-linolenic acid (ALA) to make small amounts of DHA. ALA is a member of the omega-3 fat family—it's a cousin of DHA and EPA in fish—and is an essential fatty acid, a fatty acid that is vital to our health. However, our bodies cannot make it—it must be supplied by the diet. Flaxseed oil, walnut oil, canola oil, soybeans, omega-3 eggs, and green leafy vegetables all contain ALA. With today's emphasis on low-fat and fat-free products, many experts fear we're not getting enough ALA.

You'll read later, in Chapters 12 and 13, that the omega-3 family of fats does more than prevent depression. Studies show that these fats appear to play important roles in fighting heart disease and breast cancer. So it's a good idea to get more omega-3 fats into your diet. Along with eating fish at least three times per week, buy omega-3 eggs

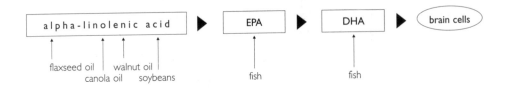

instead of regular eggs. The chickens that lay these eggs eat a diet high in flaxseed. One egg provides about 25 to 33 percent of the recommended daily intake of omega-3 fatty acids. Use flaxseed oil in salad dressings and canola oil in baking and cooking. In fact, try to get the majority of your added fats and oils from omega-3 sources. If you're allowing yourself 4 teaspoons (20 ml) of added fat a day, make sure that two or three of these (10 to 15 ml) come from omega-3 sources.

If you've never used flaxseed oil before, here are a few pointers. First, you might not be able to find this healthy oil at your local supermarket. It's likely you'll have to make a trip to a health food store, where you'll find the oil in the refrigerated foods section. Make sure you buy a brand bottled in opaque plastic or dark glass. When you take the flaxseed oil home, put it right back in the fridge; omega-3 fats are sensitive to light and heat and turn rancid quickly if not stored properly. Because of its sensitivity to heat, flaxseed oil should never be used in recipes that call for heating. Instead, use this oil in salad dressings, dips, and other unheated dishes. If you want to add it to a cooked dish such as soup, do so just before serving. Visit www.omeganutrition.com for recipes calling for flaxseed oil.

Vitamins and minerals

VITAMIN B6

Even marginal deficiencies of B vitamins have been associated with irritability, depression, and mood changes. One study found that vitamin B6–deficient mothers were less responsive to their newborns. These newborns were more likely to have older siblings care for them than were newborns whose mothers consumed adequate amounts of B6.

If you have ever suffered from PMS, chances are that you have already heard about the benefits of vitamin B6. This B vitamin has been the focus of study in more than 900 women suffering from PMS (nine clinical studies have been published at the time of this writing). A recent review of this research found that doses of vitamin B6 of up to 100 milligrams daily bring about significant improvement in premenstrual symptoms.[7] Based on the evidence available, and the relationship I've observed between the mood swings of PMS and perimenopause, a daily supplement of vitamin B6 seems likely to improve your mood and smooth out the emotional rollercoaster rides experienced by women suffering from perimenopausal depression or mood swings.

How does this vitamin affect your mood? Well, we find ourselves returning to that soothing brain chemical, serotonin. The body uses vitamin B6 to form an important enzyme needed to convert the amino acid tryptophan into serotonin in the brain. Healthy premenopausal women need 1.3 milligrams of vitamin B6 each day to prevent a deficiency of the nutrient. After menopause, women need 1.5 milligrams each day. The best sources of B6 are high-protein foods such as meat, fish, and poultry. Other good sources include whole grains, bananas, and potatoes. Below is a list of foods that will pack more B6 into your diet.

What about a vitamin B6 supplement?

If you're feeling blue and you'd like to try a supplement, reach for 50 to 100 milligrams of vitamin B6 once a day, the amount that's been used in research studies to date. However, you need to know that taking only one B vitamin in high doses can upset

VITAMIN B6 CONTENT OF COMMON FOODS (MILLIGRAMS)

MEAT AND POULTRY

Beef, flank, cooked, 3 oz. (90 g)	0.3
Chicken breast, cooked, 3 oz. (90 g)	0.2
Chicken leg, cooked, 6 oz. (180 g)	0.2
Pork centre loin, cooked, 3 oz. (90 g)	0.3

FISH

Salmon, sockeye, cooked, 3 oz. (90 g)	0.2
Tuna, canned and drained, 3 oz. (90 g)	0.4

CEREALS

100% bran cereal, 1/2 cup (125 ml)	0.5
Cereal, whole-grain flakes, 2/3 cup (160 ml)	0.5

FRUITS AND VEGETABLES

Avocado, Florida, 1/2 medium	0.4
Avocado, California, 1/2 medium	0.2
Banana, 1 medium	0.7
Potato, baked, 1 medium with skin	0.7

Source: *Nutrient Value of Some Common Foods*, Health Canada, 1999. Adapted and reproduced with the permission of the Minister of Public Works and Government Services Canada, 2003.

your body's balance, because all the eight B vitamins work together. For this reason I recommend using a B-complex supplement that contains all the Bs. I suggest a supplement that contains 50 to 100 milligrams of B6. If you do decide to take vitamin B6 alone, don't take more than 100 milligrams per day. Too much vitamin B6 taken over time can cause irreversible nerve damage.

Herbal remedies

ST. JOHN'S WORT *(HYPERICUM PERFORATUM)*

St. John's wort is a yellow-flowered plant that has been heralded for centuries for its ability to balance emotions. In its modern, standardized form, it has been used for years in Europe to treat both mild depression and seasonal affective disorder (SAD), a mood disorder related to the absence of light during the winter. In 1997, British researchers analyzed 26 controlled studies involving 1700 patients. The report concluded that the herb was as effective as certain antidepressant drugs in treating mild to moderate depression. There's no question in my mind that the evidence for this herb's effectiveness is not only strong but convincing.

Scientists are still trying to determine exactly how this herbal remedy works. Many experts believe that St. John's wort acts to keep brain serotonin levels high for longer periods of time than usual, just like the popular antidepressant drugs Paxil, Zoloft, and Prozac. The power of St. John's wort lies in two active ingredients: hypericin and hyperforin. Researchers attribute much of the herb's effectiveness to hyperforin. A large German study has found that people who take a St. John's wort extract containing a higher amount of hyperforin report better improvement in symptoms than when they take an extract containing a lesser amount. In fact, 70 percent of study participants reported their depression was much or very much improved after using high-hyperforin content St. John's wort. High hyperforin content in a St. John's wort extract has also been shown to cause greater brainwave activity, providing more evidence that it's hyperforin, not hypericin, that influences serotonin levels.[8]

As I've said before, I always try to recommend herbal extracts that are backed by scientific study. Let these research results guide you when choosing a St. John's wort supplement: look for a product standardized to contain 0.3 percent hypericin, and at least 3 percent hyperforin.

To receive the full benefits of St. John's wort, take 300 milligrams of a standardized extract three times daily. However, despite the herb's strong record of safety, it has the potential to interact with a number of medications. Do not take the herb if you are taking indinavir (Crixivan), cyclosporine (Sandimmune), theophylline (Theo-Dur), warfarin (Coumadin), oral contraceptives, or digoxin (Lanoxin). St. John's wort has been reported in a few cases to cause sensitivity to sunlight in very light-skinned individuals. The herb should not be used during pregnancy or breastfeeding.

I don't advise that you start taking St. John's wort if you're currently on antidepressant therapy without consulting your doctor. Under your physician's guidance, it is possible to taper off your use of Paxil, Prozac, or Zoloft and at the same time gradually increase the herb. If you're taking any other antidepressant drug, do not take it concurrently with St. John's wort. You must wait a week or two after stopping the medication before taking the herb. *Always consult your physician first before stopping use of any medication.*

KAVA KAVA *(PIPER METHYSTICUM)*—A GROWING CONCERN

Perhaps it's not mild depression that's plaguing you. Rather than feeling blue, you might be experiencing increased nervousness, restlessness, and the feeling that something is wrong. Increased anxiety is a mood change often reported by perimenopausal women. Anxiety is described by psychologists as a feeling of apprehension, uncertainty, and fear. It's also associated with physical changes—increased heart rate, sweating, and even tremors. Anxiety can sometimes cause insomnia, or make existing sleep problems worse.

Enter kava kava, a herb that has been touted as antianxiety and antistress. This herbal elixir is extracted from the roots of the South Pacific kava shrub. Europeans first documented the kava-drinking ceremonies of Polynesian peoples in the 18th century. Kava drinkers experienced greater tranquillity and sociability, and an overall calming, relaxing effect. If the drink was strong enough, the user went to sleep. Kava does not produce a hangover. Used in low doses, it can soothe the nerves without interfering with alertness, and in higher doses it's an effective sleeping aid. One double-blind study using a standardized kava kava extract confirmed the herb's effectiveness by measuring its antianxiety effect with the Hamilton Anxiety Scale, a standard test used by psychiatrists. Another study found that menopausal women with anxiety disorders obtained significant relief from kava after just one week; relief levels reached their plateau after one month. Women in the study did not experience the negative side effects caused by traditional drugs such as Valium.[9] Experts believe that kava's active ingredients, called kavalactones, exert their effect by acting on the limbic system of the brain, the centre of our emotions.

Until recently, kava was thought to be generally safe. It was available over the counter in virtually every health food store and pharmacy. The only side effects reported were mild stomach upset, headache, or dizziness. But that's all changed. If you are already taking kava, or have a bottle in your medicine cabinet, *read the following section carefully*. There is growing concern over reports from Europe that describe liver damage in some people taking kava. Many of these reports note liver damage in those who have taken kava concurrently with alcohol or medication. Based on current information, people at particular risk of liver damage associated with kava use include those who have compromised liver function because of liver disease, age factors, or prior or current drug or alcohol abuse.

In Canada, there have been four cases of liver toxicity associated with the use of kava-containing products. As a result of these reports and others, in August 2002, Health Canada issued a stop-sale for kava products. Canadian manufacturers, distributors, and importers were required to stop the sale of kava-containing products, and all such products were recalled from the market. This means you won't (or shouldn't) find kava at your local supplements store. Once we gain a better understanding on the benefits and risks of kava, it may be back (though more likely as a prescription drug than as a natural health supplement). *If you have a bottle at home, I advise you to throw it out.*

THE bottom LINE...

Leslie's recommendations for preventing mood swings

1   Eat three meals each day, plus one or two between-meal snacks. My general rule is to go no longer than four to five hours during the day without eating. If the gap between your meals is longer than this, plan for a snack.

2 Eat between 5 and 12 servings of grain foods and 5 to 10 fruit and vegetable servings each day to ensure you get enough carbohydrate in your diet.

3 Eliminate beverages and foods containing caffeine. Caffeine increases anxiety and irritability in some women.

4 Get more omega-3 fats into your diet. Eat fatty fish three times each week. Make sure at least one-half of your added fats and oils are rich in the omega-3 fat alpha-linolenic acid (ALA). This means that at least 2 out of 4 teaspoons (10 out of 20 ml) of your daily added fats come from omega-3 sources.

5 Eliminate alcoholic beverages, which can worsen feelings of depression and irritability.

6 Make sure you're getting enough vitamin B6 in your diet, since this nutrient is needed to convert the amino acid tryptophan to serotonin.

7 If you suffer from mild depression and you're already eating well and taking a multivitamin and mineral pill, try a daily 50- or 100-milligram B6 supplement. If you're not taking a multivitamin and mineral supplement, take a B-complex supplement every day (check the ingredients to make sure it gives you 50 to 100 milligrams of B6).

8 If you've tried B6 and it didn't help your depression, try a standardized extract of St. John's wort. Take 300 milligrams three times daily. Buy a product that is standardized to contain 0.3 percent hypericin and 3 percent hyperforin.

9 If you're experiencing anxiety or panic attacks, *don't* reach for kava kava, a herbal remedy previously recommended. In fact, if you have a bottle at home, throw it out.

10 If your mood swings do not improve with dietary changes or the recommended supplements, consult your doctor. Serious emotional problems may require medication. If perimenopausal mood changes take over your life, a psychologist can help you discover the underlying causes of your stress and teach you techniques for coping with it.

Forgetfulness and fuzzy thinking

"I have always thought my mind was pretty sharp. For the last year or so, my brain has become like peach fuzz. I have difficulty remembering the names of people I worked with less than a year ago; I constantly misplace things; I go into a room and can't remember why I was going there. It's very frustrating."

7

Can't remember where you left your wallet? Or perhaps your next-door neighbour's name has recently eluded you at the most embarrassing possible moment? We've all had memory lapses at one time or another. But there is also a definite link between brain power and hormonal fluctuations. If you have children, think back to the last time you were pregnant. If you're like many of my friends, you probably felt that your brain had turned to mush. Well, going through perimenopause can affect your ability to think and concentrate in the same way. Fortunately, this midlife brain drain is temporary. You won't continue to forget simple things (like your phone number) forever. And rest assured, minor memory lapses during perimenopause are not signs of early Alzheimer disease; this is rarely the case.

Sometimes things other than perimenopausal hormonal fluctuations may contribute to forgetfulness. For starters, we have to face the fact that there's an aging process at work. The older we get, the more short-term memory we lose. This applies to both women and men. Finnish researchers studied 70 women between the ages of 47 and 65 and found that the results of most tests of mental performance correlated with age. Older women were slower and made more mistakes than younger women. When these women were given estrogen replacement therapy for three months (short-term use), their cognitive abilities did not improve.[1] It seems that a little memory loss is a natural part of aging.

Menopausal symptoms too can cause memory problems. Certainly insomnia and fatigue can reduce your ability to think clearly. And sometimes the stress of experiencing physical changes or the emotional turmoil related to menopause can affect your mental performance.

When it comes to hormonal changes, scientists have collected a fair amount of evidence showing that estrogen affects aspects of brain chemistry and brain structures important for memory, and that the loss of estrogen associated with menopause may be largely responsible for the decline in memory that some women experience in their later years. Scientists have theorized that estrogen is needed for the transfer of nerve messages to specific regions in the brain.

Does all this mean that estrogen replacement therapy might help preserve memory and prevent senility? Some controlled studies demonstrate that short-term estrogen use in menopausal women enhances short- and long-term memory and increases the capacity to learn new material. An overview of 10 observational studies of post-menopausal estrogen use (they were not placebo-controlled trials) published in the *Journal of the American Medical Association* suggests that women on estrogen therapy have a 29 percent lower risk of developing dementia than those who don't use supplemental estrogen. Whether estrogen use lowers the risk of Alzheimer disease remains to be seen. Since June 1997, four controlled trials have investigated the effect of estrogen in women with Alzheimer disease. Although the results look promising, many of these studies were either small, of short duration, or poorly controlled.[2] The good news is that you can do a few things to sharpen your thinking and slow down the aging of your brain.

Dietary approaches

EAT BREAKFAST EVERY DAY

Time and time again, parents tell their children to eat breakfast. Well, what's good for kids is good for us, too. Studies have demonstrated that eating breakfast improves thinking power later in the morning and that a late-afternoon snack enhances performance on tasks involving prolonged concentration and memory. Many studies of both children and adults have shown that compared with breakfast eaters, people who skip the morning meal do not score as well on tests of mental performance that same morning. Breakfast-skipping appears to affect recall and memory tasks more than it does any other cognitive function.[3]

Australian researchers found that eating breakfast leads to improved mood, better memory, more energy, and feelings of calmness in overweight women. Three more experiments conducted in young men and women revealed that going without breakfast impaired the ability to recall a word list and read a story aloud. This decline in test performance associated with skipping breakfast was reversed when the study participants were given a glucose drink.[4]

One reason we don't perform well without breakfast is that, after a night of sleeping, we wake up in a fasting state. This means our blood glucose (blood sugar) levels are low, yet blood glucose is what supplies energy to the brain. Your brain's energy stores are very small, and without constant glucose replacement, your brain cells will become depleted in less than 10 minutes. Without a steady stream of glucose nourishing your brain cells, your attention span and short-term memory are likely to diminish. Breakfast foods supply carbohydrates that are converted to glucose in the bloodstream, supplying the energy needed for peak mental performance.

Breakfast also supplies key nutrients, including important B vitamins, iron, and calcium. Research has shown that when we skip breakfast, we usually don't manage to catch up on the intake of the nutrients we missed. So what's the best breakfast? I recommend having some carbohydrate to elevate blood glucose and a little protein to help sustain energy levels longer. Eating protein has this effect partly because it takes longer to digest. As a result, the carbohydrate you eat with protein is converted to glucose more slowly. In a sense, by eating a little protein with the carbohydrate, you are giving yourself "time release" energy, rather than sharply elevating your blood glucose all at once. Here are a few breakfast ideas that meet my criteria and will also help you meet your daily calcium and vitamin C requirements:

- Whole-grain cereal with low-fat milk or calcium-fortified soy beverage. Top with fruit or drink a small glass of citrus juice. To increase your fibre intake, choose a breakfast cereal that contains at least 4 grams of fibre per serving. The nutrition information panel on the cereal box will state the cereal's fibre content.
- Whole-grain toast with a poached or hard-boiled egg and a fruit salad.
- Homemade breakfast smoothie using a calcium-fortified soy beverage, orange juice, and a banana. Add soy protein isolate powder or egg whites for a protein boost.
- In a hurry? If you usually eat breakfast running out the door, grab a piece of

fruit, a low-fat granola bar, and a low-fat yogurt for protein (and calcium). You might not be able to eat the yogurt in the car or on the bus, but you can certainly eat it when you get to work.

EAT A HIGH-PROTEIN MEAL AT MIDDAY

Many of my clients complain that they feel sleepy or lethargic after lunch. If you want to be sharp and feel more energetic, eat protein, vegetables, and fruit for lunch. The body breaks down protein-rich foods such as meat, poultry, and fish into smaller units called amino acids. Amino acids are the body's building blocks for making muscle, hormones, enzymes, and brain chemicals called neurotransmitters. (If you've read Chapter 6 on mood swings, you already know all about neurotransmitters.) A high-protein meal causes a rise in blood levels of the amino acid called tyrosine. Once in the brain, tyrosine is converted to the neurotransmitters known as dopamine and norepinephrine. These neurotransmitters have been found to improve alertness, sharpen thinking, and enhance energy levels.

What does a high-protein lunch look like? Here are a few examples:
- Large green salad with 3 to 4 ounces (90 to 120 g) of tuna, salmon, or grilled chicken; glass of low-fat milk or soy beverage; piece of fruit.
- Stir-fried chicken or tofu with plenty of vegetables, piece of fruit, water.
- Omelette served with a green salad or steamed vegetables, fruit salad, water.

I'll often grill an extra piece of fish or chicken at dinner and bring it to work with me for lunch the next day. I'll also steam extra vegetables at dinner and enjoy them the next day cold, or I'll serve the protein on a bed of greens. Keep in mind, though, that a high-protein lunch doesn't give you enough energy to carry you through the rest of the day. You will need a snack to boost your blood sugar level about three to four hours after lunch. Even when you eat a starchy lunch, your blood sugar levels normally decline three to four hours later. To prevent that midafternoon drop in blood glucose and mental performance, fuel your brain with a snack combining carbohydrate and protein: fruit and yogurt, whole-grain crackers and low-fat cheese, or a low-fat decaf latte.

GET MORE OMEGA-3 FATS

As you read in Chapter 6, the type of fat we eat is important for the healthy functioning of our brain. A large proportion of the communicating membranes of the brain is made up of two omega-3 fats: docosahexaenoic acid (DHA) and eicosapentaenoic acid (EPA). Your brain cells must constantly refresh themselves with a new supply of omega-3 fats. When we eat oily fish such as salmon, trout, and sardines, we get a good supply of EPA and DHA. But a small amount of these two omega-3 fats can also be made inside the body from another omega-3 fat, alpha-linolenic acid (ALA). ALA is plentiful in flaxseed, canola, and walnut oils. It's called an essential fatty acid because it's essential to our health *and* our bodies cannot make it—it must be supplied by our diet.

While most Canadians likely eat more fat than recommended, experts are concerned that we may not be getting enough omega-3 fats for optimal brain health. To get more of these fats into your diet, aim to consume:

- 3 to 6 ounces (90 to 180 g) of fish high in omega-3 oils at least three times per week.
- 2 to 3 teaspoons (10 to 15 ml) per day of flaxseed, walnut, or canola oils. Corn, sunflower, safflower, and olive oils contain almost no omega-3 fats.

Vitamins and minerals

CHOLINE

Although not actually a vitamin, choline is a fat-like member of the B vitamin family. It's found in egg yolks, organ meats, and legumes and is one of the building blocks used to manufacture the memory neurotransmitter acetylcholine. Levels of acetylcholine increase in proportion to the amount of choline in the diet. Choline supplements have been shown to enhance memory and reaction time in animals, particularly aging animals. Currently, researchers believe that choline supplements will improve the brain's ability to do its tasks only in people who are actually deficient in the nutrient. Stress and aging can deplete choline levels.

While we don't yet know if supplemental choline will improve memory in people who have normal choline levels, it's still important to get enough of this nutrient in your diet. In fact, in 1998, the Food and Nutrition Board of the National Academy of Sciences, an organization consisting of Canadian and American experts, released for the first time a recommended daily intake for choline. There is evidence that choline may be needed in the diet because the amount synthesized by our bodies may be insufficient to meet our needs. Healthy women need 425 milligrams of choline each day (men need 550 milligrams). The best food sources are egg yolks, liver and other organ meats, brewer's yeast, wheat germ, soybeans, peanuts, and green peas.

If you don't regularly eat egg yolks, organ meats, or legumes, you can get choline from lecithin supplements. Lecithin is a natural substance consisting of phosphatidylcholine, fatty acids, and carbohydrate; it is the phosphatidylcholine that supplies the body with choline. Most lecithin supplements contain 10 to 20 percent phosphatidylcholine. Others, however, are almost pure phosphatidylcholine; they will be labelled as such. Most supplements are manufactured from soybeans. Lecithin and phosphatidylcholine supplements are considered very safe, although they may cause diarrhea, nausea, stomach upset, and a feeling of fullness.

The maximum safe dosage is 3500 milligrams (3.5 g) of choline per day. Be warned that taking large amounts of choline may cause low blood pressure and a fishy body odour. (Pass the soybeans please!) Unlike choline supplements, lecithin taken orally does not cause a fishy odour.

IRON

I am sure you are already familiar with iron's role in preventing anemia. When your diet lacks iron, your red blood cells become less efficient at transporting oxygen to your cells for energy. Iron is needed to make hemoglobin, the protein that transports oxygen to all your tissues. If your diet lacks iron, your body will make less and less hemoglobin. As your body's iron stores run low, you end up feeling tired and lethargic. A blood test that reveals a low hemoglobin level indicates iron deficiency anemia.

However, you might not have realized that iron is also used to make certain brain neurotransmitters, in particular, those neurotransmitters that regulate the ability to pay attention. It's important to keep in mind that a developing iron deficiency can affect your mental performance long before red blood cells are depleted to the point at which anemia is diagnosed by a standard blood test. And because of the neurotransmitter link, a deficiency of iron can also directly affect your mood, attention span, and learning ability. Your doctor can determine if you are iron deficient by measuring the amount of ferritin in your blood. Your ferritin level reflects the amount of iron stored in the liver. Your ferritin level can be low even if you are not yet anemic.

If you are still menstruating (and not a vegetarian), you need 18 milligrams of iron each day to prevent a deficiency. After menopause, your need decreases to 8 milligrams per day. To help you stay alert, energetic, and focused, make a point of adding a few of the following foods to your daily diet—they all top the list when it comes to iron content.

Iron in food is classified either as heme or nonheme iron. Heme iron, the form of iron found in animal foods such as red meat, poultry, and fish, is easily absorbed by

IRON CONTENT OF SELECTED FOODS (MILLIGRAMS)

Beef, lean, cooked, 3 oz. (90 g)	3.0
Chicken breast, cooked 3 oz. (90 g)	0.6
Liver, beef, cooked, 3 oz. (90 g)	5.3
Liver, chicken, cooked, 3 oz. (90 g)	7.6
Oysters, cooked, 5 medium	7.2
Shrimp, cooked, 10 large	1.7
Tuna, light, canned, 1/2 cup (125 ml)	1.2
Beans in tomato sauce, 1 cup (250 ml)	5.0
Kidney beans, 1/2 cup (125 ml)	2.5
Apricots, dried, 6	2.8
Prune juice, 1/2 cup (125 ml)	5.0
Spinach, cooked, 1 cup (250 ml)	4.0
All Bran, Kellogg's, 1/2 cup (125 ml)	4.7
All Bran Buds, Kellogg's, 1/2 cup (125 ml)	5.9
Bran Flakes, 3/4 cup (175 ml)	4.9
Just Right, Kellogg's, 1 cup (250 ml)	6.0
Raisin Bran, 3/4 cup (175 ml)	5.5
Shreddies, 3/4 cup (175 ml)	5.9
Cream of Wheat, 1/2 cup (125 ml)	8.0
Oatmeal, instant, 1 pouch	3.8
Wheat germ, 1 tbsp. (15 ml)	2.5
Blackstrap molasses, 1 tbsp. (15 ml)	3.2

Source: *Nutrient Value of Some Common Foods*, Health Canada, 1999. Adapted and reproduced with the permission of the Minister of Public Works and Government Services Canada, 2003.

the body. Foods containing significant amounts of nonheme iron include whole-grain breads and cereals, fortified breakfast cereals, beans, vegetables, and fruit. This form of iron accounts for 85 percent of our dietary intake of the mineral, but it is less well absorbed by the body. You'd have to eat 4 cups (1 litre) of raw spinach to get as much useable iron as you receive from a 3-ounce (90-g) serving of lean beef.

Maximizing iron absorption
Fortunately, you can take action to enhance your body's ability to absorb nonheme iron found in plant foods. Practice these tips to get the most from your foods:
- Add some vitamin C to foods rich in nonheme iron: top your whole-grain cereal with strawberries or have it with a glass of citrus juice.
- Include a source of heme iron with foods containing nonheme iron; a little meat or chicken tossed into your brown rice stir-fry will do nicely.
- Pull out your cast-iron cookware. During the cooking process, food will absorb some of the pan's iron.
- Don't drink coffee or tea with an iron-rich meal, as the beverage's tannins will prevent iron absorption.
- Don't take your calcium supplement with an iron-rich meal (or an iron supplement), since these two minerals compete with each other for absorption.

What about a multivitamin supplement?
You're at risk of iron deficiency if you're still menstruating; if you engage in heavy endurance exercise; if you're adhering to a low-calorie diet; or if you don't eat animal foods and are unsure about vegetarian iron sources. Vegetarians may have difficulty maintaining healthy iron stores because their diet relies exclusively on nonheme sources. If you are a vegetarian who does not eat poultry or fish, your daily iron intake must be 1.8 times greater than the RDA for nonvegetarians. For instance, if you're a 45-year-old woman eating a meat-free diet, you need 32 milligrams of iron each day (18 x 1.8 = 32 mg).

To help you meet your daily iron requirements, a multivitamin and mineral supplement is a wise idea, especially if you are still menstruating. Most formulas provide 10 milligrams, but you can find multivitamins that provide up to 18 milligrams of the mineral. Look for a "high potency" multivitamin or a "woman's" formula supplement; they should contain between 15 and 18 milligrams of iron. After menopause, switch to a formula for older adults, as it will have less iron. Iron-only supplements should be taken under supervision and only if you have an iron deficiency diagnosed by your physician.

BORON

Scientific evidence suggests that this trace mineral plays an important role in brain function. Studies have shown that a boron deficiency results in poor performance in tasks involving neuromuscular speed and dexterity, attention, and short-term memory. Study participants with low boron intakes suffered from significantly poorer performances in tests of hand-eye coordination, attention, perception, and memory, as opposed to their counterparts with high dietary boron levels. The participants with lower boron also had significantly less brain electrical activity.

Because boron has not yet been recognized as an essential nutrient for humans, no recommended daily intake has been established. A daily intake of between 1.5 and 3 milligrams is probably more than adequate to meet daily requirements, but we don't really know for sure if this amount is optimal for brain function. The main food sources for boron are fruits and vegetables, but actual content depends on the food's soil. If you want to take a supplement, 3 to 9 milligrams per day is a very safe amount. At the time of writing, boron supplements are not available in Canada. They are, however, readily available in the United States.

Herbal remedies

GINKGO BILOBA

Also known as maidenhair, ginkgo is one of the most popular herbs to hit the North American market in recent years. Ginkgo extracts are made from the fan-shaped, bi-lobed leaves of the ginkgo tree, a tree that reaches heights of over 100 feet and grows here in North America. Ginkgo is touted to improve memory loss and slow the progression of Alzheimer disease. These claims are likely true. Ginkgo is one of the most heavily researched herbs in the world. The study that made ginkgo famous was a 52-week trial with 309 patients. All had mild to moderate dementia as a result of Alzheimer disease or stroke. Patients were given either 40 milligrams of a special standardized ginkgo extract (EGb 761) at breakfast, lunch, and dinner, or a placebo pill. After one year, the placebo group showed a decline in cognitive function, whereas the group that had received ginkgo did not show an overall decline. When the researchers looked at the Alzheimer patients only, they found modest but significant improvements in memory and other brain functions.[5]

Scientists have recognized the herb's potential to slow the progression of dementia since the 1990s. But now there's evidence that ginkgo can even enhance short-term memory in healthy middle-aged adults! In a UK study, an extract combining ginkgo and ginseng improved short-term memory and mental function in healthy adults aged 30 to 59. Another study tested ginkgo in 61 healthy young adults and found significant improvements in the speed of working memory. When it comes to improving the memory of healthy adults over the age of 60, however, recent study findings on ginkgo's effectiveness are mixed. One American study found that ginkgo had no effect on memory, while another suggested the herb improved thinking power.[6]

Ginkgo may act in one of two ways to enhance memory. A number of studies suggest that ginkgo increases circulation and oxygen delivery to the brain. The herb's active ingredients also make the blood cells known as platelets less sticky. As a result, circulation becomes more efficient.[7] (Ginkgo also enhances blood flow to the extremities, and studies have found the herb to improve sex drive. Chapter 8 has more on this.)

Ginkgo has a strong antioxidant effect in the brain, the eye, and the cardiovascular system, protecting these tissues from free-radical damage. Free-radical damage to brain cells is widely accepted as a contributing factor in Alzheimer disease. Free radicals are unstable oxygen molecules that seek electrons from other molecules and, in the process, cause cellular damage. Free radicals can damage brain cells, the genetic material of cells, protein molecules in the eye, and cell membranes. Any compound able to neutralize these harmful free radicals is called an antioxidant. Antioxidant compounds, be it vitamin C in oranges, lycopene in tomatoes, or active compounds in ginkgo biloba, essentially "mop up" free radicals and, as a result, protect our cells from damage. (For more on free radicals and antioxidants, see pages 177–178, Chapter 12.) Scientists aren't sure if ginkgo's positive effect on brain function is largely due to its antioxidant ability to prevent damage to brain cells, or its power to increase blood flow to the brain.

Although no studies have been done in perimenopausal or postmenopausal women, I do recommend ginkgo to my clients to help reduce the effects of aging on brain cells. Researchers have identified the active compounds that appear responsible for ginkgo's beneficial effects: terpene lactones and ginkgo flavone glycosides. Here are some guidelines for buying a top-quality ginkgo supplement:

- Choose a product standardized to contain 24 percent ginkgo flavone glycosides and 6 percent terpene lactones.
- The EGb 761 extract used in the scientific research is available as two brands in Canada and the United States: Ginkoba (Pharmaton) and Ginkogold (Nature's Way).

Research indicates that the effective daily dose of ginkgo is between 120 and 240 milligrams, taken in two to three doses throughout the day. Start with the lower 120-milligram dose by taking a 40-milligram tablet three times daily.

Ginkgo has a slight blood-thinning effect and so could enhance the effects of other blood-thinning medications. If you take a prescription blood thinner, consult your doctor before starting on ginkgo. The herb's safety has not been established during pregnancy and breastfeeding. On rare occasions, ginkgo may cause gastrointestinal upset, headache, or an allergic skin reaction. In this case, lower your dosage, and if symptoms persist, discontinue use. You may then want to consult with your physician or other qualified health care practitioner to determine if any other herbal remedies may be helpful to you.

THE bottom LINE...

Leslie's recommendations for improving memory

1   Eat breakfast every day to provide your brain cells with their preferred fuel source—carbohydrate. To sustain your blood glucose levels, make sure your breakfast includes both carbohydrate and protein.

2   To stay alert and focused in the afternoon, eat a high-protein, low-carbohydrate lunch. A meal consisting of chicken or fish and plenty of vegetables provides your brain with plenty of tyrosine, an amino acid used to produce brain chemicals that increase alertness.

3   Make sure the fats and oils you add to your diet come mainly from the omega-3 family of fats. These special fats are used by the body to manufacture a large part

of the communicating membranes of the brain. Eat fish at least three times per week. Use flaxseed, canola, and walnut oils more often. Eat more soy foods, omega-3 eggs, and green leafy vegetables.

4   To help your brain manufacture more acetylcholine, the memory neurotransmitter, increase your intake of foods rich in choline, a fat-like member of the B vitamin family. Good sources are eggs, legumes, and organ meats. If you have difficulty incorporating these foods into your diet, consider taking a choline or lecithin supplement.

5   Reach for iron-rich foods every day. Remember, your body uses iron to make brain chemicals that regulate your ability to pay attention. It you're at risk of iron deficiency, be sure to take a multivitamin and mineral supplement that contains 15 to 18 milligrams of the mineral. If you are suffering from a lack of energy and poor concentration, ask your doctor to measure your ferritin levels (iron stores).

6   Be sure to eat 5 to 10 servings of fruits and vegetables each day to help you get more boron for brain function. While there is no official recommended intake for this trace mineral, it's extremely safe to use a supplement. If you eat plenty of fruits and vegetables but you'd still like to boost your boron intake, consider supplementing your diet. Boron supplements are available in the United States but not Canada. Try adding 3 to 9 milligrams by way of a supplement to your daily diet.

7   Consider taking the herbal remedy ginkgo biloba. A standardized extract of ginkgo might enhance your short-term memory and protect your brain cells from the effects of aging. Look for an extract that contains 24 percent ginkgo flavone glycosides. Take one 40-milligram tablet with breakfast, lunch, and dinner.

Vaginal and bladder changes

"I can't say that my interest in sex changed when going through menopause. I can say, though, that my dryness made it uncomfortable to the point of not enjoying it."

8

For women who are accustomed to enjoying regular sexual activity, experiencing sexual symptoms due to menopause can be one of the most disconcerting aspects of this life-cycle transition.

Vaginal dryness

Current estimates indicate that somewhere between 20 and 45 percent of peri- and postmenopausal women report vaginal dryness—they take longer to become lubricated during sexual arousal and intercourse may become uncomfortable. You may be at greater risk of vaginal dryness if you aren't having regular sexual intercourse, you experienced premature menopause, or you have a history of missed menstrual periods. During the perimenopausal years, vaginal dryness is often a transient condition that improves as estrogen levels increase again.

Vaginal dryness is caused by a decline in estrogen levels. As estrogen levels fall, the walls of the vagina become smaller, thinner, and less elastic. Secretion of the fluids that naturally protect the vagina from infection and lubricate it for sexual intercourse also decreases. Lack of lubrication, in turn, can make intercourse painful and cause bleeding and soreness. Regular sexual intercourse can actually help prevent these problems by stretching the vagina and increasing its blood supply and lubrication. That's right—regular sexual activity can actually help to maintain the health of vaginal tissue.

Urinary tract infections (UTIs)

These may occur more often because of the hormonal changes of menopause. Low estrogen levels and vaginal atrophy leave women more prone to infections and irritations of the vagina and urinary tract (the urinary tract comprises the kidneys, ureters, bladder, and urethra). The most common type of UTI is cystitis, commonly known as a bladder infection. If left untreated, a UTI can lead to potentially life-threatening problems; early detection and treatment are essential to prevent a serious health risk.

Any woman who has suffered through a UTI will tell you that it is a very uncomfortable condition and can make you feel miserable. In some cases, UTIs will clear up spontaneously, without any treatment. However, most UTIs are treated with antibiotics. The drugs may be given in a single, large dose or may be spread over a course of three to seven days. A repeat infection is treated with a second course of antibiotics. Treatment is usually continued until your symptoms disappear and a urine test shows no bacteria.

It is not unusual for women to experience recurrent UTIs. Some women have as many as three or four a year; others have them even more frequently. Nearly 80 percent of these cases are actually reinfections, caused by the same circumstances that produced the original infection. If you have recurrent UTIs, discuss treatment options with your doctor. Low daily doses of antibiotics for a six-month period or a single dose of antibiotic after sexual activity may prevent long-term problems. Postmenopausal women with recurrent UTIs may find some relief by using estrogen creams that are applied to the vagina.

Decreased libido

Popular beliefs hold that with menopause comes a loss of interest in sex. While researchers have not found a link between estrogen levels and libido, many women do complain that their sex drive lessens around the time of menopause. Sometimes decreased sexual desire is the result of menopausal symptoms that interfere with sexual intercourse. Libido, or sex drive, is a function of the brain. Certainly mood swings, which affect your brain, can contribute to a temporary lack of interest in sex. Insomnia can make you tired and lethargic and affect your sexual desire. Weight gain that occurs around menopause can make you self-conscious about your body and feel uncomfortable during sex; women who maintain a positive body image tend to experience greater sexual enjoyment.

Androgen (male) hormones such as testosterone may also be a factor in loss of libido. These hormones activate specific receptors in the brain to turn on sexual desire. Women who have had hysterectomies report being less interested in sex more often than do women who experience natural menopause. Studies in women who have experienced premature menopause have led researchers to theorize that a lack of testosterone due to decreased production in the ovaries may cause some menopausal libido problems. In fact, a number of studies have found that adding testosterone to estrogen replacement therapy improves sexual motivation and desire.[1] While estrogen therapy alone is effective at relieving vaginal dryness, it is less effective at enhancing sexual desire and arousal. Other medical doctors attribute a decline in progesterone production to be largely responsible for decreased libido experienced around menopause. While little research has been done in this area, the use of progesterone creams and oils is becoming more popular (for more on progesterone creams, see the discussion on pages 19–21).

So what does all this mean? Well, you certainly don't have to give up sex just because you've entered your "change of life." A healthy sexual relationship with someone you care for is important for emotional well-being. If you are experiencing serious libido problems, talk to your doctor about the possibility of hormonal therapy. If you're troubled by vaginal dryness or UTIs, you can do several things on your own to minimize this condition.

Dietary approaches

SOY FOODS AND ISOFLAVONES

If you've read Chapter 4 on hot flashes, you're already an expert on soy foods. Studies suggest that soy's natural plant estrogens, called isoflavones, can improve vaginal dryness as well as reduce hot flashes. Finnish and Israeli researchers have looked at the effect a phytoestrogen-rich diet has on hot flashes and vaginal dryness. In a study involving 145 women with menopausal symptoms, participants were randomly assigned to eat either a diet that contained 25 percent of its calories from phytoestrogen-rich foods (including tofu, soy beverages, miso, and flaxseed) or their regular diet. After 12 weeks, blood levels of phytoestrogens had increased significantly in women eating the diet rich in soy foods, but remained unchanged in the women eating their regular diet. Reductions in hot flashes and vaginal dryness were more significant in the women assigned the phytoestrogen-rich diet. Other studies have also shown that post-menopausal women report improved vaginal lubrication when regularly eating soy foods.[2]

How can soy reverse vaginal dryness? The natural isoflavone compounds in soy-beans are able to bind to estrogen receptors in the vagina and exert a weak estrogen-like effect. Acting like estrogen, although much less potent, soy's isoflavones can increase the thickness and elasticity of the vaginal walls, as well as increase vaginal secretions.

How much soy do you need?

In Chapter 4, I recommended an intake of 40 to 80 milligrams of isoflavones each day. Many experts believe that this is the amount of phytoestrogens needed to achieve the desired effects. Keep in mind that noticeable improvement in vaginal dryness may not be felt for weeks.

Also in Chapter 4, you'll find a list of soy foods that demystifies soy products and explains how to use them, as well as a list of 10 ways to enjoy more soy (see pages 29–33). Appendix 3 offers some tasty recipes that will help you experiment with soy in the kitchen. To ensure a daily dose of at least 40 milligrams of isoflavones, I recommend you also try one of the following strategies:

- Enjoy, every morning, a breakfast smoothie made with a soy beverage, fruit, and soy protein isolate powder (see pages 33–34 for a list of high-quality brands).
- Add 2 tablespoons (25 ml) of soy protein isolate powder to your morning orange juice (although not nearly as tasty as a breakfast smoothie, a few of my clients do this religiously).
- Munch on 1/4 cup (50 ml) of unsalted roasted soy "nuts" as a regular midday snack. You'll find these nuts at supermarkets and health food stores. They come in plain and flavoured varieties and are quite tasty. And don't worry, they contain less fat than real nuts. Just stick to a small serving. You can also sprinkle them

over green salads, frozen yogurt, and hot breakfast cereal, or add them to stir-fried dishes made with vegetables and tofu, chicken, or lean meat, or in a home-made snack mix of shredded wheat squares, raisins, dried cranberries, and low-fat granola.

WATER AND FLUIDS

I can't emphasize enough the importance of drinking enough fluids. Keeping your body adequately hydrated at all times is a critical component of a healthy lifestyle. We all know the effects of dehydration—dry skin, chapped lips, and lower energy levels. Well, a lack of fluids can affect your vagina in the same way. Dehydration decreases natural body secretions and can exacerbate vaginal dryness caused by an estrogen deficiency. Drinking plenty of water each day also helps flush infection-causing bacteria out of your system, reducing your risk of bladder infection.

To maintain fluid balance, women need to drink 9 cups, or 2.25 litres, of non-caffeinated, nonalcoholic fluids each day. If you exercise, work in an air-conditioned building, or spend time outside in hot, humid weather, then you need more than this.

Water, vegetable juice, unsweetened fruit juice, milk, herbal tea, soup, and high-water-content fruits and vegetables all contribute to your daily fluid intake. In fact, for people with an average diet, high-water-content foods can actually contribute as much as 4 cups (1 litre) of fluids daily. But to be sure you're getting enough fluids, always drink at least eight glasses of water daily. Minimize caffeine and alcohol, which can cause your body to lose water. Here are a few strategies to boost your fluid intake:

- Drink fluids with each meal and snack.
- Keep a bottle of water on your desk at the office. The water cooler may be close at hand, but how many times do you actually get up to fill your glass?
- When you travel—by car, plane, or train—always carry a bottle of water with you.
- If you don't like drinking plain water, add a splash of white grape juice, cranberry juice or blackcurrant concentrate. Or try a glass of sparkling mineral water with a slice of lemon.
- If you deprive your body of fluids because you don't like the taste of tap water, buy a water pitcher with an activated carbon filter. Always keep a full pitcher in the fridge. (And don't forget to replace the filter periodically.)

- Have a bottle of water with you when you exercise. Drink 1/2 to 1 cup (125 to 250 ml) of fluid every 15 minutes.

Cranberry juice

If you suffer from repeated UTIs, this is one fluid you should add to your daily diet. Studies show that a daily glass of the juice may not only prevent these infections but may also be effective at treating them. In a 1994 landmark study, researchers from the Brigham and Women's Hospital/Harvard Medical School in Boston studied 153 women for six months. The women were given either 10 fluid ounces (300 ml) of cranberry juice or a placebo drink once daily. At the end of the study, women drinking the cranberry juice were only about one-quarter as likely as the placebo group to continue to have UTIs. This improvement was seen after two months of treatment.[3]

Natural chemicals in cranberries, known as proanthocyanins, treat a UTI by preventing the adherence of E. coli bacteria to the wall of the urinary tract. Instead of hanging around to multiply, bacteria are flushed out in the urine. To treat and prevent a UTI, drink 1 1/4 cups to 4 cups (300 ml to 1 litre) of cranberry juice per day.

Cranberry juice may not be for everyone, though. Drinking large quantities—4 cups (1 litre) or more—of the juice may aggravate kidney stones in some people. Stones made from oxalate and uric acid are more likely to form in acidic urine. Women with irritable bowel syndrome may experience diarrhea if they drink too much cranberry juice. If you are at risk for such problems, limit your intake to 1 1/4 cups (300 ml) per day. Also, you may not want (or need) the extra calories from the added sugar in the juice. If this is the case, try cranberry capsules, which contain anywhere from 300 to 800 milligrams of dried cranberry powder. They are available in health food stores and pharmacies. Take two 500-milligram capsules to get the equivalent of 1 1/4 cups (300 ml) of cranberry juice.

Herbal remedies

ASIAN GINSENG (PANAX GINSENG, PANAX QUINQUEFOLIUS)

If you've ever been to a health food store in search of an energy boost, chances are you've come across ginseng. Among the five top-selling herbal remedies in North America, *Panax ginseng* (Asian, Korean, and Chinese) is best known for its ability to help the body deal more effectively with stress. Probably for this reason, users report that they experience more consistent energy levels. Now it also appears that the health benefits of ginseng include improving vaginal dryness associated with menopause. One study reported in the *British Medical Journal* found that *Panax ginseng* had a protective effect on vaginal tissue in postmenopausal women. Women who took the herb for six weeks noticed an improvement in vaginal dryness.[4] Ginseng does not have an estrogenic effect. Rather, it encourages the pituitary gland to increase the body's production of hormones that affect vaginal tissue.

Ginseng's benefits can be attributed to active compounds called ginsenosides. Two in particular, Rg1 and Rb1, have received the most attention from researchers. Most studies have focused on ginseng extracts standardized to contain 4 to 7 percent ginsenosides. When buying ginseng, look for a statement of standardization, or, better yet, choose a product whose label specifies "G115." This designation indicates that the product contains a special extract of ginsenosides that has been used in research.

The usual daily dosage of a standardized extract is 100 or 200 milligrams once daily. Take ginseng in cycles—two to three weeks on, one week off. Some experts believe that over time, your body can get used to the effects of ginseng, and its effectiveness is then reduced. Taking it in cycles helps prevent this. According to the German Commission E, an expert committee established in 1978 by the German government to evaluate the safety and efficiency of over 300 herbal supplements sold in that country, ginseng is safe to use for up to three months at a time in this cyclical way.

Ginseng is relatively safe at the 100- or 200-milligram dosage. In some people, it may cause mild stomach upset, irritability, and insomnia. To avoid overstimulation, start with 100 milligrams a day. If you experience overstimulation at this dose, avoid using caffeine while you're on ginseng. Ginseng should not be used during pregnancy or breast feeding, and it's not suitable for people with uncontrolled high blood pressure. There have also been a few reports of ginseng causing spotting in postmenopausal women. If you experience this side effect, stop taking the herb. If spotting continues, consult your physician.

SIBERIAN GINSENG *(ELEUTHEROCOCCUS SENTICOSUS)*

Siberian ginseng has much milder effects than *Panax*, or Asian, ginseng, and few reported side effects. Pregnant and nursing women can safely take Siberian ginseng, and it's much less likely to cause overstimulation in sensitive individuals. But keep in mind that in the research to date, the type of ginseng shown to improve vaginal cell maturation is *Panax* ginseng, not Siberian.

To ensure that you are buying a high-quality extract, choose one standardized to contain eleutherosides B and E. The usual dosage is 300 to 400 milligrams once daily for six to eight weeks, followed by a one- to two-week break. It is safe to use Siberian ginseng for up to three months and also safe to take repeated courses of the herb.

DONG QUAI (ANGELICA SINENSIS)

Herbalists often recommend dong quai as an all-purpose herb for gynecological complaints, including menopausal symptoms. However, if you're taking this herb to treat vaginal dryness or hot flashes, you might want to think twice. When researchers from the Kaiser Permanente Medical Center in Oakland, California, assessed the herb's effects in 71 postmenopausal women over 24 weeks, they found no difference between the groups taking dong quai or placebo in terms of vaginal wall thickness, rate of vaginal cell maturation, or hot flashes. The researchers concluded that when used alone, dong quai does not have an estrogen-like effect on vaginal tissues and is no more helpful than placebo in relieving menopausal symptoms.[5]

The results of this study are a little surprising, given dong quai's long tradition of use in Asia. However, practitioners of traditional Chinese medicine (TCM) usually prescribe dong quai in combination with other herbs. While the herb might not reduce certain menopausal symptoms by itself, it might as part of a combination of herbs. If you're interested in learning more about dong quai, I recommend you consult a practitioner well trained in the use of traditional Chinese herbs.

GINKGO BILOBA

In Chapter 7, you learned that ginkgo might be effective in enhancing memory, but did you know that it also can help with sexual dysfunction? California researchers made this startling discovery after a patient taking ginkgo biloba for memory problems reported improved erections. The researchers decided to investigate whether there was any substance to the patient's story. Each day, they gave between 60 and 120 milligrams of standardized ginkgo extract to a group of 63 men and women who complained of sexual dysfunction as a result of using antidepressant medication. And guess what? Ginkgo was found to be 84 percent effective in treating sexual dysfunction. Women were more responsive than men, with a success rate of 91 percent versus the men's rate of 76 percent.[6] It appears that ginkgo's ability to increase blood and oxygen delivery to the tissues may not only help your brain function better but may also improve your sex life! So if you are taking Prozac, Effexor, Paxil, Zoloft, or Serzone for depression and are experiencing sexual dysfunction, research suggests that ginkgo may be an effective remedy.

Buy a ginkgo product standardized to 24 percent ginkgo flavone glycosides.

Other ways to prevent vaginal dryness

In addition to the dietary and herbal suggestions I've provided, here are other ways to combat vaginal dryness:

1   *Use a vaginal lubricant.* Many women find that vaginal lubricants (gels and liquids) replenish moisture to the vaginal lining and eliminate general itchiness and discomfort during sexual intercourse. If you decide to try an external lubricant, be sure to buy a water-based product such as Replens, Vagisil, Gyne-Moistrin, or KY Long Lasting Vaginal Moisturizer. Water-based lubricants are less likely to cause bacterial growth or infection than oil-based products. Depending on the severity of vaginal dryness, these products may be used anywhere from daily to once every three days.

2   *Try vitamin E suppositories.* These suppositories can be made by a compounding pharmacist (to find such a pharmacist in your community, refer to Appendix 5). Each suppository contains 120 international units (IU) of vitamin E. After insertion into the vagina, the suppository softens and dissolves in the cavity. Some vitamin E will be absorbed into the body through the vaginal lining, but most of the oil-based vitamin will act to lubricate the vagina. Vitamin E suppositories can be used once daily or less often as needed.

Other ways to prevent urinary tract infections (UTIs)

While drinking plenty of fluids, including a daily dose of cranberry juice, can certainly help prevent a urinary tract infection, other lifestyle modifications are necessary too. One of the most important methods of preventing a UTI is to practise good personal hygiene.

1   *Wipe gently from front to back* whenever you urinate or have a bowel movement. This will avoid spreading bacteria from the rectum into the urethra. When you

feel the urge to urinate, try not to resist. A regular release of fresh, sterile urine will often wash harmful bacteria out of the urethra before it has a chance to travel into the urinary tract.

2   *Clean your genital area before having intercourse,* as this will remove harmful bacteria that may be accidentally transferred into the urethra. Urinating before and after intercourse will help to wash out any bacteria that has migrated into the urinary tract. If you are experiencing UTIs and are using a diaphragm or spermicide-coated condoms, you may want to consider another method of birth control. Always check the fit of your diaphragm and only leave it in for short periods of time.

3   *Wear cotton.* Bacteria grow best in a warm, moist environment. Cotton is a fibre that provides good ventilation, so wear cotton underwear or pantyhose with cotton liners whenever possible. Avoid tight-fitting pants or other types of clothing that may trap heat, irritate tissues, and promote bacterial growth. Washing your underclothes in strong soaps or bleach may cause irritations that could lead to an infection.

4   *Avoid irritants.* If you are susceptible to UTIs, avoid the chemical irritants in bubble bath, perfumed soaps, douches, feminine hygiene deodorants, and deodorant tampons and pads.

5   *Use heat to ease discomfort.* If you are experiencing a UTI, many women find that a heating pad, a hot water bottle, or a warm bath will go a long way to relieve the pain and discomfort caused by a UTI (but be sure also to see your doctor to determine whether you need antibiotics).

THE bottom LINE...

Leslie's recommendations for minimizing vaginal and bladder discomfort

1   Start adding soy foods to your daily diet; experiment to find a few of these foods that you like. Aim to consume at least 40 milligrams of isoflavones from a combination of these foods each day.

2   If soy foods aren't for you, try a protein powder made from isolated soy protein, preferably made from Supro soy protein isolate, which contains plenty of

isoflavones and is the soy protein isolate used in most scientific studies. (For a list of products made with Supro, see Chapter 4, pages 33–34.) Add soy protein powder to a breakfast milkshake or glass of juice.

3   Be sure to consume enough fluids. Aim to drink at least 8 glasses of water each day. Avoid beverages and medications that cause your body to lose water. Dehydration can make vaginal dryness worse and increase your risk of getting a UTI.

4   If you're prone to urinary tract infections, drink 1 1/4 cups (300 ml) of cranberry juice each day. Natural chemicals in the berry have been proven to prevent and treat an infection. Or consider taking an extract of cranberry powder.

5   Consider trying a daily dose of 100 to 200 milligrams of *Panax ginseng* to help restore vaginal epithelial tissue. Buy a standardized extract containing 4 to 7 percent ginsenosides or look for a statement of "G115" on the label. Take ginseng cyclically: two to three weeks on, one week off.

6   If you're experiencing sexual dysfunction as a side effect of antidepressant medication, consider taking 60 milligrams of standardized ginkgo twice daily.

7   Vitamin E suppositories and other vaginal lubricants are helpful in providing moisture and easing milder cases of vaginal dryness.

Menstrual cycle changes

"My periods became a real worry. I'd never had such heavy flow before. On a few occasions, I felt so drained I could barely make it through the day. Thankfully, this didn't go on too long."

9

More than 75 percent of women will experience some change to their monthly cycle during their mid- to late 40s or early 50s. For many women, this is the first sign that menopause is approaching. A number of years before her "last" period, a woman may notice that her cycle becomes less frequent or that periods arrive closer together. And often her period shortens in duration because of fluctuating estrogen production. While an erratic menstrual cycle can be annoying, what's more distressing is the heavy bleeding that can occur during the perimenopausal years.

Heavy bleeding in perimenopausal women is usually the result of an imbalance of estrogen and progesterone. When ovulation does not occur and your ovaries don't release an egg, progesterone is not produced. Since progesterone counters the effects of estrogen, this means that in its absence, estrogen is allowed to continue to build up beyond normal limits within the uterine lining. The lining becomes very thick and laden with more capillaries than usual, releasing a great deal of blood when it is finally shed during your next period (a naturally orchestrated, sharp decline in both estrogen and progesterone each month catalyzes menstrual bleeding). As your estrogen levels decline with approaching menopause, heavy bleeding will become less of an issue.

While heavy bleeding is a common symptom in the years leading up to menopause, it can still be scary. In some cases, heavy bleeding is a sign of something else going on in the uterus—polyps, a fibroid, or, less commonly, cancer. *Always alert your gynecologist if* your periods last more than seven days, if you bleed between your periods, if your menstrual flow becomes much heavier than usual, or if bleeding from the vagina occurs after intercourse.

Heavy menstrual bleeding may cause you to experience chills, dizziness, fatigue, and anemia caused by blood loss. To minimize these side effects, make sure you pay attention to your diet.

Dietary approaches

GET ENOUGH IRON

Now, more than ever, it's important to eat a diet rich in iron. Iron is used by red blood cells to form hemoglobin, the molecule that transports oxygen from your lungs to your cells. If your diet is deficient in iron, or if your body loses iron faster than your diet replaces it, red blood cell levels drop and less oxygen is delivered to your tissues. Symptoms of iron deficiency include weakness, lethargy, and fatigue on exertion (for example, during exercise). Iron deficiency is a progressive condition, which means that even if your iron stores aren't low enough to warrant a formal diagnosis of anemia, you can still be deficient and feel symptoms.

While you're still menstruating, you need 18 milligrams of iron each day. In Chapter 7, I mentioned iron's role in your ability to think and pay attention and discussed ways to increase your intake. You may remember that iron in food comes in two forms: heme iron and nonheme iron. Heme iron is the form most efficiently absorbed by the body and is found in red meat, chicken, eggs, and fish. Nonheme iron comes from plant foods such as whole grains, legumes (lentils, chickpeas, kidney beans), fruit, and vegetables. The body has a harder time absorbing nonheme iron from foods. Eating foods rich in vitamin C along with food sources of nonheme iron will allow your body to absorb much more of the nonheme iron. If you include a little heme iron (for example, meat) with your meal, you'll also increase the absorption of nonheme iron. As you can see by the numbers on page 71, the best iron sources are lean beef, legumes, enriched breakfast cereals, whole-grain breads, raisins, dried apricots, prune juice, spinach, and peas.

What about an iron supplement?

To ensure you get 18 milligrams of iron each day, a multivitamin and mineral supplement is a wise idea. Most formulas provide 10 milligrams, but you can find multivitamins that provide up to 18. If you're experiencing persistent heavy bleeding, however, the recommended daily intake of 18 milligrams might not be enough to meet your needs. Sometimes 100 to 300 milligrams of supplemental iron daily is needed to rebuild your iron stores. Because iron is toxic in large doses, take iron pills only if your doctor has determined that you have low enough iron levels to warrant this level of supplementation. If you are advised to use an iron supplement, take it on an empty stomach to enhance absorption. Many people find that taking their iron supplement just before going to bed reduces stomach upset. Iron can be constipating, so I recommend that you boost your fibre and your water intake when using an iron supplement. Here are 10 strategies for boosting your fibre intake that are easy to implement and that increase your intake of tasty and healthy foods to boot.

1   Strive to consume five or more servings of fruits and vegetables each day.

2   Eat the skin of the fruits and vegetables you consume whenever possible. Just be sure to wash beforehand.

3   Eat at least five servings of whole-grain foods each day.

4   Buy breakfast cereals high in fibre. Aim for at least 4 grams of fibre per serving. (Check the nutrition information panel to find out how much fibre the cereal contains.)

5   If you're looking for a real fibre boost at breakfast, choose a 100 percent bran cereal, which packs 10 grams of fibre per 1/2-cup (125-ml) serving.

6   Top your breakfast cereal with dried apricots, berries, or raisins.

7   Add 2 tablespoons (25 ml) of natural wheat bran, oat bran, or ground flaxseed to hot cereals, yogurt, casseroles, and soup.

8   Eat legumes more often—add white kidney beans to pasta sauce, black beans to tacos, chickpeas to salads, lentils to soup.

9   Add a handful of nuts, seeds, raisins, or dried cranberries to salads.

10   Reach for high-fibre snacks such as popcorn, dried apricots, or dried or fresh dates.

Herbal remedies

CHASTEBERRY (VITEX AGNUS-CASTUS)

Extracts of the berries of the Mediterranean chaste tree have been used in Europe for more than 40 years for female menstrual cycle disorders and menopausal complaints. This herb was first mentioned as a medicinal plant some 2000 years ago when a Greek physician noted the ability of a drink made from the plants' seeds to reduce sexual desire. The herb was also reported to help medieval monks keep their vow of chastity. Accordingly, its Latin name, *agnus castus*, means chaste lamb. Today, chasteberry is most often used in women with premenstrual syndrome, though the herb has also been shown to help women manage irregular menstrual periods. Studies have found the herb effective in normalizing menstruation in women with infrequent periods, short cycles, and long periods. It's thought that chasteberry may be most effective in women with low levels of progesterone.

Chasteberry contains about 0.5 percent volatile oils, along with two compounds, agnuside and aucubin. Studies have shown that an extract of chasteberry is able to lower blood levels of a hormone called prolactin. Scientists believe that the herb acts on the brain's pituitary gland to curb prolactin production and slow down its daily secretion. Chasteberry's ability to lower prolactin levels is important because high prolactin levels lead to decreased progesterone. Remember that without progesterone opposing its action, estrogen builds up your uterine lining unimpeded throughout the month, resulting in heavy bleeding during your period.

If you are experiencing erratic periods and want to try chasteberry, buy a product that's standardized to contain 6 percent agnuside. Some clinical studies have used a specific extract of chasteberry standardized to contain 6 percent of the constituent agnoside. In Canada and the United States, this formulation is found in the brand product Femaprin (Nature's Way). The recommended dosage is 175 to 225 milligrams taken once a day. If you prefer to use a tincture, take 1/2 to 1 teaspoon (3 to 5 ml) once a day. Some experts believe the herb works best if taken in the morning on an empty stomach. A few herbal supplements for menopause combine chasteberry with other herbs, such as black cohosh and dong quai. You can certainly try these, but if you don't find them effective, it may be because they offer too little of each ingredient.

Chasteberry is not fast acting; plan on using it for at least eight weeks before noticing significant improvement. The herb has been used safely in studies lasting up to one and a half years.

Side effects are rare. A few cases of gastrointestinal upset, headache, and mild skin rash have been reported. Also, be sure to let your doctor know that you are taking chasteberry if you're on any medication that interacts with dopamine receptors in the brain. Two common drugs that do this are the antidepressants Wellbutrin and Effexor, but other drugs also influence dopamine levels; ask your doctor or pharmacist. If you are taking chasteberry at the same time as these drugs, your doctor will want to monitor you closely to make sure that the herb doesn't make your medication less effective. If you are taking birth control pills or hormone replacement therapy, use caution. Although there have been no case reports, theoretically, chasteberry could interfere with the effectiveness of these medications because of its hormone-regulating activity. (Although there's no reason to take this supplement if you're on these medications, as they both help regulate your period.) Discontinue use if you become pregnant.

THE bottom LINE...

Leslie's recommendations for managing heavy menstrual flow

1   If you experience heavy flow during your periods, increase your intake of iron-rich foods. Every day, choose at least two iron-rich foods.

2   Make sure that your multivitamin and mineral supplement contains 15 to 18 milligrams of iron. A multivitamin containing this amount of iron will likely be sold as a "woman's" supplement. At menopause, when you are no longer menstruating, switch to a regular formula containing no more than 8 milligrams of iron.

3   If heavy flow has plagued you for some time and your energy levels are down, ask your family doctor to measure your iron level. If iron-deficiency anemia is diagnosed by your blood test, take 100 milligrams of elemental iron one to three times a day two hours after meals. After six to twelve weeks, your doctor will retest your blood to determine your iron levels. Once iron supplements are

discontinued, continue taking your multivitamin and mineral supplement. Since iron supplements can cause stomach upset and constipation, they are often better tolerated when taken later in the day (afternoon and evening). Iron-only supplements should be taken *only* if your doctor has diagnosed anemia or low iron stores (ferritin levels).

4   If iron pills are warranted, aim to consume 25 grams of fibre each day (along with plenty of fluids) to help prevent the constipation often associated with iron supplements.

5   Consider taking a standardized extract of chasteberry to alleviate erratic or prolonged periods. Take a 175- to 225-milligram dose once a day. Keep in mind that this herb does not work overnight: take it for at least eight weeks before making a decision as to whether it helps or not. Use caution if you're taking birth control pills or hormone replacement therapy.

Part three

Protecting your long-term health

"The approach of menopause was a real wake-up call. It forced me to evaluate my habits—and make a few changes for the better."

Preventing weight gain

"I used to be able to just add a little exercise or cut back a little to manage my weight. Now I have to exercise at least three or four times a week and watch what I eat all the time. It's a real struggle!"

10

For many women, myself included, weight control is a major concern. Since I was a teenager, I've had to watch what I eat and exercise regularly in order to maintain a healthy weight. Some women, on the other hand, find that staying trim comes naturally, and they don't have to work very hard at it. But as menopause approaches, many of these same women find that, for the first time in their lives, it becomes more difficult to take off a few unwanted pounds. Or they complain about a "softening around the middle" even with their best efforts at weight control. Over the years, many of my clients have also found that weight gain is an annoying side effect of hormone replacement therapy. One reason is that hormone therapy causes fluid retention. Yet, despite its uncomfortable side effects of bloating and fluid retention, estrogen replacement may actually prevent the accumulation of body fat around the waist that postmenopausal women often report.

Israeli researchers studied 63 early postmenopausal women for one year; one-half of these women took estrogen and progestin replacement therapy, the other half refused hormone therapy. At the end of 12 months, body weight and body fat had increased significantly in both groups. However, there was a significant shift from lower body fat to abdominal fat in the women who did not take hormones. This redistribution of body fat from the hips to the waist was not seen in the women taking hormone replacement therapy.[1] It would seem that at menopause, some women see a shift in body fat, but necessarily an increase on the scale. Others definitely experience weight increases and difficulty keeping the extra pounds off.

There is some evidence to support the notion that menopause itself is partly to blame for increasing waistlines. Recently, scientists from the University of Maryland in Baltimore discovered that enzymes needed to store fat are more active in post-menopausal women compared with perimenopausal women. What's more, the breakdown of stored body fat was reduced in the postmenopausal women.[2] It's thought that the lower levels of estrogen after menopause and factors secreted by fat cells affect fat cell metabolism and result in the shifting body fat experienced by many women during the transitional years.

Menopausal weight gain

What other factors contribute to perimenopausal weight gain? We know that our metabolic rate, which determines the speed at which our bodies burn calories, slows with aging. I have always maintained, however, that regular workouts consisting of aerobic exercise and weight training can prevent much of this age-related slowdown. In fact, the most common cause of weight gain—at any age—is inactivity. But here's something that you might not have known: A woman's metabolic rate increases during the last 14 days of her menstrual cycle (just in time to help us handle those chocolate cravings!). With menopause, then, comes a loss of this cyclic increase in metabolic rate. It's possible that this accounts for some weight gain.

For the most part, though, midlife weight gain is a result of lifestyle choices—poor eating habits and too little exercise. The most common dietary mistakes I see women make include:

• Eating too much starch—bagels, pasta, bread, low-fat muffins, and the like.
• Enjoying desserts and sweets too often.
• Not eating at regular intervals throughout the day.
• Drinking too many alcoholic beverages.
• Not exercising regularly.

All these habits will have an impact on your ability to manage your weight. I have helped scores of peri- and postmenopausal women lose weight, both women taking hormone replacement and those not doing so. Making smart changes with respect to *what* you eat, *how* you eat, and *how* you exercise can help you fit comfortably into your clothes once again.

CALORIES OR FAT?

I'm sure you're familiar with the notion that if you cut back on fat and don't worry about counting calories, you'll lose weight. Cutting back on fat isn't all you need to do to lose weight, but there is some truth to this idea. The foods we eat contain three basic nutrients: carbohydrate, protein, and fat. All three provide our bodies with calories. Some foods, such as milk and yogurt, are made up of a combination of all three nutrients, whereas other foods—oils or grains, for example—are predominantly made up of one nutrient (in this case, fat and carbohydrate, respectively). One gram (less than one teaspoon) of protein gives your body four calories, one gram of carbohydrate also provides four calories, and the same amount of fat packs nine calories, more than double.

That's the rationale for cutting back on fat to help lose weight. Calories from fat add up quickly, and reducing the amount of fat you eat can make a big difference in your calorie intake. So, at the end of the day, it still comes back to eating fewer calories. Note also that the strategy of cutting back on fat will work only if you're actually eating a high-fat diet; these days many of us are careful when it comes to fat (we overeat other types of foods instead!).

Indeed, you've probably heard nutritionists quoted in the media lamenting the fact that, even though we are eating less fat than we did 20 years ago, we are heavier than ever. In fact, 50 percent of Canadian women aged 55 to 64 are overweight, and 35 percent of those overweight are obese. Besides not exercising enough, what are we doing wrong? For starters, we are eating more carbohydrate than ever. In our state of fat phobia, whether in an effort to shed a few pounds or to lower our cholesterol, we're eating baked potato chips, fat-free cookies, and muffins, bagels, and plenty of pasta with tomato sauce. We seem to think that as long as it doesn't contain fat, it's free for the taking. Yet, all nutrients, whether they're fat, carbohydrate, or protein, have calories. If you eat too much of any of them, your body stores the excess as fat. For instance, eating that low-fat bagel (it certainly seems like a better choice than a fat-laden muffin) is the same, calorie-wise, as eating four or five slices of bread. When's the last time you sat down to five pieces of toast for breakfast? By the time you've finished your Italian meal of pasta and bread, you've probably had the equivalent of six (or more) slices of bread! In other words, even though your calories aren't coming from fat, they are still adding up. What's more, the refined carbohydrates we are eating today may actually be triggering us to overeat.

We're also eating more because restaurants and fast food outlets are serving larger portions than ever before. Back in 1916, a serving of Coke at a restaurant was 7 ounces (207 ml). Today, some single-size servings are 20 ounces (590 ml)—that's almost 17 teaspoons worth of sugar!

Today's fad diets

The question remains, how should you eat to successfully lose weight? Should you eat a high-carbohydrate, low-fat diet? Or should you try one of the high-protein, low-carbohydrate diets? Is there any truth to food combining? To choosing foods based on your blood type? I can understand if you're confused. These days there is certainly no shortage of diet books on the market, each claiming that its own special formula is guaranteed to make those readers who diligently follow the protocols given become thin and healthy. To help you sort out the useless from the useful, I've summarized today's popular (but not necessarily sound) weight-loss diets. And in Appendix 1, I'll give you my own weight-loss diet plan. Now, let's take a look at some of the most popular diets on the market today.

DR. ATKINS' DIET AND THE PROTEIN POWER PLAN

Both these diets are high in protein, fairly high in fat, and contain almost no carbohydrate. They restrict your daily carbohydrate intake to 20 to 30 grams—the amount found in one and one-half regular slices of bread or one-half of a medium-size banana. These diets promote "ketosis," an abnormal metabolic state. The brain and central nervous system rely on carbohydrate as a fuel source; after two days without carbohydrate, they must adapt to a new energy source. That adaptation is called ketosis. In this state, the body breaks down fat into ketones, which the brain and central nervous system then use as fuel.

These diets are intended for short-term use only. Research suggests being in ketosis for a long period of time increases the risk of heart disease by damaging low-density lipoprotein (LDL) cholesterol. Once LDL cholesterol is damaged, it is more likely to stick to artery walls. You'll find more detailed information on LDL cholesterol in Chapter 12, Reducing Your Risk of Heart Disease.

DR. ATKINS' NEW DIET REVOLUTION

This diet involves a strict two-week "induction" (induction of ketosis), then a gradual reintroduction of carbohydrate. Most people who come off this diet regain their weight quickly. This is because when you start eating carbohydrate again, your body rebuilds its glycogen (carbohydrate) stores in your liver and muscles. For every gram of carbohydrate stored, you store 3 grams of water. The net result? Rapid weight gain. The Atkins' diet is not the answer for long-term weight control. It's a diet you go "on and off." It doesn't change your eating habits over the long term. Furthermore, no studies have been published on the *long-term* success of high-protein, very-low-carbohydrate diets.

PROTEIN POWER

Written by medical doctors Michael and Mary Eades, Protein Power is another plan that puts you into ketosis. In the first phase of the diet, you are not allowed to eat more than 30 grams of carbohydrate each day (the equivalent of two regular slices of bread). This phase lasts four to six weeks. In the second phase, you're allowed to eat a little more carbohydrate (a measly 55 grams a day). This level of carbohydrate intake is followed until you reach your weight and health goals. In the next phase, the maintenance phase, you gradually increase your carbohydrate intake at each meal.

So, like the Atkins' diet, the Protein Power is not a diet for life. It does, however, encourage you to eat more fibre and healthier types of fat than the Atkins' diet discussed above. It also recommends taking a multivitamin and daily potassium supplement; the authors recognize that ketosis is a powerful diuretic and causes your body to lose fluid and minerals, especially potassium and sodium. Not replacing lost potassium can have serious health consequences. While a pill might take care of your potassium needs for a time, does this high-protein approach sound like a healthy way to lose weight?

There are other health risks associated with high-protein diets. To prevent dehydration while on these diets, you must drink plenty—and I mean plenty—of water. As I just mentioned, ketosis causes your body to excrete large amounts of water, sodium, and potassium. If you choose fatty meats and cheese as your main protein foods, you run the risk of high blood cholesterol levels. Your liver uses saturated fat in animal food to manufacture blood cholesterol. And because you're allowed virtually no fruit or dairy products on these diets, you won't be meeting your needs for certain nutrients, especially vitamins C, D, and folic acid, or the mineral calcium. What's more, these diets often cause constipation because of the lack of fibre.

If you take medication for high blood pressure, high cholesterol, or diabetes and you decide to try a high-protein diet, ask your doctor to monitor you. These diets are definitely not appropriate for people with kidney problems, as high amounts of protein stress the kidneys. And if you exercise regularly, these diets won't provide fuel for your muscles. It's carbohydrate that fuels your workouts—whether you weight train, jog, or play tennis.

THE ZONE

The Zone is a low-carbohydrate, moderate-protein, low-fat diet developed by Dr. Barry Sears. The Zone diet does not cause ketosis because it doesn't eliminate carbohydrates (I'll give it points for this). Rather, Dr. Sears advocates eating meals and snacks made up of 40 percent carbohydrate, 30 percent protein, and 30 percent fat. This combination of nutrients supposedly promotes the right balance of two hormones important in blood sugar regulation: insulin and glucagon. If your diet encourages you to produce less insulin, says the author, your body will burn your fat stores and cause you to lose weight.

While no clinical study has proven that the Zone diet results in weight loss attributable to achieving a certain balance of hormones in your bloodstream, the plan does have nutritional merits. For one, the diet recommends you eat those starchy foods that are *slowly* converted to blood glucose, called low glycemic index (GI) carbohydrates. (Eating such foods results in lower insulin secretions after a meal.) And researchers are finding that the type of carbohydrate you eat just might affect your ability to lose weight. See diet-friendly foods, pages 111–112 and page 114, for details on low glycemic foods.

The Zone diet also encourages the consumption of protein foods lower in fat, such as chicken breast and fish, and it promotes the use of healthy fats and oils. Sounds fine so far. Are there any drawbacks to this diet? I'll warn you right now that the Zone is a complicated diet to understand, and you may find the instructions highly impractical and time-consuming, since you must measure out all food portions. A Zone lunch might include 3 ounces (90 g) of lean protein, one-quarter of a pumpernickel bagel, and low GI vegetables. Following this diet also means, for the most part, preparing your meals yourself, rather than buying them prepared.

Many people find that the carbohydrate portions from bread, grains, fruits, and vegetables are very limiting. For instance, you might be allowed three carbohydrate servings (called blocks) at a meal. A carbohydrate serving could be 1/4 cup (50 ml) kidney beans, half an apple, 1/5 cup (30 ml) of brown rice, or 1/4 cup (50 ml) of pasta. It's easy to see that you'll be eating much less carbohydrate from starchy foods and fruit.

This diet also lacks calcium. A small 1/2-cup (125-ml) portion of plain yogurt or low-fat milk is allowed only as a daily snack, not at meals. According to my calculations, this diet provides at most 500 milligrams of calcium per day. If you decide to follow this diet, you'll definitely need to take a supplement to reach your daily requirement of 1000 (perimenopause) or 1500 milligrams (postmenopause).

SUGAR BUSTERS!

Sugar Busters! was created by four medical doctors: H. Steward, M. Bethea, S. Andrews, and L. Balart. Like the Zone diet, this diet is based on the concept of eating foods that minimize the amount of insulin your body secretes. The authors contend that if you produce less insulin, you won't store body fat and, even better, you'll mobilize your fat stores. This diet limits portions of starchy foods and recommends only those carbohydrates with a low GI. This means that if you follow this diet, you can't eat white bread, white rice, white pasta, watermelon, potatoes, corn, or even beets. That leaves you with brown rice, whole-grain pastas, pita bread, rye bread, high-fibre cereals, sweet potatoes, legumes, most fruits, and green vegetables as choices.

Unlike the Zone, this diet does not require you to eat carbohydrate, protein, and fat in specific proportions at each meal. Starchy foods are eaten at only one or two meals daily, never at all three. On the suggested two-week meal plan, you're allowed only three servings of starch or grains each day (most balanced weight-loss programs allow at least four to six servings of grain, depending on your exercise level). Although the authors do mention that portion control is important, serving sizes are not given for any of the plan's acceptable foods, not even in the 14-day meal plan.

If you're trying to lower your cholesterol level, the Sugar Busters! plan might not be the best to follow, as consumption of cheese, pâté, bacon, and plenty of red meat are encouraged. This diet also incorporates the concept of food combining (for more details on food combining, see the Fit for Life section following). For example, fruit is allowed only before or after a meal, never with a meal. The authors say that eating fruit separately leads to improved digestion, less heartburn, and less bloating. So you can forget those berries on your bowl of cereal! Calcium is another concern if you follow this diet—the daily menus provide nowhere near the recommended daily intake.

EAT RIGHT FOR YOUR TYPE

This diet is based on the theory that your blood type reflects the diet and behaviour of your ancestors. The author, naturopathic physician Dr. Peter D'Adamo, says that the ancestors of Type O individuals were hunters and gatherers and therefore should eat animal protein, especially red meat. Type O people are told to limit grain and legume consumption, as these are said to encourage weight gain. The ancestors of people with Type A blood, says D'Adamo, were cultivators and supposedly do best on a vegetarian diet. They're told to limit their meat, wheat, and dairy consumption. If you have type B blood, your ancestors were nomads, so you can eat a more varied diet. But corn, lentils, peanuts, sesame seeds, and wheat will apparently cause you to gain weight.

On what does Dr. D'Adamo base his advice? He believes that all foods contain protein molecules called lectins, which are capable of "sticking" to the structures found on the surfaces of cells. When you eat a food that contains lectins incompatible with your blood type, the lectins cause blood cells to clump together, usually in the vicinity of a particular organ or tissue. D'Adamo says that because of these "sticky" effects, food incompatible with your blood type can interfere with digestion, slow down your metabolism, affect insulin levels, and cause water retention. I certainly agree that the wrong foods can cause these problems in sensitive people, but until I see studies that validate this theory of how food lectins interact with blood type, it's a stretch for me to believe that such reactions have to do with blood type.

Dr. D'Adamo's diet is based on observations made by his father (also a naturopathic physician) with patients. In my view, people experience weight loss on the blood-type diets because they tend to eat fewer calories—all blood-type diets eliminate wheat. This means no bread, pasta, bagels, crackers, cookies, or cereal. If you don't make an effort to incorporate the grain foods for your blood type, which might be rice, buckwheat, or spelt, you may very well lose weight on a blood-type diet.

FIT FOR LIFE

Harvey and Marilyn Diamond were, in the early 1980s, the first to popularize food combining for weight loss, with their book *Fit for Life: A New Way of Eating*. In a nutshell, here's the rationale of food combining: Your body uses certain enzymes to digest starch and other enzymes to break down protein. When you eat protein and starch together in the same meal, these enzymes neutralize each other and can't digest the food. So the meal ends up sitting in your stomach, rotting and forming toxins. These toxins, in turn, cause you to gain weight. On this diet, then, starchy foods can be combined only with vegetables, never with protein foods such as meat and chicken. Only fruit is allowed throughout the morning, and after noon, it must be eaten on an empty stomach. Dairy products are forbidden because they are a combination of protein and carbohydrate. Food combining was originally intended as a way to maximize a person's digestion and energy, and, of course, weight loss is an inevitable side effect for most people. Doesn't it sound as though you'd be eating less food on this program? The *Fit for Life* diet is also low in calcium, and potentially deficient in protein.

I wonder what the next "breakthrough diet" will be. It seems we've come full circle. From the high-protein Atkins' diet of the 1970s to the Protein Power surge of the late 1990s. And food combining has resurfaced in Michel Montignac's *Eat Yourself Slim* and Suzanne Somers' *Get Skinny*. Is there any truth to any of these diet prescriptions? I'm not talking about the high-protein diets, which put you into ketosis. (They're a whole different ball game from the other diets, one I don't recommend.) But does minimizing insulin levels, combining the proper foods, or eating meals to match your blood type hold the key to long-term weight control?

Well, people do lose weight on these programs. But usually this is simply because once they start following these diets, they eat less food. All these diets eliminate junk food and often one whole food group. If you can no longer have a bagel for breakfast or a plate of pasta for dinner, you will be consuming fewer calories because you'll be eating a lot less starch (not to mention less peanut butter, cream cheese, and pesto sauce!). If you can no longer combine tuna or turkey with bread, you're going to be eating a sandwich lower in calories. With the exception of the diet outlined in *Eat Right for Your Type*, the magic of these diets lies in the fact that most of them provide about 1200 to 1400 calories each day. And that's a weight-loss diet. They work because they force people to eat less food, period.

And many people do report feeling healthier and more energetic on these programs. When you cut back your food intake and make healthier choices, you will feel better.

And that's a good thing. If you do decide to try one of these diets (but not the ketosis diets!), ensure you make up for any missing nutrients. It might be wise to consult a dietitian on what supplements you might take. If you have access to the internet, visit the Dietitians of Canada website (www.dietitians.ca) to locate a consulting dietitian in your community.

If you're thinking about spending money on a commercial weight-loss program, whether it's Weight Watchers, Jenny Craig, or a program at your local hospital, first determine if the program is right for you. The questions I've outlined on pages 108–109 will help you decide if the program is credible and if it will suit your needs.

Before I give you my advice on how to lose weight or prevent weight gain, let me say that I don't for one minute believe that one diet or one way of eating is right for all people. When I develop weight-loss plans for clients, I ask about their food preferences, frequency of food cravings, exercise routine, past weight-loss attempts, and other lifestyle issues. This information helps me determine the best type of diet for my client. In some cases, high-carbohydrate/low-fat works well, and in other situations a higher protein diet is a better approach. In Appendix 1, you'll find my recommended meal plan for achieving and maintaining a healthy weight. But before you decide to cut back on your food intake, take a minute to read the following section and assess your current weight.

Assess Your Body Weight

DO YOU REALLY NEED TO LOSE WEIGHT?
While being overweight can increase your risk of heart disease and breast cancer, your risk is only partially determined by the number you see on the bathroom scale. Once you complete this assessment, you'll have a more complete picture of how your weight is likely to affect your health. Don't worry, the meanings of the calculations will be explained once you've done them (you will need a calculator).

What's your body mass index (BMI)?
Calculate your body mass index (BMI) as follows:
1   Determine your weight in kilograms.
    (Divide your weight in pounds by 2.2)   _____

2   Determine your height in centimetres.
    (Multiply your height in inches by 2.54) _____

3   Determine your height in metres.
    (Divide your height in centimetres by 100) _____

4   Square your height in metres.
    (Multiply your height in metres by your height in metres.) _____

5   Your BMI.
    (Divide your weight in kilograms by your height [in m^2]) _____

Long-term studies show that the overall risk of developing heart disease, diabetes, or high blood pressure is generally related to your BMI in this way:

BMI under 20	You may be more likely to develop certain health problems, including anemia, osteoporosis, and irregular heart rhythms, because of malnutrition.
BMI 20–24.9	Healthy range. Your risk of health problems is low.
BMI 25–29.9	Overweight. Having a BMI in this range is a call to action. Your risk of future health problems is increasing.
BMI 30 or higher	Obese. You are at high risk of weight-related health problems

If your BMI is at the upper end of the healthy zone, say at 24 or 25, you might still be carrying extra weight. A little extra body fat has generally not been thought to affect long-term health, although new research begs to differ. According to researchers from the Brigham and Women's Hospital and Harvard Medical School, adults who weigh in at the high end of the healthy range of the BMI scale may be at increased risk of type 2 diabetes, gallstones, high blood pressure, heart disease, stroke, colon cancer, and high cholesterol. The study revealed that people not traditionally considered to be overweight (those with a BMI of 22 to 24.9) were also at greater risk of developing at least one of the chronic diseases, compared with their slimmer peers. Based on their findings, the scientists recommend that adults maintain a BMI of between 18.5 and 21.9.[3]

What's your waist-hip ratio?

The waist-hip ratio indicates where fat is accumulated on your body. An accumulation of fat in the abdomen is closely related to increased health risks. Statistics clearly show that being overweight, especially if excess weight is carried around the waist, significantly increases the risk of heart disease and stroke, type 2 diabetes, osteoarthritis, sleep apnea, gout, and gallbladder disease. Calculate your waist-hip ratio as follows:

1   Using a tape measure, measure the circumference of your waist at its narrowest point, when your stomach is relaxed.
Waist = _____ inches

2   Next, measure the circumference of your hips at their widest. (Sorry, girls, this is where your buttocks stick out the most!)
Hips = _____ inches

3   Finally, divide your waist measurement by your hip measurement.
Waist ÷ hip = _____ inches

A healthy waist-hip ratio for women is less than 0.8. At this ratio, you're not carrying excess weight around your waist. It is fat especially around the abdomen that can lead to health problems. You might not appreciate hefty hips and thighs, but at least they don't increase your health risk.

You must remember that there are factors other than weight that increase your risk of disease. Poor diet, excessive alcohol consumption, a lack of exercise, smoking, and high blood pressure are other important risk factors for disease.

Is the time right?

So you've done the calculations, and it seems that losing some weight would be a good idea. But you need to take one more step before embarking on a weight-loss program. You need to determine if this is a good time for you to make a lifestyle change. Otherwise your chances of success are slim. Think about these questions:

•   How motivated are you this time? Compare your present level of motivation with your state of mind during previous unsuccessful attempts to change your eating habits and exercise patterns. Are you feeling differently now?

•   Are you looking at a long-term commitment? Can you envision yourself continuing to cook healthy foods and to work out a year from now?

•   Is your life full of stress? If so, now is probably not the time to start a lifestyle change.

•   How much weight do you expect to lose? How quickly? Are your goals realistic?

•   How do you feel about fitting exercise into your daily schedule?

- Do you have friends, family members, or co-workers who will support you in your efforts? If not, would you consider joining a support group or starting one?
- Are you easily swayed from your healthy habits by social occasions?
- Do you eat when you feel lonely, bored, anxious, or depressed? If so, do you feel ready to come up with alternative responses to these feelings?
- When you go off your plan or miss a workout, how quickly can you get back on track?
- If you binge, use laxatives or diuretics, or induce vomiting, do you have strategies for changing this behaviour by yourself? If not, would you consider seeing a therapist or eating-disorder specialist?

Choosing a commercial weight-loss program

Before you sign up for a commercial weight-loss program, ask yourself the following questions. Check off the ones that apply. When you're finished, take a look at how the pros and cons of the program you're interested in stack up. Another point to keep in mind is whether the program offers one-on-one or group sessions, and which type would suit you best.

Pros
☐ Does the program include a nutrition-education component?
☐ Will I learn healthy eating skills?
☐ Does the program emphasize weight maintenance?
☐ Does the program emphasize exercise?
☐ Does the program incorporate behavioural therapy or stress-management techniques?
☐ Does the program address how to create social-support systems that will back your attempt at weight loss?
☐ Are the counsellors well qualified?

Cons
☐ Does the program exclude any one food group?
☐ Does the program rely on any type of meal supplement?

- ☐ Does the program rely on specially purchased foods?
- ☐ Is the same approach used for both men and women?
- ☐ Do the counsellors seem unqualified or inexperienced?

Leslie's strategies for weight loss

If you're still reading, it's likely that the numbers say you need to lose weight—and that you feel ready to tackle the challenge. Here are the key strategies I encourage clients to implement so that they will successfully lose weight and keep it off.

SET A REALISTIC GOAL

Take a look at what your weight has been for the past 10 to 15 years. If you want to weigh 130 pounds, but you haven't weighed that since your early 20s, keep in mind that your goal might be more difficult to achieve. In fact, depending on your lifestyle, it may be unrealistic. Also, don't think you need to rely on the scale to set a goal. Many of my clients choose a size of clothing as their target. Others prefer to measure their success by improvements in physical fitness or improvements in blood cholesterol or blood pressure readings. If you do decide to use a number on the scale as your goal, pick a 5-pound (2.2-kg) weight range that you want to stay within. It's not realistic to expect yourself to remain a constant weight. You need a little room for holidays and entertaining.

HAVE THE RIGHT MINDSET

Think long-term lifestyle change instead of short-term quick fix. I can tell you right now that people who approach losing weight with this attitude are far more likely to be successful. Before you embark on a weight-loss program, ask yourself what your motivation is. Are you trying to fit into a dress for your son's wedding next month? Or do you want to be healthier and have more energy? The right mindset also means being comfortable with slow and steady weight loss. No weight-loss plan should cause you to lose much more than 2 pounds (1 kg) per week. Weight lost at a faster rate likely means you're losing muscle and water. And the more muscle you lose, the slower the rate at which your body burns calories.

GET SOCIAL SUPPORT

If you need help from a spouse, family member, co-worker, or friend, ask for it. It often helps to have a workout partner, especially if you're just beginning an exercise program. If your partner pulls out potato chips every night after dinner, ask him or her to be mindful of your attempt to change your eating habits. If you want positive reinforcement from someone, let that person know.

START AN EXERCISE PROGRAM

If you're not already active, it's time to get moving. Exercise burns calories, and by building up muscle, it helps your body burn more calories while at rest. To help you lose body fat, aim to get four cardiovascular workouts each week (brisk walking, jogging, stair climbing, swimming, cross-country skiing, aerobics classes). Start exercising for 20 minutes per session, gradually building up to a minimum of 30 minutes each session. When you're ready, add two or three weight-training sessions per week. Studies have found that adding weight training to a weight-loss program speeds up weight loss. If you're currently completely sedentary, consult your doctor before starting an exercise program.

EAT AT REGULAR INTERVALS

Eating a meal or snack every four to five hours will help boost your metabolism, improve your energy level, and maintain a consistent blood sugar level. Eating regularly prevents hunger and helps eliminate unwanted nibbling or overeating at the next meal.

DON'T EAT DINNER LATE

Finish eating dinner no later than eight o'clock or, if possible, by seven o'clock. As the evening approaches, your body's metabolism naturally slows down. Dinner is actually the time your body needs the smallest meal, even though this is when most of us eat the bulk of the day's calories. And after an evening meal, most of us are sedentary, watching television, reading, or sleeping. This practice increases the odds that a late meal will be stored as body fat. If you get home late, tell yourself that you've missed dinner. Just because you walk in the door doesn't mean you have to have dinner; have a light snack instead—some yogurt, a piece of fruit, or a bowl of soup.

SNACK WISELY

If any two of your day's meals will be more than five hours apart, plan to snack between them. Between-meal snacks are important to help keep your energy levels up and prevent snacking on sweets (or some other unhealthy food). Depending on the meal, your blood sugar will drop three to four hours later. Since your blood sugar is the only source of fuel for your brain, a post-meal dip can make you feel sluggish and tired. Often this is when people go in search of a pick-me-up. So instead of letting a blood sugar low push you into rash action, plan to give yourself the needed energy boost at the right time. Here's my rule: No snacking on refined starchy foods such as bagels, pretzels, low-fat cookies, low-fat crackers, or fat-free muffins. Because these foods are quickly converted to blood glucose (remember, they're high glycemic index foods), they're more likely to lead to more hunger and sweet cravings. (For an overview of the glycemic index of various foods, see the section on low glycemic carbohydrates, page 112.) Better snacks include low-fat yogurt, milk, soy beverages, homemade smoothies, nuts, and whole fruit, which will also help you get more fibre and calcium into your diet.

SATIETY VALUES OF SELECTED FOODS

Food	Value	Food	Value
Potato, boiled	323	Cookies	120
Fish, baked	225	Banana	118
Oatmeal	209	French fries	116
Orange	202	Bread, white	100
Apple	197	Muesli	100
Pasta, whole-wheat	188	Ice cream	96
Beef steak	176	Potato chips	91
Grapes	162	Peanuts	84
Popcorn	154	Candy bar	70
Bran cereal	151	Doughnut	68
Cheese	146	Cake	65
Crackers	127	Croissant	47

Diet-friendly foods

Feeling hungry but don't want to sabotage your healthy eating plan? Researchers at the University of Sydney have created what they call a satiety index of various foods. They tested the ability of 240 calories worth of particular foods to satisfy one's appetite. All foods were compared with white bread, which was given a satiety index rating of 100. As you'll see on page 111, 240 calories' worth of some foods were only half as satisfying as white bread, while others were three times more satisfying.[4]

EAT ENOUGH PROTEIN

To meet your protein needs, be sure to get at least six servings of protein-rich foods each day. Protein will also help maintain your blood sugar levels longer. I recommend splitting your protein servings between lunch and dinner. Some people prefer to include protein at breakfast, too. See Appendix 2 for what constitutes one serving of protein.

CUT BACK ON CARBS, ESPECIALLY REFINED STARCHY FOODS

When you have pasta, avoid the bread basket. If you have a meal that includes rice or potatoes, don't eat bread. Too much starch adds extra calories to your day. Even though plain bread is low in fat, it still has calories, and it all adds up. For example, one large bagel is equivalent in carbohydrate to four to five slices of bread. Here are a few tips to help prevent you from overeating starchy foods:

- Say no to the bread basket in restaurants.
- When you have pasta, rice, or potatoes, skip the bread.
- At breakfast, have cereal or toast, not both.
- Keep your pasta portion to one cup (250 ml) when cooked (appetizer size).
- If you tend to overeat foods such as pasta, rice, or potatoes, consider skipping the starch altogether at dinner. Enjoy grilled fish, chicken, or lean meat with plenty of vegetables.

EAT MORE LOW GLYCEMIC CARBOHYDRATES

Make sure your carbohydrate intake is more heavily weighted toward low glycemic carbs. Nutritionists assign carbohydrate foods a glycemic index (GI) ranking based on how quickly they increase blood sugar levels. In this system, foods are compared with pure glucose, which has a reference value of 100 (fast acting). A high GI food (for example, white and whole-wheat bread, sugar, white rice, mashed potatoes, muesli, puffed rice, bananas, raisins) is converted to blood glucose quickly. A rapid rise in blood glucose causes your pancreas to secrete a large amount of insulin into your bloodstream. Insulin's job is to lower your blood sugar and store carbohydrates as glycogen or, if you've overeaten, as fat. The end result of high insulin production is that your blood sugar will drop off sooner and you'll soon feel hungry again. Foods with a low GI (for example, oatmeal, yogurt, dried beans, citrus fruit) take longer to digest and lead to a gradual rise in blood glucose. You don't get a surge of insulin production, and the energy from the food circulates in your bloodstream longer. This means you don't feel hungry as soon after eating foods with a low GI.

An American study confirms this point. In the study, overweight teenage boys were offered, on three different days, unlimited snacks for five hours after eating meals with foods with a low GI (vegetable omelette and fruit), a medium GI (regular oatmeal), or a high GI (instant oatmeal). The boys ate nearly twice as much in snacks after the high GI meal as compared with after the low GI meal. The researchers also found that the boys' blood sugar and insulin rose the highest and fastest after a high GI meal but then crashed.[5] A crash in blood sugar, as I mentioned, leads to hunger, carbohydrate cravings, and possibly overeating, as well as less energy for your brain.

In the list on pages 114–115, French bread has a GI ranking of 95; chickpeas 42. That means the bread increases blood sugar as quickly as pure glucose, whereas chickpeas boost sugar levels only half as quickly. To stay satisfied longer after a snack or meal and to aid weight loss, choose more foods with lower GI values (less than 55), such as legumes, barley, brown rice, sweet potatoes, new potatoes, whole-grain rye bread, whole-wheat pasta, All Bran cereal, oatmeal, brown rice, apples, oranges, milk, or yogurt. Studies also show that eating low GI foods at two meals daily can help lower elevated blood sugar, cholesterol, and triglyceride levels.

DON'T ELIMINATE FAT

Our current nutrition guidelines emphasize the importance of cutting back on total fat to help control weight and stay healthy. But researchers are learning that the *quality* of fat you consume is also very important to your health. Focus on reducing your intake of *saturated fat* by making a habit of choosing lower-fat animal foods, such as lean meat, poultry breast, and low-fat dairy products. Eliminate sources of *trans fat* from your diet by avoiding foods that list "hydrogenated fat" or "shortening" as an ingredient. Fried fast food, French fries, doughnuts, store-bought bakery goods, and snack foods are prime culprits.

GLYCEMIC INDEX (GI) OF SELECTED CARBOHYDRATE FOODS

Here's a list of foods ranked by their GI value. When using this table to help plan your meals, use the following scale: < 55 = low GI; 55–70 = medium; GI; >70 = high GI.

BREAD AND CRACKERS

Baguette, French	95
Kaiser roll	73
Melba toast	70
Pita bread, whole-wheat	57
Pumpernickel, whole-grain	51
Rice cakes	82
Rye bread	65
Soda crackers	74
Sourdough bread	52
Stoned Wheat Thins	67
White bread	70
Whole-wheat bread	69

BREAKFAST CEREALS

All Bran, Kellogg's	51
All Bran Buds with Psyllium, Kellogg's	45
Bran Flakes	74
Corn Bran, Quaker	75
Corn Flakes	84
Oat bran	50
Oatmeal	49
Raisin Bran	73
Shredded Wheat, spoon-size	58
Special K	54

COOKIES, CAKES, AND MUFFINS

Angel food cake	67
Arrowroot	69
Banana bread	47
Blueberry muffin	59
Graham crackers	74
Oat bran muffin	60
Oatmeal cookies	55
Social Tea biscuits	55
Sponge cake	46

PASTA, GRAINS, AND POTATO

Barley	25
Bulgur	48
Corn, sweet	55
Couscous	65
Fettuccine, egg	32
Potato, French fries	75
Potato, instant, mashed	86
Potato, new, unpeeled, boiled	62
Potato, red-skinned, boiled	88
Potato, red-skinned, mashed	91
Potato, sweet, mashed	54
Potato, white-skinned, baked	85
Rice, basmati	58
Rice, brown	55
Rice, converted, Uncle Ben's	44
Rice, instant	87
Rice, long-grain, white	56
Rice, short-grain	72
Spaghetti, white	41
Spaghetti, whole-wheat	37

LEGUMES

Baked beans	48
Black beans	31

Black bean soup	64	**DAIRY PRODUCTS AND ALTERNATIVES**	
Chickpeas, canned	42	Ice cream, low-fat	50
Kidney beans	27	Milk, chocolate	34
Lentils	30	Milk, skim	32
Lentil soup, canned	34	Milk, whole	27
Soy beans	18	Soy beverage	31
Split-pea soup	66	Yogurt, flavoured, low-fat	33

FRUIT

SNACK FOODS

Fruit		Snack Foods	
Apple	38	Corn chips	72
Apricot, dried	31	Peanuts	14
Banana	55	Popcorn	55
Cantaloupe	65	Potato chips	54
Cherries	22	Pretzels	83
Dates, dried	103	Sports bar, PowerBar, chocolate	58
Grapefruit	25	**SUGARS**	
Grapes	46	Fructose (fruit sugar)	23
Mango	55	Glucose	100
Orange	44	Honey	58
Peach, canned	30	Lactose (milk sugar)	46
Pear	38	Sucrose (table sugar)	65
Raisins	64		
Watermelon	72		

Reproduced with permission by the *American Journal of Clinical Nutrition.* © Am J Clin Nutr. American Society for Clinical Nutrition.

Now for the good fats to include in your diet! To meet your daily requirements for essential fatty acids, use oils rich in *alpha-linolenic acid*. The best sources include flaxseed oil, walnut oil, and canola oil. And don't forget about those heart healthy *monounsaturated* fats—use extra-virgin olive oil in salad dressings and sauces. Aim to get four to six fat servings per day. (See Appendix 2 for what constitutes one fat serving.)

AVOID EXCESS SUGAR

A little jam on your toast or a teaspoon of sugar in your coffee is certainly okay. But drinking beverages such as regular pop, fruit drinks, and fruit juice only add extra calories to your day. I'd rather you quenched your thirst with water and got your fruit servings in the form of whole fruit. You'll cut back on calories, and you'll also boost your fibre intake.

LIMIT ALCOHOL

Keep your alcohol intake to no more than seven drinks per week. I explained to you earlier that one gram of pure fat has nine calories, more than double the amount in one gram of protein or carbohydrate. A gram of alcohol in beer, wine, or liquor has seven calories—and they add up. Perhaps even more important, I also find that alcohol consumption tends to lower one's willpower, making it more difficult to stick to a healthy meal plan. If you do drink alcohol, one drink per day is not considered to increase your risk of disease. If you're out for an evening, try drinking only one alcoholic drink and rounding out your evening with a low-calorie, alcohol-free beverage such as mineral water, club soda, Clamato juice, or cranberry and soda. One drink is equivalent to 6 ounces (175 ml) of wine, one bottle (375 ml) of light beer or 1.5 ounces (45 ml) of liquor.

TREAT YOURSELF

Treat yourself to a serving of sweets, dessert, or candy once a week. Enjoy a "real" serving of whatever you really want once a week. If sweets aren't your thing, it can be French fries, nachos, or chicken wings. Make this weekly treat part of the plan, and don't feel guilty for enjoying it. Remember that any changes you make to lose weight need to be sustainable. Can you really see yourself giving up your special treats for good?

DEAL WITH LAPSES

We're all human. That means our weight is not intended to always measure one particular number on the scale. When you have a busy social calendar or you're spending three wonderful weeks enjoying the wine and food of Italy, you're bound to put on a few pounds (I did!). The key to long-term weight maintenance is nipping small weight gains in the bud. That's why I advised you earlier to choose a weight *range* to stay within. If you want to stay trim, you've got to catch that 3-pound gain before it becomes 10. And if you're not watching things carefully, that 10 pounds can quite easily turn into 20. I'm sure that many of you know just what I mean.

I recommend monitoring your weight on a weekly basis. When you see a few pounds creep on, have a plan of action to take them off. You might decide to keep a food diary for a few weeks. When you have to write down all the foods you eat, you're more likely to make healthy choices. And keeping a daily record of the food you eat gives you focus and serves as a reminder of your goals. Or you might add an extra workout to your week for a month. Some people give up sweets until the pounds are back down. Do whatever will work for you.

Keeping your weight off—for good!

Over the past 15 years, I have helped scores of people successfully lose weight. I have done so by teaching them *what to eat* and *how to eat*. My philosophy is very straightforward: *Everything you do to lose weight must be everything you do to keep it off.* It just doesn't make sense to give up your favourite food or exercise fanatically seven days per week. It just won't stick.

By studying the habits of successful dieters, researchers have now learned which key strategies help keep the weight off. The National Weight Control Registry is a database of more than 2000 people from all over the United States who have successfully maintained a 30-pound (14-kg) weight loss for at least one year.[6] Most registrants have kept off 60 pounds (27 kg) for a minimum of five years. About half of these people lost weight on their own without any type of formal program. What makes these people so successful? As you'll see below, many of the strategies I recommended above for losing weight are just as important for maintaining that loss.

1 *Eat a low-fat, high-carbohydrate diet.* The average registrant consumes 1400 calories per day, with 24 percent of those calories coming from fat. Registrants say they don't use fat as a seasoning, avoid frying foods, and substitute low-fat for high-fat foods. Whole grains, legumes, fruit, vegetables, and low-fat dairy products make up the bulk of their diets.

2 *Keep high-fat foods out of the house.* To stay on track, almost all say they stock their kitchen with plenty of healthy foods, and about one-third say they eat in restaurants less often.

3 *Eat five times per day.* Instead of devouring three big meals, successful dieters eat more often. Spreading out their food over the day keeps their stomach always partly full and prevents overeating at any one time.

4   *Don't deny yourself.* People in the National Weight Control Registry say they don't give up their favourite foods. They continue to enjoy them, just not as often as they did when they were overweight.

5   *Keep a food diary.* One-half of all successful weight-loss participants say they record their daily food intake and workouts. Doing so provides focus and motivation.

6   *Weigh yourself often.* Almost 80 percent of the registrants weigh themselves on a regular basis, some even in their sixth year of maintaining their loss. Monitoring your progress provides motivation and impetus to keep on going. It also allows you to nip small weight gains in the bud.

7   *Learn about nutrition.* Seventy-five percent of successful dieters say they buy books and magazines related to nutrition and exercise, and they continue to do so years after they have lost the weight. When you create an environment that fosters healthy eating, you're more likely to stay on track and make these changes permanent.

8   *Get planned exercise.* Nine out of 10 registrants report getting one hour of scheduled exercise each day. Many participants get their calorie burn from brisk walking. Exercise makes you feel good about yourself, making you want to eat healthy. And you can enjoy more food if you work out regularly!

9   *Sneak in activity.* Small things like taking the stairs instead of the escalator, parking at the end of the lot and then walking, and getting off the bus a few stops early all add up.

10 *Expect failure, but keep on trying.* People who are successful at losing weight don't expect to be perfect. They consider lapses as momentary setbacks, not the ruin of all their hard work. Whether you've had a busy social schedule or you've just returned from a food-laden business convention, you're bound to have put on a few pounds. As I mentioned above, the key to long-term weight maintenance is dealing with small weight gains when they occur. By telling yourself that you're human and it's okay to have slipped a little, you'll be amazed at how easy it is to return to your usual healthy routine.

YOUR WEIGHT-CONTROL CHECKLIST

Following is a list of the major behaviours associated with successful weight control. Place a checkmark next to those behaviours that are a regular part of your life. Then comes the hard part. Take a look at the behaviours that aren't yet part of your daily routine. Choose one and begin practising it until it is. Then choose another behaviour you're currently not practising and do the same thing, until every behaviour on this list is part of your life!

- [ ] I maintain a positive, optimistic attitude about my ability to control my weight.
- [ ] I set small, bite-sized goals on the way to my weight target.
- [ ] I keep a food and activity record, so I always know how well I'm doing and why my weight is fluctuating the way it is.
- [ ] I recognize and reward my successes.
- [ ] I monitor my weight by how my clothes fit, not only by what the scale reads.
- [ ] I make healthy eating choices that are consistent with my lifestyle needs.
- [ ] I select low-fat meat and milk products.
- [ ] I eat breakfast every day.
- [ ] I go no longer than five hours at a time without eating.
- [ ] I spend at least 20 minutes eating each meal.
- [ ] I stop eating when I feel satisfied, not when I feel stuffed.
- [ ] I stay aware of the portion sizes I am eating.
- [ ] I enjoy eating meals with family and friends.
- [ ] I recognize when I eat for reasons other than hunger.
- [ ] I reserve high-fat or sweet treats for special occasions, rather than vowing never to eat them again.
- [ ] I include a variety of physical activities in my life.

Vitamins and minerals

MULTIVITAMIN AND MINERAL SUPPLEMENTS

Should you take a "multi" if you're on a lower-calorie diet? Yes! If you are following a low-calorie diet (less than 1500 calories daily), you are very likely experiencing a shortfall of vitamins and minerals. Even when you aren't cutting back on calories, it is a challenge to meet your requirements for certain nutrients important for long-term health. For instance, each day, women need 400 micrograms of folate (folic acid), a B vitamin that plays a role in protecting us from heart disease and cancer. To get the minimum

400 micrograms, you'd have to make sure you eat plenty of whole grains, and a serving of spinach, lentils, or orange juice on a daily basis. A low-calorie diet also presents a challenge meeting your iron requirements. And if you're over 50, you need to get vitamin B12 from a supplement or from fortified foods. That's because as we get older, our stomachs produce less hydrochloric acid, making it more difficult to absorb B12 from our foods.

So you can see that a multivitamin and mineral supplement offers you a little extra nutritional insurance. A good one will provide you with the recommended daily amounts of all the key vitamins and minerals, except for your daily requirements of calcium, magnesium, vitamin E, and possibly iron. Here's what you should look for when choosing a product:

- Premenopausal women should buy a supplement containing at least 10 milligrams of iron, but preferably 15 to 18 milligrams. Postmenopausal women have lower iron requirements and can choose a multi containing 8 milligrams or less.

- Look for a supplement that offers from 0.4 to 1.0 milligrams of folic acid.

- A multivitamin and mineral supplement should contain beta carotene, vitamin A (see page 162 for more on this), and vitamins D, B1, B2, B6, B12, and folic acid. Biotin and pantothenic acid aren't important since they're easily supplied by food.

- In terms of minerals, a supplement should contain iron, copper, zinc, magnesium, iodine, selenium, and chromium. Don't worry if you don't see phosphorus or potassium since these minerals are widely available in food.

- Take your supplement with food to allow for better breakdown and absorption of the pill. Plan to take your supplement at the meal you are most likely to remember it. For me, that's breakfast, the meal I am always at home for unless I'm travelling. Once a week, I put my supplements—a multivitamin, vitamin C, vitamin E, and calcium—in a pill container I bought at the drugstore. It has a compartment for each day of the week. This saves me the hassle of opening up a number of bottles every morning. And if I do travel, the pill container helps keeps me on track.

- Don't pay a lot of attention to terms such as "natural" or "slow release." (You should, however, seek out "natural source" vitamin E.) Don't be impressed by the addition of amino acids, ginseng, or other herbs. Some multivitamins contain small amounts of protein, other nutrients, or herbs. The tiny dosage of these that you'll receive from a multivitamin supplement won't give you any benefit, however. The main purpose of such additions is to add market appeal to the product.

IRON

You've already heard me say that if you're following a low-calorie diet, chances are you're not getting enough iron. If you are still getting a period, you need 18 milligrams of iron each day; if you've hit menopause, 8 milligrams daily is sufficient. A daily multivitamin and mineral pill will help you meet your needs. But also make an effort to boost the iron content of your diet. See page 71 for a list of foods rich in iron.

Only iron found in animal foods (heme iron) is well absorbed by your body. That's why red meat is such a good source. Not only does it pack a fair amount of the mineral, but what it contains is also well absorbed. Ironically, the iron-rich foods we eat the most of—whole grains, beans, dried fruit, and vegetables—offer nonheme iron, a less available form of iron. If this is the first chapter of this book you've read, I'll bet you didn't know that if you have a source of vitamin C with plant foods rich in iron, your body will absorb up to four times more of the iron! Here are a few iron-boosting combinations:

- Whole-grain cereal with strawberries
- Stone-ground toast with orange juice
- Cream of Wheat cereal with dried cranberries
- Whole-wheat waffles topped with kiwi slices and blueberries
- Spinach salad with orange segments
- Broccoli and red pepper stir-fry with brown rice
- Whole-wheat spaghetti with rapini, chili flakes, and olive oil
- Brown beans in tomato sauce

Here are a few more tips to help you enhance your body's absorption of nonheme iron:

- Include a little animal protein with your meal. The presence of heme iron in a meal will enhance the absorption of the nonheme iron eaten at that same meal. It takes only a few ounces of meat, fish, or eggs to achieve this.
- Don't drink coffee or tea with meals rich in iron. The tannins in these beverages

interfere with iron absorption. Drink coffee or tea one hour before or one hour after a meal.

- Foods high in calcium and phosphorus (dairy products) can slightly inhibit iron absorption. Don't combine foods rich in iron with large quantities of milk or yogurt.

CALCIUM

This is another important mineral that's often missing in a diet designed for weight loss. The even sadder truth is that this bone-building mineral is often lacking in high-calorie diets too. You'll read all about calcium in Chapter 11, but I do want to make sure you know here how to make up for what you might be missing. To start, you need to know that most women require 1000 milligrams of calcium each day; if you're over 50, you should be aiming for 1500 milligrams. Here are a few of the top calcium sources in the average diet:

CALCIUM CONTENT OF COMMON FOODS (MILLIGRAMS)

Milk, 1 cup (250 ml)	300
Milk, calcium enriched, 1 cup (250 ml)	420
Yogurt, plain, 3/4 cup (175 ml)	300
Yogurt, fruit-flavoured, 3/4 cup (175 ml)	250
Cheese, hard, 1.5 ounces (45 g)	300
Calcium-fortified soy or rice beverage, 1 cup (250 ml)	300
Calcium-fortified orange juice, 1 cup (250 ml)	300
Tofu, raw, firm (with calcium sulphate), 4 oz. (120 g)	260
Blackstrap molasses, 2 tbsp. (25 ml)	288
Bok choy, cooked, 1 cup (250 ml)	158
Swiss chard, cooked, 1 cup (250 ml)	102
Broccoli, cooked, 1 cup (250 ml)	94

Source: *Nutrient Value of Some Common Foods.* Health Canada, 1999. Adapted and reproduced with the permission of the Minister of Public Works and Government Services Canada, 2003.

For every 300 milligrams of your daily calcium target missing from your diet, take a 300-milligram calcium citrate supplement with magnesium (2:1 ratio) and vitamin D added. Calcium citrate is much more easily absorbed than calcium carbonate.

Calcium carbonate requires a lot of stomach acid to be well absorbed. If you take acid-blocking medication for ulcers or heartburn, don't give the carbonate form a second thought. Calcium citrate is your best bet. If you need to take more than one calcium pill (most calcium citrate supplements don't have more than 350 milligrams of calcium per pill), split your dose over two or three meals. For those of you who don't like to swallow pills, chewable calcium citrate supplements are available.

CHROMIUM

You may have heard that this trace mineral helps burn fat and build muscle, certainly a winning combination if you're trying to lose weight. While a few studies have found that chromium supplements aided weight loss in people who exercise, most found chromium to have no effect.[7] But that doesn't mean you shouldn't worry about chromium. A few studies do point to chromium's ability to change body composition. One large study measured the effect of chromium supplementation (200 micrograms daily) in 123 obese men and women. Study participants were assigned to either a diet-exercise-supplement combination protocol or a diet-exercise-only protocol. All participants consumed 1500 calories a day and went for five brisk 45-minute walks each week. At the end of four weeks, while there was no difference in body weight between the two groups, there was a significant difference in body composition. Those people taking the supplement lost more body fat and gained more muscle mass.

Another study found that overweight women who exercised and took 400 micrograms of chromium daily lost significant weight and lowered the amount of insulin their body produced in response to a carbohydrate meal. Interestingly, nonexercising women who took the same amount of chromium showed significant weight *gain*. This study suggests that chromium supplementation may help improve body composition, increasing the ratio of muscle to fat, when combined with regular exercise.[8]

Chromium works hand in hand with insulin, the hormone that helps regulate your blood sugar level and your body's energy stores. With adequate amounts of chromium present, your body uses less insulin to do its job. A deficiency of chromium causes impaired blood sugar balance, increased levels of potentially harmful blood fats and cholesterol, and decreased levels of high-density lipoproteins (HDLs), the good form of cholesterol. And if you go to the gym a lot, you might want to know that heavy exercise causes chromium to be excreted from the body.

Healthy women need to consume 25 micrograms of chromium per day—a tiny amount. Good food sources include apples with the skin, green peas, chicken breast, refried beans, mushrooms, oysters, wheat germ, and brewer's yeast. Processed foods and refined starchy foods such as white bread, white rice, white pasta, sugar, and sweets all contain very little chromium. So if you're a runner who loads up on white bagels, regular pasta, and white rice, you're probably falling short of meeting your chromium needs. If you're concerned that you're not getting enough through food, check your multivitamin and mineral supplement to see how much it contains. If it's less than 25 micrograms, consider taking a separate 200-microgram supplement each day. Chromium supplements are extremely safe.

Herbal remedies and other weight-loss supplements

Herbal remedies advertised to promote weight loss are extremely popular items in supplements stores. These products are generally touted to boost metabolic rate, the speed at which calories are burned, and break down body fat. Most herbal weight-loss formulas contain a few herbs combined with other nutrients. Will these products help you permanently lose weight? This question remains to be answered. No clinical studies have evaluated their long-term success.

But some research does support the use of a few of the individual ingredients added to certain products. But before you run off to the health food store, keep supplementation in perspective. As you know, there are no quick fixes or magic bullets when it comes to weight loss. If you want to lose weight permanently, you must learn how to change your eating habits, and you need to exercise regularly. While the supplements listed below might *assist* your weight-loss effort, you still need to change your eating habits and get up off the couch. Think of these supplements as aids to weight loss, not a means to losing weight.

If you want to try a weight-loss supplement, you need to know what's safe and what's not. Here's a look at the more popular ingredients added to products.

SUPPLEMENTS THAT MIGHT BE HELPFUL

Citrus aurantium

Advantra Z is one of the latest "thermogenics" to hit the herbal supplement market. It is an extract made from the dried fruit of *Citrus aurantium*, also known as bitter orange (or Seville orange). It is touted to burn fat, enhance physical performance, and increase muscle, and apparently works as effectively as ephedra without any negative effects on the heart or nervous system. The herb stimulates the body's beta-3 receptors, which in turn elicit the breakdown of fat and catalyze an increase in the body's metabolic rate.

To explain in more detail, every cell in the body has receptor sites called alpha-1, alpha-2, beta-1, beta-2, and beta-3. The hormones we naturally produce to counter stress, adrenaline, and noradrenaline, interact with these receptors to elicit a response. When these hormones interact with beta-3 receptors, fat breakdown in the body is promoted and the resting metabolic rate is increased. (Ephedra has a wider range of action than Advantra Z because it affects both the alpha and beta receptors. It is its impact on the alpha receptors that can cause dangerous side effects.)

Sounds good so far, but does Advantra Z work? A 1999 study evaluated the combined effect of bitter orange, caffeine, and St. John's wort on weight loss in 20 overweight adults. All the participants exercised three times per week and ate an 1800-calorie diet. At the end of a six-week period, the group receiving the herbal supplement had lost significantly more weight and body fat than the group on a placebo. The combination of substances given in the study did not affect heart rate or blood pressure.[9] So it appears that bitter orange just might speed up weight loss when used in conjunction with diet and exercise. You'll find the standardized extract of *Citrus aurantium* (Advantra Z) in a few products, including Quest Vitamin's TrimFit, Twinlab's Diet Fuel, and Interactive Nutrition's Metabolean (all three products contain a little caffeine). TrimFit and Diet Fuel also contain St. John's wort. *Citrus aurantium* is also sold on its own.

Conjugated Linoleic Acid (CLA)

This is a naturally occurring fatty acid found in dairy products and meat. It's also found in pork and chicken, though in lesser amounts. It's estimated that nonvegetarians consume about one gram each day through their diet. The body does not manufacture CLA, so the only way to get it is through foods or supplements. In supplemental doses, CLA is thought to promote weight loss by inhibiting the action of lipoprotein lipase, an enzyme that breaks down dietary fat so it can be absorbed by the body. It's also thought that CLA increases the activity of the enzyme responsible for breaking down body fat stores.

A handful of studies suggests CLA helps people lose body fat. Two studies presented at the Research Conference of the American Chemical Society (August 2000) found that CLA supplements helped people lose weight and keep the extra pounds off. In one, Norwegian researchers studied 60 overweight individuals. Half were given CLA, the others took a placebo. After three months, the CLA users lost more weight than those in the placebo group. Another study from the University of Wisconsin followed 80 overweight people for six months. Subjects received either daily CLA supplements or a placebo. All dieted and exercised, and most lost weight. Once the study was completed, the people who were not taking CLA regained weight in the typical pattern: 75 percent of their weight gain was as fat. But the people who were taking CLA put weight back on very differently—only half as fat, the other half as muscle.[10]

Based on the studies done so far, the recommended dose is 1000 milligrams of CLA taken three times per day with meals (3 grams per day). Look for supplements that contain Tonalin CLA, a branded CLA that has been used in the research and manufactured under high-quality standards. Keep in mind that no long-term safety studies have yet been done: CLA has been used in studies only for up to six months. CLA may cause mild stomach upset.

SUPPLEMENTS THAT AREN'T HELPFUL

Hydroxycitric Acid (HCA)

Here's yet another ingredient you'll find in certain weight-loss formulas. It is also sold on its own. Hydroxycitric acid (HCA) is an active compound found in the herb *Garcinia cambogia*. You'll find HCA sold as "Citrimax" in weight-loss products. In the lab, HCA acts by inhibiting the action of a cellular enzyme and thereby increasing the breakdown of fat. But just because HCA does this in a test tube doesn't mean it works the same way in the body.

I can find only two published studies that evaluated the effectiveness of this herb in humans. Both were well controlled and found that people who took HCA burned body fat no differently from those taking the placebo. The larger of the two studies measured weight and fat loss in 135 overweight men and women who took either 1500 milligrams of HCA or a placebo. Both groups exercised and followed a high-fibre, low-calorie diet. After 12 weeks there was no significant difference between the two groups. HCA or not, both lost a significant amount of weight.[11] From what I've seen to date, there's no good evidence that HCA assists weight loss—another reason to stick to your diet and exercise routine!

Apple cider vinegar

This product is used for everything from weight loss to leg cramps. Cider vinegar is fermented juice from crushed apples. Like apples, it contains some pectin (a fibre), B vitamins, vitamin C, and certain minerals. Does it work? We don't know; no studies have been published. But it is not harmful in small amounts. It may be unsafe, however, when taken in amounts greater than one cup (250 ml) per day. One case reports someone's developing low potassium blood levels and osteoporosis by taking one cup (250 ml) per day for six years. A typical dose for weight loss is one ounce of apple cider vinegar plus one teaspoon (5 ml) honey in 1/4 cup (50 ml) of water, taken before each meal.

SUPPLEMENTS TO AVOID

Ephedra, or Ma Huang

Over the past few years, ephedra, also known as Ma huang, has received a lot of bad press. After issuing a public warning in 2001, Health Canada finally recalled all weight-loss products containing ephedra in January 2002. So far in Canada there have been at least 60 reported adverse reactions and one death due to ephedra abuse.

The plant contains an active ingredient called ephedrine, which stimulates the central nervous system, speeds the heart rate, and increases blood pressure. When combined with other stimulant ingredients such as caffeine, it increases the metabolic rate. However, taking ephedra in high doses with other stimulants can cause serious side effects, including stroke, heart attacks, heart rate irregularities, and seizures. People who suffer from heart conditions, high blood pressure, and diabetes are among those particularly at risk. Because of its negative side effects, some companies were one step ahead of the government. They had reformulated their weight-loss products and removed ephedra before the stop-sale was ordered. Many manufactures replaced ephedra with *Citrus aurantium* (Avantra Z).

THE bottom LINE...

Leslie's recommendations for managing your weight

1   Stay away from fad diets. Any diet that excludes one or more food groups or relies on specially purchased foods or supplements is not healthy. Nor will it teach you how to implement the long-term behavioural changes needed for ongoing weight control.

2   Consult a registered dietitian for advice. Visit www.dietitians.ca.

3   Follow my meal plan for weight loss, outlined in Appendix 1.

4   Take a multivitamin and mineral supplement every day. Low-calorie diets often don't provide enough iron, calcium, or B vitamins.

5   To help you meet your iron requirements, add two iron-rich foods to your diet each day.

6   Depending on your age, you need 1000 or 1500 milligrams of elemental calcium each day. For every 300 milligrams missing from your diet, take 300 milligrams of elemental calcium in citrate form with vitamin D added.

7   If you have problems keeping your blood sugar levels stable and your diet lacks the mineral chromium, you might consider taking a 200-microgram chromium supplement. But first check how much chromium is in your multivitamin and mineral supplement. That amount, combined with what's available in your diet, might be all you need.

8   If you've decided to take an herbal supplement to help you lose weight, choose an ephedra-free product that contains Avantra Z. Avantra Z is a standardized extract of *Citrus aurantium* (bitter orange) and has been shown to increase the metabolic rate, without the side effects of ephedra. *Avoid* products that contain ephedra (Ma huang). And remember that supplements are not a magic bullet.

9   Be sure to exercise. Gradually build up to four cardiovascular workouts weekly, each 30 to 60 minutes in duration. Consider adding a weight-training component two or three times a week. To get started, consult a certified personal trainer. Consult your doctor if you are starting an exercise program for the first time.

Reducing your risk of osteoporosis

"All my life I have never had a problem drinking plenty of milk. That's why I was shocked when my first bone density test showed bone loss. I've always been told that when it comes to preventing osteoporosis, calcium is what matters. I guess there's more to it than that."

11

It's not uncommon to think that fragile, brittle bones are an inevitable part of the midlife change. In fact, osteoporosis is often viewed as a natural result of menopause. But the truth is that only 25 percent of postmenopausal women get osteoporosis. As you'll come to understand as you read this chapter, just because your bone density test score is low doesn't mean you'll end up with fractured bones or a hunched posture. Now don't get me wrong. I certainly don't mean to trivialize this debilitating condition. It is true that 1.4 million Canadians have osteoporosis and that the rate at which bone fractures occurs among Canadians is increasing faster than ever. What's more, the fact that we're an aging population doesn't account for our higher rate of fractured bones. It seems there's something else at play here. What I want to emphasize is that while menopause is a natural part of aging, osteoporosis is not. And if you begin taking preventive measures right now, you can lower your odds of getting this painful bone disease.

Osteoporosis defined

Osteoporosis is usually a silent disease, until a fracture occurs. It's characterized by low bone mass and deterioration of existing bone tissue. The thinning and deterioration of bones that occurs in osteoporosis means that they become more fragile and the risk of fracture increases. In other words, if your bones are weaker, they're more likely to break.

Studies do tell us that the lower the bone mass a woman (or man) has, the higher the risk of fracture. You've probably noticed that this definition of osteoporosis emphasizes *fracture risk*, not only low bone density. By the age of 50, the average Caucasian woman has a 40 percent chance of suffering at least one fracture caused by brittle bones.

While many bone fractures are not life-threatening, consider this: The risk of getting a fracture is at least five times the risk of developing breast cancer. The impact that fractures have on health is often not fully appreciated. Did you know that having a hip fracture increases the risk of dying by 16 percent? Or that close to half of elderly women who fracture their hips lose their ability to live independently? I told you earlier that not every woman ends up with osteoporosis. Nor does every woman with low bone density end up with bone fractures. To help you better understand the factors that shape your risk of osteoporosis and subsequent bone fracture, we need to take a look at bones themselves.

PEAK BONE MASS

Your bones grow in length and density until you finish your growth spurt in your teens (sometime between the ages of 11 and 14 years for girls). After the growth spurt, your bones continue to increase in density but at a slower rate. Most bone density is achieved between the ages of 8 and 16 years. Then, sometime in your 20s, your bones achieve what's called their *peak mass*. Once this occurs, they stop increasing in density. This happens any time between the ages of 20 and 30. Some experts say that our bones may even continue to build density up until the age of 35. In any case, when you reach your peak bone mass, you have the densest bone you're ever going to have. Think of peak bone mass as the maximum bone density that you are physically able to develop. An individual's peak mass is pretty much determined by genetics, but nutrition and other lifestyle factors (such as type and frequency of exercise) determine whether or not you ever achieve your body's genetically programmed peak bone mass.

After you achieve your peak bone mass, natural bone loss begins. Before menopause, women lose bone at a rate of 1 percent per year, the same rate at which men lose bone. Within the first five years after menopause, women lose bone two to six times faster than do premenopausal women. By about 10 years after menopause, the rate of bone loss returns to 1 percent per year. During the 10-year period of rapid bone loss following menopause, some women have the potential to lose bone very quickly. Others are slow bone losers and won't lose as much bone mass.

BONE BUILDING

Despite its "dead" appearance, bone is very active tissue. Two important types of cells keep it that way. *Osteoclasts* break down bone. They go to work, for example, when your diet lacks calcium. Calcium is vital to all cells, not just bone cells. When there's not enough calcium available to maintain important body functions, the osteoclasts break down bone cells to release calcium into the blood. *Osteoblasts*, on the other hand, are responsible for building bone. These cells secrete a collagen protein compound that provides the support matrix for the bones. The collagen matrix is then filled in with bone mineral also secreted by the osteoblasts. When this bone mineral matures, this cement-like substance that gives the bones their hardness and strength is known as hydroxyapatite. Calcium is the chief ingredient of hydroxyapatite.

The osteoclasts and osteoblasts constantly remodel your bones, breaking them down cell by cell, and then rebuilding them. This is how bone density is increased in response to weight-bearing exercise, like brisk walking. The physical pounding of bones stimulates osteoblasts to rebuild bone in a particular area. But before new bone can be built, some old bone must be broken down by the osteoclasts. During childhood and adolescence, osteoblast (building) activity exceeds osteoclast (breakdown) activity. In young adults, up to 30 percent of the skeleton is rebuilt every year. More bone is added to areas put under stress. For example, a right-handed golfer or tennis player will have greater bone mass in his or her right arm than in the left. After you've achieved your peak bone mass in your 20s or 30s, osteoclast (breakdown) activity wins out.

HORMONES AND BONE HEALTH

Many different hormones influence whether bones are being broken down or rebuilt at any given time. The three main players in calcium and bone metabolism are parathyroid hormone, vitamin D, and calcitonin. It's important that you know how these hormones affect your bones because, as you'll see later, your diet can affect their actions.

Parathyroid hormone (PTH)

Parathyroid hormone (PTH) is secreted by your parathyroid gland. Its job is to keep your blood calcium levels stable. Because calcium is critical for blood clotting, muscle contraction, and the transmission of nerve impulses, a constant amount of the mineral must be circulated throughout your body at all times. When blood calcium falls too low (because you're not consuming enough in your diet), PTH tells your kidneys to stop excreting calcium. PTH also activates vitamin D in your body, and vitamin D in turn causes your intestines to absorb more dietary calcium. Finally, PTH instructs your osteoclasts (the cells that break down bone) to release calcium from your bones into your bloodstream. The net result? Your blood calcium rises to normal at the expense of bone loss. Now you can see why getting plenty of calcium and vitamin D in your diet is so important for strong bones. (More on that subject later.)

Calcitonin

Your thyroid gland secretes calcitonin in response to a high calcium level in the bloodstream. This hormone lowers calcium to a normal level by inhibiting the action of the osteoclasts and stimulating the osteoblasts to build new bone. However, calcitonin levels decline with age and at menopause.

A number of other hormones and drugs with hormonal effects also influence the bones:

Thyroid hormone

Too much thyroid hormone from an overactive thyroid gland (hyperthyroidism) causes a higher rate of bone breakdown. I have many clients with an underactive thyroid (hypothyroidism) who take thyroid medication. If you take levothyroxin (Synthroid), it is important to have your doctor check your thyroid hormone levels regularly. If they are too high, you'll need to adjust your medication. Keeping your thyroid hormone dose in check is an important way to prevent accelerated bone loss.

Steroid drugs

Doctors use steroid drugs such as glucocorticoids (for example, prednisone) to treat inflammatory conditions such as rheumatoid arthritis, lupus, and colitis. These drugs unfortunately increase the rate of bone loss because one of their side effects is their ability to enhance the action of PTH. If you think back to how PTH works, you'll realize that this means your bones will mobilize more calcium into your bloodstream. Anyone who takes this type of medication must be sure they're getting plenty of calcium and vitamin D.

Estrogen

Estrogen acts to protect bones. This hormone seems to be able to prevent osteoclasts from releasing calcium from the bone into the bloodstream. Estrogen also causes calcitonin and vitamin D to be released, stimulating new bone growth to occur. In other words, your premenopausal estrogen level helps vitamin D efficiently perform its jobs of increasing calcium absorption in your intestine and preventing excess calcium loss through your kidneys.

Risk factors for osteoporosis

You may already have some idea of what can increase your risk of osteoporosis. Simply put, the strength of your bones is determined by their density, their rate of healing, and the integrity of their support structures (collagen proteins). Any factor that jeopardizes your bones' density, integrity, or ability to heal themselves can increase the odds of getting osteoporosis.

Here's a list of known factors that put your bones at risk:
- older age
- low bone density
- being female
- slender or petite body structure (slender people have less bone to start with than do heavier-set people)
- deficiency of estrogen (early menopause further increases the risk)
- low calcium and vitamin D intake
- cigarette smoking
- excessive alcohol intake
- excessive caffeine intake
- sedentary lifestyle
- use of certain medications (see the discussion about bone density testing on pages 134–138)
- prolonged immobilization (bones need to work against the pull of gravity to maintain their density)
- family history of maternal hip fracture
- previous bone fracture of any type after the age of 40
- certain health conditions (kidney failure, hyperthyroidism, poor digestion or absorption)

I want to draw special attention to one of the risk factors mentioned above—cigarette smoking. Studies have shown that cigarette smoking reduces bone density and increases the risk of fracture. The U.S. Nurses' Health Study revealed that women who smoked 25 or more cigarettes a day had a 60 percent higher risk of hip fracture than women who never smoked. Two other American studies reported cigarette smoking to significantly decrease bone density in the hip and lower spine of older women (and men).[1] Smoking affects bone health by causing increased production of inactive estrogens, leading to estrogen deficiency. Studies find that women who smoke have early natural menopause and an increased risk of bone fractures. If you currently smoke and would like to quit, look for a smoking-cessation program in your community. A good program will offer group support, stress-management techniques, and strategies to help prevent relapse.

Measuring bone density

Your overall risk of osteoporosis depends on how much bone you currently have, how strong that bone is, and how fast you're losing it. The only way doctors can get a sense of what's happening in your skeleton is by taking repeated measures of your bone density. Today, the best tool available to determine your bone density is dual-energy X-ray absorptiometry (DEXA). The machine that creates DEXA readings uses an X-ray tube attached to a computer to measure bone density in the lower spine and the hip, two places where fractures are likely to occur. DEXA is very accurate. The test can detect a change in bone density of as little as 1 percent. What this test can't do, however, is detect bone fractures. And it doesn't measure bone density in the upper spine, where a series of small fractures can result in shrinking and "dowager's hump," the characteristic hunching of the spine seen in osteoporosis. Doctors use X-rays to detect these types of fractures in your upper spine.

The DEXA test is simple, fast, and painless. A complete scan can take as little as 10 minutes. You don't even have to undress. To have your lower spine or hip scanned, you'll lie comfortably on your back on a flat padded table. You don't have to worry about fasting before your test; since food doesn't interfere with the test results, you can eat right before you go, if you like. However, don't take a calcium supplement right before the test. An undigested pill might be measured as part of your bone density because, when you're lying on your back, your intestines lie on top of your spine. So skip your calcium pill on the day you're having a bone density test.

INTERPRETING TEST RESULTS

To help you understand your test results, you'll see below the results of a DEXA bone density scan done on Nancy, a 58-year-old woman. The test begins by creating a computer-generated image of four vertebrae in Nancy's lumbar, or lower, spine (L1, L2, L3, and L4). The computer then calculates how much bone mineral is present in each vertebra and calculates an average bone mineral density (BMD) for three vertebrae. The more densely packed the bone mineral crystals are, the stronger the bone. In Nancy's report, you can see that the average density is calculated from the bone densities of L2, L3, and L4. The average density is represented in the last row of the chart and visually in the graph; in both places these three vertebrae are called L2–L4. Nancy's BMD for L2–L4 is 0.944 grams per square centimetre (g/cm^2). You're probably wondering what this number means: Is it good or bad?

Luckily, you don't have to depend on this number alone to understand your test results. On the DEXA report, your bone density is compared with the bone density of a healthy 30-year-old woman. You can see these results under the "Young-adult" column in the chart. In Nancy's case, the young-adult comparison for her lower spine (L2–L4) is 79 percent. That means Nancy's bone density is 79 percent of the average 30-year-old woman's density. In other words, she has lost 21 percent of her bone density. Every 10 percent loss of bone density, as measured against the benchmark set by a 30-year-old woman, doubles the risk of bone fracture.

AP SPINE BONE DENSITY RESULTS

Region	BMD (g/cm^2)	Young-adult (%)	(T)	Age-matched (%)	(Z)
L1	0.868	77	-2.2	86	-1.2
L2	0.969	81	-1.9	90	-0.9
L3	1.039	87	-1.3	96	-0.3
L4	0.840	70	-3.0	78	-2.0
L2–L4	0.944	79	-2.1	88	-1.1

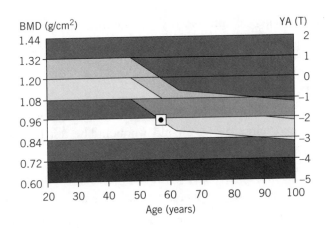

Bone density results are also presented in the form of T scores. The T score shows the number of levels (standard deviations) between your bone density and that of a healthy 30-year-old woman. In other words, your T score represents how far you deviate from what is considered normal. If you score one level away (-1 standard deviation), you are considered to have *osteopenia,* or decreased bone mass. If your test shows that your bone density is more than 2.5 levels away (-2.5 standard deviations) from the healthy standard, you have *osteoporosis.* If your score is higher still and you have one or more tiny fractures, you are considered to have *severe osteoporosis.* In Nancy's case, her T score is 2.1, which would classify her as osteopenic. How do these results influence the risk of bone fracture? Well, if you're over 65 years old, osteopenia doubles the risk of fracture, osteoporosis quadruples it, and severe osteoporosis increases the risk of bone fracture 20-fold.

You'll also notice that Nancy's DEXA results include something called an "age-matched" comparison. This means that Nancy's results have been compared with what is expected for women of her age. Nancy's age-matched comparison is 88 percent. This means her bone density is 88 percent of what is expected for a woman her age. If your age-matched comparison is unusually low, your doctor endeavours to determine what is causing such severe bone loss.

SHOULD YOU HAVE A BONE DENSITY TEST?

In November 2002, the Scientific Advisory Council of the Osteoporosis Society of Canada issued new recommendations for bone density testing.[2] All adults 65 years of age or older and younger people with certain risk factors should be screened for osteoporosis. You should get tested if you have *one* of the following major risk factors:

- You're 65 years or older.
- You have a family history of osteoporosis or multiple bone fractures.
- You have premature menopause (younger than 45).
- You have had a bone fracture after the age of 40.
- You've been on corticosteroid drugs (for example, prednisone) for a medical condition for three months or longer.
- You've experienced one or more episodes of long-standing malnutrition or malabsorption (for example, you have a history of anorexia nervosa, celiac disease, or Crohn's disease).
- You have hyperparathyroidism.
- You have a propensity to fall.
- You have had an X-ray that shows bone loss.
- You have hypogonadism.

You should get a DEXA bone density test if you have *two* of the following minor risk factors:

- You have rheumatoid arthritis.
- You have a history of hyperthyroidism.
- You are on long-term anticonvulsant therapy.
- You are on long-term heparin therapy.
- You lost more than 10 percent of your body weight when under the age of 25.
- You currently weigh less than 125 pounds (57 kg).
- You are a smoker.
- You are a heavy alcohol drinker.
- You consume excessive amounts of caffeine (more than 450 milligrams per day).
- You don't consume enough calcium.

Your first bone density test serves as the baseline to which future test results will be compared. If at the age of 50 your first bone density test comes back low (osteopenia), you're not necessarily heading for osteoporosis. It may be that you're a "slow loser" and later tests will find that your bone mineral content hasn't changed much. The rate of bone loss is greater in early postmenopause than in older women. This brings up an important point: To establish your actual bone loss trends, bone density tests must be repeated every two years. If there is concern about rapid bone loss, your doctor may recommend an annual bone mineral test. If future tests show that your bone density has declined rapidly between tests, your doctor will likely recommend drug treatment to slow the rate of bone loss. Here's a brief look at your options.

Drug-based osteoporosis treatments

ESTROGEN THERAPY

There is no doubt in the medical and scientific community that estrogen replacement therapy reduces postmenopausal bone loss and reduces the risk of fractures. Many studies have shown that hormone replacement therapy (HRT) protects the bones. Back in the 1980s, the famous Framingham Heart Study reported that among 3000 Boston women, those who took estrogen when postmenopausal had a 35 percent lower risk of hip fracture as compared with those who never took hormones.[3]

More recently, the Women's Health Initiative (WHI) Hormone Study also reported that combined HRT (estrogen plus progestin) lowered the risk of osteoporotic bone fractures. Sponsored by the National Institutes of Health, WHI followed more than 27,000 healthy women, aged 50 to 79, taking either combined HRT or estrogen only. The goal was to determine whether HRT protected from heart disease and osteoporosis, as well as increased the risk of cancer and blood clots. While there was good news, there was also bad news. Despite the benefits to bone health, combined HRT increased the risk of heart disease, blood clots, stroke, and breast cancer.[4]

The study arm investigating combined HRT was halted in July 2002. While the increased health risks were small, the concern was that a drug taken by millions of women over many years could result in a large number of women developing breast cancer or heart disease. The bottom line: The risks of this hormone regime outweighed the benefits, and HRT is no longer considered the gold standard to prevent osteoporosis and bone fractures.

If you are taking combined HRT solely to prevent osteoporosis, consider stopping. As you will read below, many other medications can help lower the odds of osteoporosis and bone fracture, with fewer risks to your health. However, combined HRT may be appropriate if you are also taking it for the short-term relief of hot flashes and other menopausal symptoms. To decide if HRT is right for you, you must consult with your doctor. If you and your doctor decide there are good reasons for you to stay on HRT, you should know that a lower dose of estrogen, in combination with calcium and vitamin D supplementation, has bone-preserving effects. The following study supports this point.

Researchers at the Osteoporosis Research Center at Creighton University in Omaha, Nebraska, studied 128 women over 65 years old with low bone density. The women were given either low-dose estrogen (0.3 milligrams/day) along with progesterone or a placebo pill (no hormones were given to the placebo group). Both groups were given supplemental vitamin D and enough supplemental calcium to bring their calcium intake to over 1000 milligrams daily. After three and a half years, bone density in the spine increased by 5.2 percent in women who adhered to the combined hormone and nutrient-supplementation treatment. This increase was roughly equivalent to that seen in women on higher dose HRT. (Women in the placebo group maintained their bone density, but it did not increase.) Symptoms related to low-dose HRT were mild and short-lived. Based on their results, the researchers concluded that low-dose HRT with estrogen and progesterone, combined with adequate calcium and vitamin D, offers bone-sparing effects similar or superior to that provided by higher dose HRT regimes.[5]

BIPHOSPHONATES

This class of nonhormonal drugs offers postmenopausal women with low bone density or osteoporosis a useful alternative to HRT. Biphosphonate drugs prevent bone loss by binding to the bone surface and inhibiting the activity of the osteoclasts, the cells that strip down old bone. In a nutshell, these drugs work by preventing bone breakdown. It seems that biphosphonates can actually decrease the number and lifespan of osteoclasts. The result is that the balance between bone breakdown and formation tips in favour of bone formation.

Didrocal (Etidronate and calcium carbonate)

This bisphosphonate-calcium combination treatment is taken in three-month cycles. For the first two weeks, a 400-milligram tablet of etidronate (the biphosphonate drug) is taken. A 500-milligram calcium carbonate pill is then taken for the remainder of the three-month period (76 days). Etidronate interferes with the osteoclast cells to reduce bone breakdown, and the calcium provides the raw material the body uses to form bone. Studies have shown that cyclic treatment with etidronate and calcium increases spinal bone density and decreases the risk of spine fractures.[6] However, there is no evidence that the drug prevents hip fractures. Etidronate is given in an on-off cycle because it is known that daily, long-term use can cause structural abnormalities in bone.

Common side effects associated with this drug regime include nausea and diarrhea. Postmenopausal women who are taking Didrocal must make sure they get at least 1500 milligrams of calcium daily from their diet and supplements (including the calcium supplied by the Didrocal regime), as well as 800 international units (IU) of vitamin D.

Fosamax (Aldendronate)

Chances are you've heard about this biphosphonate drug, or perhaps you're already taking it. Studies of women who are within five years of menopause show that 5 milligrams of Fosamax each day can maintain bone density in 85 percent of treated women. Fosamax and estrogen appear equivalent in their ability to preserve bone in the hip, spine, and throughout the body after two years of treatment.[7] In Canada, a daily Fosamax dose of 5 milligrams is given to prevent osteoporosis, and 10 milligrams is used to treat the disease.

This biphosphonate drug has been studied extensively for the treatment of osteoporosis. In one large study of postmenopausal women with existing spinal fractures, treatment with Fosamax reduced the incidence of spine, hip, and wrist fractures by 50 percent over three years.[8] The drug has also been shown to increase bone density and prevent fractures in postmenopausal women with no prior bone fractures but low bone density scores. While Fosamax does prevent bone loss in healthy postmenopausal women, whether it reduces fracture risk remains to be seen.

Many of my clients who take Fosamax are pleased with their bone density results. There are, however, a couple of disadvantages to taking Fosamax. First, you must take the drug on an empty stomach, with a glass of water—so you generally must take it first thing in the morning and then wait at least 30 minutes before eating breakfast. If you take Fosamax with food, coffee, or juice, you won't absorb any of the medication. The second drawback is that you have to stay upright after taking the pill (you can't go back to bed!). Staying upright prevents the pill from coming back from your stomach into your esophagus, where it can cause severe irritation and possibly ulcers. However, in view of the positive benefits to bone health achieved with Fosamax, most women consider these small sacrifices.

SELECTIVE ESTROGEN RECEPTOR MODULATORS (SERMS)

Considerable effort has been applied to the development of what might be called designer estrogens. These drugs offer all the beneficial effects of estrogen (bone protection, cholesterol lowering, hot flash reduction), without causing any of its negative effects (increased breast cancer risk, endometrial bleeding). In other words, they act like estrogen in certain parts of the body, such as the bones, while leaving other parts of the body unaffected. The first of these drugs to be developed was tamoxifen, which has been used for many years to help prevent the recurrence of breast cancer in women. While tamoxifen acts as an anti-estrogen in the breast, it acts like an estrogen in bone and does increase bone density in postmenopausal women, though to a lesser extent than do estrogen and Fosamax. However, it also acts like an estrogen in the uterus and stimulates the growth of endometrial tissue, which may increase the risk of endometrial cancer. For this reason, tamoxifen is not used to prevent osteoporosis. It may, however, offer women with breast cancer some bone protection.

Newer SERMs such as raloxifene act as anti-estrogens in the breast and uterus. That means they don't stimulate the growth of breast or uterine cells. And they do appear to offer some of the favourable effects of estrogen on bone and blood cholesterol levels. Unlike estrogen, however, SERMs don't relieve hot flashes or vaginal dryness. Clinical studies in postmenopausal women indicate that a daily raloxifene dose of 60 milligrams prevents bone loss without stimulating endometrial tissue.[9] The Multiple Outcomes of Raloxifene Evaluation (MORE) has determined that the drug, when taken by postmenopausal women with osteoporosis, increases bone density in the lumbar spine and neck and prevents fractures.[10] It has not yet been shown to reduce the risk of hip fractures. Raloxifene is available as Evista in Canada. Possible side effects include an increase in hot flashes and leg cramps.

Ideally, every woman's goal should be to slow down, as much as possible, age-related bone loss during her 30s, 40s, and 50s so that bone-sparing medication is not necessary after menopause. Unfortunately, some women, because of medical problems, lack of knowledge, or difficult life circumstances, are not able to take effective action during the premenopausal years and so develop low bone density. These women require drugs to halt bone loss and reduce the risk of bone fracture. Yet, even if you are taking medication now, diet and nutritional supplements can still influence your bone density. Indeed, calcium and vitamin D are essential adjuncts of osteoporosis treatment. Earlier in this chapter you learned that adding calcium supplements to low-dose estrogen therapy is as effective at preserving bone as higher-dose hormone regimens are. Here's a look at the nutritional strategies that can help slow down bone loss before and after menopause. Remember, it's never too late!

Dietary approaches

SOY FOODS

Once again, the humble soybean makes an appearance. By now you might be wondering if there's anything that soybeans can't do. I must admit, I'm hard pressed to come up with an example (wait until you read about their cholesterol-lowering ability in Chapter 12!). If you've read Chapter 4, on hot flashes, you've already learned a lot about the medicinal properties of soy foods. Soybeans contain naturally occurring compounds called isoflavones, a type of plant estrogen. Genistein and daidzein are the most active isoflavones in soy and have been the focus of much research. Isoflavones have a chemical structure similar to that of estrogen and because of this they are able to bind to estrogen receptors in the body. In fact, genistein has a very strong affinity for certain estrogen receptors called beta-receptors. It is the action of isoflavones on estrogen receptors in the bone that scientists believe may be responsible for soy's potential bone-preserving effect. As well, soy isoflavones may reduce the activity of osteoclasts, the cells that break down bone.

The interest in soybeans and osteoporosis began when researchers observed that populations that consume soy foods on a regular basis report much lower rates of hip fracture. Since then, soy foods and their naturally occurring phytoestrogens have been the focus of many studies. While some studies find that soy consumption has no effect on bone loss, others show soy to have a significant bone-saving effect. Both soy protein and soy isoflavones have been found to preserve bone density in animal studies.

There is some evidence that soy protects a woman's bones too. One six-month trial conducted at Iowa State University investigated the effect of soy in 66 postmenopausal women aged 49 to 73. The researchers found that 40 grams of soy protein (90 mg of isoflavones) significantly increased bone density in the spine of the soy users. On the other hand, women in this study who were given whey protein powder (a protein made from milk) instead of the soy showed bone loss in the lower spine.

Another study from the Department of Obstetrics and Gynecology, Internal Medicine and Pediatrics at the University of Cincinnati's College of Medicine found that 60 to 70 milligrams of soy isoflavones consumed daily from a soy beverage and soy nuts significantly decreased bone turnover in postmenopausal women. The researchers found that in these women, osteoblast activity (bone building) increased by 10.2 percent and osteoclast activity (bone breakdown) activity decreased by 13.9 percent. Reduced bone loss was seen after only four weeks of eating soy foods.[11]

The studies that have found a bone-sparing effect are those that give participants enough soy foods to supply a minimum of 50 milligrams of isoflavones daily. It is also important to note that in these studies, isoflavones are usually consumed in two doses (twice daily). Depending on what kind of soy food you eat, your blood level of genistein will peak anywhere from four to eight hours later. If you want to keep your blood genistein levels high, it makes sense to eat soy foods in the morning and once again in the afternoon or evening. Soy foods vary with respect to the amount of isoflavones they contain. Even the same type of food made by different manufacturers can differ in isoflavone content. You'll find a general guide to soy foods and their isoflavone content on pages 29–32.

PROTEIN FOODS

Eating too much protein may be part of the reason North American women have high rates of osteoporosis, despite our moderate to high calcium intakes. Studies have shown that high levels of dietary protein cause calcium to be excreted by the kidneys. The effect of eating large quantities of protein is rapid, and it appears that the body doesn't correct for it by absorbing more calcium from food. People who consume very little calcium or who absorb very little calcium because of intestinal problems may find it especially important to take the protein effect into account.

It's estimated that the average North American overshoots the recommended daily intake for protein by more than 50 percent. That doesn't take into account all those people following faddish high-protein weight-loss diets! I hate to think how those diets impact on calcium loss and bone health. But while eating very large amounts of protein may not be good for your bones, eating too little isn't healthy either. Protein is an important structural component of bone, and studies have shown that eating too little might increase the risk of hip fracture. The Iowa Women's Health Study found that dietary protein protected postmenopausal women from hip fracture. And it appeared that animal protein, rather than vegetable protein, accounted for this protection. Women who ate the most protein, while staying within the recommended daily intake levels, had a 69 percent reduced risk of hip fracture compared with women who ate the least.

Extra protein may also help women who have hip fractures. A Swiss study of 82 patients with recent hip fractures showed that a 20-gram protein supplement taken daily reduced bone loss and shortened hospital stay. In addition, the study participants experienced lower complication and death rates immediately after surgery and for six months afterward. This effect is not seen in hip fracture patients who are not given extra protein.[12]

Although the protein issue is controversial, it does seem clear that it's important to be getting enough. Women at risk of protein deficiency include:

- Those who don't often eat meat, chicken, or fish.
- Those who frequently grab a quick meal—a bagel, pasta, a low-fat frozen dinner—during the day, as these meals lack protein.
- Vegetarians who do not regularly incorporate high-quality vegetable protein sources into their diet.
- Those who engage in heavy exercise and fall into any of the above categories.

So, how much protein *do* you need? Start by reading the table on the following page.

Then find out how much protein you need to eat each day, first calculate your daily protein needs by multiplying your weight by your recommended protein intake. For example:

- A 125-pound woman who does not exercise: $125 \times 0.36 = 45$ grams protein
- A 140-pound woman training for a marathon: $140 \times 0.6 = 84$ grams protein
- A 150-pound woman who takes aerobics classes: $150 \times 0.5 = 75$ grams protein

RECOMMENDED DAILY PROTEIN INTAKES FOR HEALTHY ADULTS[13]

Adult, sedentary (no regular exercise)	0.8 grams per kg body weight (0.36 grams per lb)
Adult, recreational exercise	1.1–1.5 grams per kg body weight (0.5–0.7 grams per lb)
Adult, endurance athlete	1.2–1.4 grams per kg body weight (0.5–0.6 grams per lb)
Adult, strength trainer	1.6–1.7 grams per kg body weight (0.7–0.8 grams per lb)
Elderly	0.8–1.0 grams per kg body weight (0.36–0.45 grams per lb)
Maximum for healthy adults	2.0 grams per kg body weight (0.9 grams per lb)

Here's a look at how much food you need to eat to get this much protein:

PROTEIN CONTENT OF FOODS (GRAMS)

Meat, 3 oz. (90 g)	21–25
Poultry, 3 oz. (90 g)	21
Salmon, 3 oz. (90 g)	25
Sole, 3 oz. (90 g)	17
Tuna, canned and drained, 1/2 cup (125 ml)	30
Cheese, cheddar, 1 oz. (30 g)	10
Egg, 1 whole	6
Milk, 1 cup (250 ml)	8
Yogurt, 3/4 cup (175 ml)	8
Legumes, 1/2 cup (125 ml)	8
Vegetables, 1/2 cup (125 ml)	2
Bread, 1 slice	2
Rice, pasta, cooked, 1/2 cup (125 ml)	2

Source: *Nutrient Value of Some Common Foods*. Health Canada, 1999. Adapted and reproduced with the permission of the Minister of Public Works and Government Services Canada, 2003.

ALCOHOL

Here's another dietary factor that can have both a positive and negative effect on bone health. Many studies have determined that chronic alcohol abuse causes low bone density. Alcohol acts directly on your bones and suppresses bone formation. Consuming alcohol also increases the risk of falls in postmenopausal women and is associated with an increased incidence of hip fractures.

However, evidence also suggests that moderate alcohol drinking (one or two drinks a day) may actually increase bone density. Many population studies have found that a moderate pattern of drinking is linked with higher bone densities. It does seem odd that alcohol might actually stimulate bone building. It turns out that alcohol increases estrogen levels in the blood, and estrogen, as you know, has a bone-sparing action. The Nurses' Health Study conducted by Harvard University researchers investigated alcohol use and bone health in 188 postmenopausal women. They found that women who consumed 75 grams of alcohol each week (about five drinks) had significantly higher bone density in the lower spine than did nondrinkers. The study showed that as alcohol intake rose from none to 75 grams, bone density increased in proportion. This suggests that women may benefit from taking less than 75 grams of alcohol per week.[14]

If you want to keep your weekly alcohol intake below 75 grams, it helps to know just how much of it is present in the popular beverages.

ALCOHOL CONTENT OF COMMON BEVERAGES (GRAMS)

Beer, regular, 12 oz (375 ml) bottle	14–16
Beer, light, 12 oz (375 ml) bottle	11
Wine, red or white, 6 oz (187 ml)	16
Liquor, 80 proof, 1.5 oz (45 ml)	14

Considering that a moderate intake of alcohol (one or two drinks daily) increases the risk of breast cancer (read Chapter 13 for more on this topic), I certainly don't recommend that nondrinkers start drinking. There are plenty of other bone-building factors you can incorporate into your life (calcium, vitamin D, and exercise, for starters). But if you do enjoy no more than a drink each day, you'll be pleased to know that it might help preserve your bone density.

CAFFEINE

Drinking coffee, tea, or cola increases the amount of calcium your kidneys excrete in the urine. Increased calcium excretion continues up to three hours after consuming caffeine. It's been estimated that every 6-ounce (175-ml) cup of coffee leaches 48 milligrams of calcium from your body.

One study found a significant relationship between increasing caffeine intakes and lower bone density in 980 postmenopausal women. The effects of caffeine are likely most detrimental for women who are not meeting their calcium requirements. A study from Tufts University in Boston found that women who consumed less than 800 milligrams of calcium *and* 450 milligrams of caffeine (about three small cups of coffee) daily had significantly lower bone densities than women who consumed the same amount of caffeine but more than 800 milligrams of calcium.[15] Coffee drinking has also been associated with a greater risk of hip fracture in older women.

The bottom line on caffeine is quite simple:

- If you drink coffee, make sure you're meeting your calcium requirement of 1000 or 1500 milligrams daily.
- Don't consume more than 450 milligrams of caffeine a day.
- Add 3 tablespoons (45 ml) of milk or calcium-fortified soy beverage to every cup of coffee you drink. This amount contains 58 milligrams of calcium.

Here are a few tips to help you decaffeinate your day:

- Eliminate caffeine-containing beverages after noon (this means you can still enjoy your morning wake-up cup). Instead, try water, herbal tea, vegetable juice, milk, or a glass of soy beverage.
- Replace coffee with tea, which has substantially less caffeine.
- Instead of plain coffee, try a calcium-rich latte made with milk or calcium-fortified soy beverage.

SODIUM

Like caffeine, sodium causes your kidneys to excrete calcium. For every 500-milligram increase in your sodium intake, you must eat an additional 40 milligrams of calcium to make up for the increased loss. A study of postmenopausal women determined that

ADDED SODIUM CONTENT OF COMMON COMMERCIAL FOODS (TEASPOONS)

SOUPS

Chicken noodle soup, 1 cup (250 ml)	1/2
Cup of Noodles	3/4
Low-sodium soups	1/20

CRACKERS

Soda crackers, 8	1/4

PROCESSED MEATS

Bologna, beef, 2 slices (46 g)	1/5
Ham, Black Forest, 3 oz. (90 g)	1/2
Smoked turkey, 3 oz. (90 g)	1/3
Wiener, 1	1/4

SNACK FOODS

Pretzels, 1 cup (250 ml)	1/3
Popcorn, salted, 3 cups (750 ml)	1/4
Potato chips, plain, 8 oz. bag (227 g)	1/2

CANNED FOODS

Peas, canned, 1/2 cup (125 ml)	1/8
Pasta sauce, 1/2 cup (125 ml)	1/2
Pork and beans, canned, 1 cup (250 ml)	1/2

PACKAGED FOODS

Peas, frozen in sauce, 1/2 cup (125 ml)	1/4
Rice & Sauce, 1 cup (250 ml)	1/2
Pasta & Sauce, 1 cup (250 ml)	1/2

FAST FOOD

Big Mac, McDonald's	1/2
Crispy Chicken Breast, KFC, 1	1/2
Spicy Chicken Burger, Wendy's	1/2
French fries, large order	1/4
Pizza, pepperoni, 2 medium slices	1/5

a maximum daily intake of 2000 milligrams of sodium and 1000 milligrams of calcium minimized bone loss.[16] (By the way, 2000 milligrams of sodium is the amount that's found in about 3/4 teaspoons [3 ml] of salt.)

Although we do need some salt every day, we require very little. Salt is made of sodium and chloride, both of which are needed to help maintain water balance in our body. We continually lose sodium through sweat and urine. The more active we are or the warmer the weather, the more sodium we must replace from the diet. But here's the kicker—it takes only about 500 milligrams (or 1/5 teaspoon) of sodium to meet the daily needs of sedentary people living in temperate climates. The average Canadian consumes about 1 3/4 teaspoons (4500 mg) of sodium each day, almost 10 times more than needed! (One teaspoon of salt provides 2400 milligrams of sodium.)

Experts recommend that we consume no more than 2400 milligrams of sodium per day. To cut back on sodium, avoid the salt shaker at the table, minimize the use of salt in cooking, and try to buy commercial food products that are low in added salt. Eating fewer processed foods is one of the best things you can do to cut back on sodium. That's because most of the salt we eat every day comes from processed and prepared foods. It might surprise you to learn that for most of us, only one-quarter of our daily sodium intake comes from the salt shaker.

The chart on page 148 shows how much salt is found in commercial foods (remember, you're aiming to consume less than 1 teaspoon [5 ml] daily).

Vitamins and minerals

CALCIUM

That calcium is the most abundant mineral in the body and that 99 percent of it is housed within the bones and teeth underlines the importance of dietary calcium to bone health. During the bone-building process, the osteoblast cells secrete bone mineral (consisting of calcium and phosphorus), which strengthens the bone. This mineral matures into hyroxyapatite, a compound responsible for the strength and rigidity of bones. By making it possible for the osteoblasts to provide structural integrity to bones, dietary calcium plays a critical role in preventing osteoporosis.

Think back to what happens to your bones if your diet is low in calcium. One percent of your body's calcium circulates in your bloodstream and is vital to your heart, nervous system, and muscles. Your body keeps this circulating pool of calcium at a constant level. If your diet is lacking calcium and your blood calcium level drops, your parathyroid gland releases parathyroid hormone (PTH). This hormone then goes to work to return calcium to your blood. It makes your kidneys stop excreting calcium, and it works with vitamin D to release calcium from your bones into your blood. So when you shortchange your diet, you shortchange your bones too.

How much calcium do you need?

Here's a look at how much calcium you and your family members need.

DAILY RECOMMENDED CALCIUM INTAKES (MILLIGRAMS)

Children, 1–3 years	500
Children, 4–8 years	800
Children, 9–2 years	1300
Teenagers, 13–18 years	1300
Adults, 19–50 years	1000
Adults, over 50 years	1500
Pregnant women	1000
Daily upper limit	*2500*

Source: *Nutrient Value of Some Common Foods.* Health Canada, 1999. Adapted and reproduced with the permission of the Minister of Public Works and Government Services Canada, 2003.

Getting more calcium into your diet

I encourage clients to get as much calcium as possible from food. Unlike calcium pills, many calcium-rich foods provide other important bone-building nutrients, such as vitamin D, magnesium, and potassium. One study found that spinal bone loss was significantly lower in premenopausal women who used milk products to raise their calcium intake from 900 milligrams to 1500 milligrams.[17] If you suspect you may not be getting as much calcium as you need, use the list of calcium-rich foods on the next three pages to help you boost your intake.

Here are more ways to boost your calcium intake:

- If you use dairy products, aim for three servings daily.
- Cook hot cereal, rice, and grains in low-fat milk or a calcium-fortified soy beverage.

- Add milk instead of water to condensed cream soups, puddings, and egg dishes.
- Add skim milk powder to casseroles, soups, shakes, meatloaf, French toast, muffin batters, breads, mashed potatoes, and dips—1/4 cup (50 ml) of skim milk powder packs 210 milligrams of calcium!
- Use evaporated 2 percent or evaporated skim milk instead of regular milk in pudding, cream soups, and cream sauces—1 cup (250 ml) of the evaporated milk contains 700 milligrams of calcium.
- Top a baked potato with 1/4 cup (50 ml) low-fat sour cream for an additional 70 milligrams of calcium.
- Try an instant breakfast drink made with 1 cup (250 ml) skim milk to gain 400 milligrams of calcium.
- Eat *at least* two servings of calcium-rich vegetables every day—one serving is 1/2 cup (125 ml) of cooked vegetables.

CALCIUM CONTENT OF CALCIUM-RICH FOODS (MILLIGRAMS)
DAIRY FOODS

Milk (Lactaid or plain milk), 1 cup (250 ml)	300
Milk (Neilson TruTaste), 1 cup (250 ml)	360
Milk (Neilson TruCalcium), 1 cup (250 ml)	420
Carnation Instant Breakfast, with 1 cup (250 ml) milk	540
Chocolate milk, 1 cup (250 ml)	285
Cheese, cheddar, 1.5 oz (45 g)	300
Cheese, Swiss or Gruyère, 1.5 oz. (45 g)	480
Cheese, mozzarella, 1.75 oz (50 g)	269
Cheese, cottage, 1/2 cup (125 ml)	75
Cheese, ricotta, 1/2 cup (125 ml)	255
Evaporated milk, 1/2 cup (125 ml)	350
Skim milk powder, dry, 3 tbsp. (45 ml)	155
Sour cream, light 1/4 cup (50 ml)	120
Yogurt, plain, 3/4 cup (175 ml)	300
Yogurt, fruit, 3/4 cup (175 ml)	250
Pudding, low-fat Healthy Choice, 1/2 cup (125 ml)	110

SOY AND LEGUMES

Soybeans, cooked, 1 cup (250 ml)	175
Soybeans, roasted, 1/4 cup (50 ml)	60
Soy beverage, 1 cup (250 ml)	100
Soy beverage, fortified, 1 cup (250 ml)	300–330
Baked beans, 1 cup (250 ml)	150
Black beans, cooked, 1 cup (250 ml)	102
Kidney beans, cooked, 1 cup (250 ml)	69
Lentils, cooked, 1 cup (250 ml)	37
Tempeh, cooked, 1 cup (250 ml)	154
Tofu, raw, firm, with calcium sulphate, 4 oz. (120 g)	260
Tofu, raw, regular, with calcium sulphate, 4 oz. (120 g)	130

FISH

Sardines, Atlantic, with bones, 1/2 tin (45 g)	175
Salmon, sockeye, with bones, 1/2 can (180 g), drained	440

VEGETABLES

Bok choy, cooked, 1 cup (250 ml)	158
Broccoli, raw, 1 cup (250 ml)	42
Broccoli, cooked, 1 cup (250 ml)	94
Collard greens, cooked, 1 cup (250 ml)	357
Kale, cooked, 1 cup (250 ml)	179
Okra, cooked, 1 cup (250 ml)	176
Rutabaga, cooked, 1/2 cup (125 ml)	57
Swiss chard, raw, 1 cup (250 ml)	21
Swiss chard, cooked, 1 cup (250 ml)	102

FRUIT

Currants, 1/2 cup (125 ml)	60
Figs, 5 medium	135
Orange, 1 medium	50

NUTS

Almonds, 1/4 cup (50 ml)	100
Brazil nuts, 1/4 cup (50 ml)	65
Hazelnuts, 1/4 cup (50 ml)	65

OTHER FOODS

Molasses

Blackstrap molasses, 2 tbsp. (25 ml)	288
Fancy molasses, 2 tbsp. (25 ml)	70

FORTIFIED ORANGE JUICE

Oasis Florida Premium Orange Juice, 1 cup (250 ml)	300
Oasis Health Break (juice & milk cocktail), 1 cup (250 ml)	300
Tropicana Calcium Fortified Orange Juice, 1 cup (250 ml)	300
Minute Maid Calcium Fortified Orange Juice, 1 cup (250 ml)	300

Source: *Nutrient Value of Some Common Foods*. Health Canada, 1999. Adapted and reproduced with the permission of the Minister of Public Works and Government Services Canada, 2003.

Boosting calcium absorption

On average, we absorb about 30 percent of the calcium we consume in our diet. In other words, if you are getting 1000 milligrams of calcium from food each day, your body is absorbing about 300 milligrams of that. But you needn't worry. The scientists who set the recommended dietary allowance (RDA) for calcium took into account that our bodies absorb calcium inefficiently. What you should worry about, however, are factors in your diet that make your body absorb calcium even less effectively. Here's a list of dietary factors that limit calcium absorption:

- Large amounts of phytates (a type of fibre). Phytates in wheat bran and other grains can bind with calcium and limit its absorption.
- Oxalic acid in spinach and some other vegetables. (You may have noticed in the chart of calcium-containing foods above that cooking green vegetables boosts their calcium content. That's because cooking releases some calcium that's bound to oxalic acid.)
- Too much phosphorus in the diet.
- Taking iron with calcium-rich foods (iron competes with calcium for absorption).
- Drinking tea with a meal rich in calcium. Tannins, natural compounds in tea, inhibit calcium absorption.
- A lack of vitamin D (as you've read above, vitamin D stimulates the intestines to absorb dietary calcium).

Calcium absorption is also affected by our body's need for the mineral. During the rapid growth of childhood, the body absorbs about 75 percent of dietary calcium. During pregnancy, absorption may be as high as 60 percent. In general, the younger we are, the more calcium we absorb. After menopause, calcium absorption can be as low as 20 percent.

What about a calcium supplement?

Studies support the idea of using calcium supplements to minimize your odds of osteoporosis. Researchers at the University of Texas Southwestern Medical Center in Dallas found that a 400-milligram calcium citrate supplement taken twice daily increased bone density in healthy postmenopausal women. Women taking the calcium pills experienced no loss of bone density in the radial shaft (one of two bones in the forearm), neck, or lower spine after two years of treatment. In contrast, women in the placebo group experienced a 2.38 percent reduction in the bone density of the lower spine.

Other studies have found that calcium supplements can prevent bone loss in premenopausal women. Scientists at the University of Massachusetts studied 98 premenopausal women (average age 39) for three years. Those who received 500 milligrams of calcium carbonate increased their bone density by 0.3 percent per year. The women in the placebo group lost bone at a rate of 0.4 percent per year in the hip and 0.7 percent per year in the neck. According to the researchers, if this rate of bone density loss occurred throughout the years between ages 30 and 50, the total loss would be between 8 and 14 percent—a loss that translates into a doubled or tripled risk of hip fracture. A number of studies have also shown that older women (and men) who take calcium and vitamin D supplements have a lower incidence of nonvertebral fractures.[18]

By now you're probably thinking you'd better visit your local pharmacy to pick up a calcium supplement. Chances are, you're probably right. Recent surveys have found that most Canadians get a mere 1.6 servings of milk products each day. That translates into 480 milligrams of calcium—a far cry from the recommended 1000 or 1500 milligrams. Sure, there's broccoli and almonds and tofu. But let's be truthful: Do you really eat tofu on a daily basis? Are you willing to eat five cups of cooked broccoli to make up for your missing 500 milligrams of calcium? The truth is, many women are not meeting their daily calcium needs and should be taking a calcium supplement. It can be especially difficult to meet your calcium goals if you're lactose intolerant (that is, you can't digest lactose, a sugar found in milk), following a vegetarian diet, or have poor eating habits. I frequently recommend calcium supplements to my clients, as they represent the best way for me to ensure a woman will meet her calcium needs.

To help determine your need for a calcium supplement, use my 300 Milligram Rule: One milk serving gives you about 300 milligrams of calcium. If you are a post-menopausal women, this means that, to get 1500 milligrams of calcium, you need to get five servings of dairy or calcium-fortified beverage every day! I have yet to meet a woman who achieves this goal. For every serving you don't get and don't replace with other calcium-rich foods, you need to take 300 milligrams of elemental calcium in supplemental form. But before rushing off to the health food store, keep in mind a few things to look for when buying a supplement.

Choosing a quality supplement

If you've been to the pharmacy or health food store and found yourself overwhelmed by all the different types of calcium supplements, you're not alone. Many of my clients have described their frustration about calcium supplements. Should you choose calcium carbonate or calcium citrate? Is a 600-milligram pill better than two 300-milligram tablets? What about added vitamin D and magnesium? I'm sure that many of you know what I mean. To help make your next calcium shopping experience stress-free, follow these guidelines for choosing a high-quality supplement.

Look at the source.   Many types of calcium supplements are available. These are the most common types:

- *Calcium carbonate*   Only about 10 to 30 percent of this form of calcium is absorbed. The amount you absorb depends on how much stomach acid you have. As you age, your stomach produces less hydrochloric acid. Always take calcium carbonate supplements with meals to increase their absorption. Do not take calcium carbonate at bedtime, unless you take it with a nighttime snack. Calcium carbonate is not the best choice for older adults or people on medications that block acid production. On the plus side, calcium carbonate is the most inexpensive type of calcium, and it packs 500 milligrams of elemental calcium per tablet.

  Since a calcium carbonate supplement needs to break down completely before it can be absorbed, I recommend that you test your brand to determine how quickly it disintegrates. Drop the calcium carbonate tablet into a glass of vinegar. If most of the tablet hasn't disintegrated within 30 minutes, you should switch to another brand that will disintegrate more quickly. However, if you're using a chewable calcium supplement, disintegration is not a big concern, since the act of chewing helps to break the pill down.

- *Calcium citrate* About 30 percent of the calcium in a calcium citrate pill is absorbed by the body, so this form is more available to your bones than calcium carbonate. Calcium citrate is therefore a better choice for anyone over the age of 50. Calcium citrate malate is one of the most highly absorbable—and expensive—forms of calcium. Calcium citrate supplements are well absorbed with meals or on an empty stomach. Each tablet usually supplies 300 milligrams of elemental calcium.

- *Calcium chelates (HVP chelates)* These supplements contain calcium that's bound to an amino acid (the most basic forms of protein). The amino acid in HVP chelate is extracted from vegetable proteins. Some manufacturers claim that up to 75 percent of the calcium in chelate form is absorbed by the body; however, I have yet to see research supporting this claim.

- *Effervescent calcium supplements* These contain calcium carbonate and often other forms of more absorbable calcium. For this reason, they may be better absorbed by some people. And because the calcium in these supplements starts disintegrating before it reaches the digestive tract, it may be absorbed more quickly. Dissolve effervescent calcium supplements in water or orange juice.

- *Bone meal (hydroxyapatite, dolomite, or oyster shell)* Taking a calcium supplement made from any of these sources is not recommended because some products have been found to contain trace quantities of contaminants such as lead and mercury.

Look at the amount of elemental calcium. The list of ingredients will alert you to how much elemental calcium each pill will give you. This is important because it is the amount of *elemental calcium* that should be used to calculate your daily intake. The label on the supplement's bottle may state it is a 500-milligram supplement, but when you look at the ingredient list on the bottle, you may find the product contains only 350 milligrams of elemental calcium. This amount, and not the 500-milligram amount, will determine how many tablets you need to take to get your recommended calcium dose. For instance, if you need to supplement your diet with 1000 milligrams of calcium daily, you would take three of these pills, rather than two.

Look for vitamin D and magnesium. Choose a calcium formula that includes vitamin D and magnesium. These nutrients work in tandem with calcium to promote optimal bone health. For instance, vitamin D increases calcium absorption in your intestines by as much as 30 to 80 percent.

How much calcium is too much?

The daily upper limit for calcium intake is 2500 milligrams. In most healthy people, this amount will not cause any side effects. The major risks you run from getting too much calcium include kidney stones, constipation, and gas. To lower your risk of kidney stones, take your calcium supplements with a large glass of water. Drinking sufficient water with the supplement helps to prevent calcium buildup in the kidneys.

You might be interested to learn that people who take 1300 milligrams of calcium daily in supplemental form, as compared with people who take 500 milligrams, have *fewer* kidney stones made from oxalate (oxalic acid). High amounts of calcium in the intestines can bind to oxalates in the diet (found in spinach, rhubarb, and other vegetables), preventing its absorption and reducing the amount that eventually reaches the kidneys to cause stones. But in people who have a history of kidney stones, excessive intakes of calcium can increase the risk of stone formation. At intakes higher than 2500 milligrams, too much calcium can reach the kidneys for excretion in the urine.

Very high intakes of calcium from milk, fortified beverages, and supplements can cause a condition called milk-alkali syndrome. In this condition, the level of calcium in the bloodstream becomes so high that calcium "leaches" into body tissues and destroys them. As long as you stay at or below the daily upper limit of 2500 milligrams of calcium, you needn't worry about milk-alkali syndrome.

What if you have a lactose intolerance?

If you suffer gastric distress after drinking a glass of milk, you're not alone. In my private practice, it's not uncommon for me to hear people complain of difficulty digesting lactose, the natural sugar found in dairy products. The fact that 70 percent of the world's population has difficulty digesting lactose has led some researchers to believe that lactose intolerance is normal and that it is lactose tolerance that is the abnormal condition.

Lactose intolerance is caused by low levels of lactase, the enzyme in the small intestines that breaks down the milk sugar and makes it ready for absorption. If lactose remains undigested in the gut, it draws water into the intestines, which can lead to diarrhea. Also, bacteria in the intestinal tract will begin to ferment the undigested lactose, causing bloating, gas, and discomfort.

Lactose intolerance is more common among people of Asian, African, and South American descent. Many individuals with these origins lose the ability to produce lactase when they're children. Difficulty digesting lactose can also occur when other gastrointestinal problems are present, such as celiac disease, irritable bowel syndrome, Crohn's disease, or a gastrointestinal infection. In these cases, the intolerance is often temporary, disappearing when bowel health returns to normal.

Just because you have a lactose intolerance doesn't mean you have to give up calcium-rich dairy products. Most people with a mild to moderate lactose intolerance can handle yogurt quite well and can tolerate milk in 1/2-cup (125-ml) servings. The bacteria in yogurt actually digest some of the lactose, so you end up with a food that has considerably less lactose than a glass of milk.

Here's a ranking of foods according to their lactose content. If you have a severe lactose intolerance, be sure to read ingredient lists on packaged and processed food labels. If you see milk, milk solids, cheese flavour, or whey curds in the list of ingredients, lactose is present.

High lactose
- Condensed milk
- Evaporated milk
- Processed cheese

Moderate lactose
- Cottage cheese, 2%
- Feta cheese
- Fluid milk
- Goat's milk
- Ice cream
- Mozzarella cheese
- Ricotta cheese
- Swiss cheese
- Yogurt, low-fat

Low lactose
- Brie cheese
- Butter
- Cheddar cheese
- Cottage cheese, 1%
- Cream cheese
- Lactaid milk

Lactose free (nondairy products)
- Calcium-fortified orange juice
- Calcium-fortified rice-based beverages
- Calcium-fortified soy beverages

People with severe lactose intolerance must avoid all sources of lactose. While a diet without dairy products can still offer plenty of calcium, getting enough vitamin D, which is so important for adequate calcium absorption, is often a problem. Calcium-fortified orange juice, tofu, broccoli, leafy greens, almonds, and legumes are all good sources of calcium, but none of them contains vitamin D. Continue reading to find out how to get your vitamin D.

VITAMIN D

By now you've likely heard and read from many sources besides this book that too little dietary calcium makes bones brittle and increases the risk of osteoporosis. But experts also blame a silent epidemic of vitamin D deficiency. The main reason for this nutrient deficiency is that most foods have little or no natural vitamin D, and only a few foods are actually fortified with the vitamin.

Vitamin D acts like a hormone in your body (remember from Chapter 1 that a hormone is any compound manufactured in one part of the body that affects another part). The active form of vitamin D is made in your liver but acts on your intestines, kidneys, and bone. As I mentioned earlier, vitamin D raises blood levels of calcium in three ways: it stimulates your intestines to absorb more dietary calcium, it tells your kidneys to retain calcium, and it withdraws calcium from your bones. Vitamin D works alone in the intestinal tract and, in the kidneys and bones, in tandem with parathyroid hormone. The result of vitamin D activity is that more calcium and phosphorus become available for bone growth; these minerals are supplied to the bones via the blood and deposited as new bone hardens, or mineralizes.

As you can see, vitamin D's main job is to maintain your blood calcium in the normal range. If you're not eating enough calcium-rich foods, vitamin D will remove calcium from your bones to keep your blood level constant. Simply put, if you're lacking vitamin D, you are not absorbing enough calcium to meet your needs, regardless of how much calcium you consume. A vitamin D deficiency will speed up bone loss and increase the risk of fracture at a younger age.

Vitamin D is different from other essential nutrients in that our bodies synthesize it with the help of sunlight. When ultraviolet light from the sun reaches your skin, it becomes possible for your body, through a special chemical reaction, to convert a vitamin D precursor that's made from cholesterol into previtamin D3.

This compound then makes its way to your liver, where it's transformed into the active form of vitamin D (25-hydroxy vitamin D3). As you can see from the diagram below, vitamin D in food must also be converted to an active form by the liver before it can go to work.

VITAMIN D SOURCES AND ACTIVATION

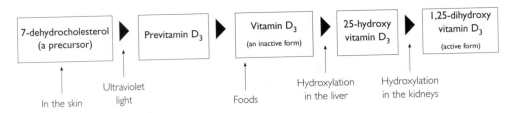

While exposing your skin to sunlight can provide most, if not all, of the vitamin D your body needs, very little vitamin D synthesis occurs in the skin of many Canadians for months at a time because of our long winters. The situation is exacerbated by most of us working indoors. Researchers from Tufts University in Boston have demonstrated that blood levels of vitamin D do indeed fluctuate throughout the year. They are at their lowest point in February and March and at their highest in June and July.[19] But even during the summer, your body might not be making enough vitamin D. Did you know that the sunscreen that protects you from skin cancer also blocks the production of vitamin D? Suntan lotion with a sun protection factor (SPF) as low as 8 prevents 95 percent of your skin's vitamin D production. Because of this, when it is sunny, you should expose—without sunscreen—your hands, face, and arms for 10 to 15 minutes two or three times a week to help meet your vitamin D needs. You can also now see how important it is to get plenty of vitamin D from food, not only in the winter but also in the summer months.

How much vitamin D do you need?

In November 2002, vitamin D intake recommendations for Canadians were increased. The requirements were doubled for all age groups in view of the fact that sun exposure does not appear to be sufficient to replace dietary sources of vitamin D. Here's how much you should be striving to get every day:

DAILY RECOMMENDED VITAMIN D INTAKES (INTERNATIONAL UNITS)[20]

0–50 years	400
51+ years	800
Daily upper limit	*2000*

As you can see, the need to obtain vitamin D from food increases with age; older adults make less vitamin D from sunlight. By the time the average person reaches the age of 70, the vitamin D precursor levels in the skin are three to four times lower than in that of a person younger than 50.

Unfortunately, good food sources of vitamin D are few and far between. Vitamin D occurs naturally in egg yolks, liver, butter, and oily fish. Foods fortified with the vitamin include fluid milk, margarine, and some brands of soy and rice beverages. Take at look at how these foods affect your vitamin D intake.

VITAMIN D CONTENT OF FOODS (INTERNATIONAL UNITS)

Cod liver oil, 1 tsp. (5 ml)	450
Salmon, canned, 3.5 oz (100 g)	360
Sardines, canned, 3.5 oz (100 g)	270
Mackerel, cooked, 3.5 oz (100g)	345
Milk, fluid, 1 cup (250 ml)	100
Fortified soy beverage, 1 cup (250 ml)	100
Fortified rice beverage, 1 cup (250 ml)	100
Egg, 1 whole	25
Margarine, 1 tsp. (5 ml)	20

Source: US Department of Agriculture, Agricultural Research Service, 2001. USDA Nutrient Database for Standard Reference, Release 14, Nutrient Laboratory Home Page, http://www.nal.usda.gov/fnic/foodcomp.

What about a vitamin D supplement?

If you're over 50, or if you don't drink at least two glasses of a fortified beverage every day, or if winter means little exposure to sunshine, you should reach for a good-quality multivitamin and mineral supplement to supply your vitamin D. The daily upper limit for vitamin D is 2000 international units (IU). Most supplements give you 400 IU. If you take calcium supplements, buy a product with vitamin D added (most will provide 100 IU of vitamin D per tablet). Although fish liver oil supplements are another way to get your vitamin D, I don't recommend them. Fish liver oil capsules contain high amounts of both vitamin D and vitamin A. And as you'll read below, too much vitamin A may be harmful to your bones.

Instead, buy single supplements of vitamin D from health food stores and pharmacies. Vitamin D3 (cholecalciferol) is preferred over vitamin D2 (ergocalciferol). Vitamin D is usually sold in 400, 800, and 1000 IU doses. Keep in mind that vitamin D is fat-soluble. This means a risk of vitamin D toxicity because it is stored in the body. Be sure you don't exceed 2000 IU of vitamin D per day from diet and supplements combined.

OTHER BONE-BUILDING VITAMINS AND MINERALS

There's no doubt that calcium and vitamin D both play a crucial role in bone health. Without adequate calcium, your bones cannot make an effective mineral complex (hyroxyapatite) that lends strength and rigidity to bones. And without enough vitamin D, your body cannot absorb the calcium it needs. But the story doesn't end there. Other nutrients are important for bone building as well. Together with calcium and vitamin D, they make up the nutrient team your body needs to orchestrate the continual process of bone remodelling.

Vitamin A

One of this vitamin's important jobs is to support growth and development, especially bone development. I told you earlier that to build new bone, the osteoclast cells must first undo parts of old bone. To accomplish this task, osteoclasts contain a sac of degradative enzymes. With the help of vitamin A, these enzymes break down old bone. That bone growth relies on vitamin A is witnessed by the fact that children deficient in vitamin A fail to grow properly. However, while we need some vitamin A for good health (0.7 mg/2331 IU per day for women; 0.9 mg/3000 IU for men), too much may actually increase the risk of hip fracture. That's what researchers from Harvard University learned when they studied almost 73,000 postmenopausal women. Those women who consumed more than 3 milligrams (10,000 IU) of vitamin A each day had a significantly higher risk of hip fracture compared with women who consumed less than 1.2 milligrams (4160 IU) each day. This increased risk was mainly due to retinol, the form of vitamin A found in animal foods and fortified foods. When it came to supplements users, women who took a vitamin A supplement had a 40 percent higher risk of hip fracture compared to non–pill poppers.[21]

A recent study from Sweden found similar results with respect to the harmful effects of too much vitamin A. In this study, 2322 men were followed for an average of 24 years. The researchers learned that men who consumed more than 1.5 milligrams (5000 IU) of vitamin A each day were twice as likely to suffer a bone fracture compared to men who got much less.[22] What's more, compared to men with the lowest levels of vitamin A in their blood, those who had the highest levels had a seven-fold higher risk of bone fracture.

High blood levels of vitamin A stimulate bone breakdown and, based on a growing body of evidence, increase the risk of bone fracture. Researchers from California learned that a daily vitamin A intake of 0.6 milligrams to 0.9 milligrams (2000 to 2800 IU) was associated with optimal bone density.[23]

The main food sources of vitamin A include dairy products, fish, and liver as well as fortified foods such as milk. Currently the upper daily limit for safe vitamin A intake is set at 3 milligrams (10,000 IU). But based on these studies, this might be too high. I recommend that you avoid consuming more than 1.5 milligrams (5000 IU) per day.

VITAMIN A (RETINOL) IN FOODS

Food	Vitamin A (mg)	(IU)
Liver, beef, cooked, 3 oz (90 g)	9.2	30,689
Liver, chicken, cooked, 3 oz (90 g)	4.4	14,730
Kidneys, cooked, 3 oz (90 g)	0.3	1116
Cod liver oil, 1 tsp (4.5 g)	1.4	4500
Salmon oil, 1 tsp (4.5 g)	0	0
Salmon, Atlantic, 3 oz (90 g) cooked	0.01	37
Milk, 1%, 1 cup (250 ml)	0.16	530
Yogurt, 1-2%, fruit bottom, 2/3 cup (175 ml)	0.04	141

U.S. Department of Agriculture, Agricultural Research Service, 2001. USDA Nutrient Database for Standard Reference, Release 14. Nutrient Laboratory Home Page, http://www.nal.usda.gov/fnic/foodcomp.

Unless you eat liver regularly, it's unlikely you'll get too much vitamin A from your diet. The real concern rests with vitamin A supplements. Make sure your multivitamin contains no more than 2500 IU of vitamin A. Some brands don't contain any vitamin A at all. And I certainly recommend that you avoid taking single supplements of vitamin A.

We also get some vitamin A by eating bright orange and green fruits and vegetables. The beta-carotene in these plant foods is converted to vitamin A in the body. Fortunately, research suggests that beta carotene—from food or supplements—does not increase the risk of bone fracture. The best sources of beta-carotene include carrots, winter squash, sweet potatoes, spinach, broccoli, rapini, Romaine lettuce, apricots, peaches, mango, papaya, and cantaloupe.

Vitamin K

You've probably heard very little about this fat-soluble vitamin. One of the reasons for its low profile is that vitamin K deficiency is rarely seen. That's because the billions of bacteria in our intestinal tract synthesize this vitamin. Once our bodies absorb this bacteria-manufactured vitamin K, it is stored in the liver. The vitamin is not a part of the bone mineral complex. Instead, our bodies need it to make osteocalcin, a bone protein. Doctors can measure the amount of osteocalcin in your blood. A high level indicates that your osteoblasts are busy making new bone. Without enough vitamin K, the bones produce an abnormal protein that cannot bind to the minerals that give the bones their strength and defined form. The best food sources of vitamin K are leafy green vegetables, cabbage, milk, and liver.

When it comes to bone health, do not underestimate the importance of vitamin K. The Nurses' Health Study from Harvard University found that women with the highest intake of vitamin K had a significantly lower rate of hip fracture as compared with women who consumed the least. And guess what? Eating lettuce was also linked with fewer hip fractures, because lettuce accounted for most of the vitamin K in the diet of the women with stronger bones. Those women who ate one or more servings of the leafy green each day (versus one or fewer servings a week) had a 45 percent lower risk of hip fracture.[24]

Phosphorus

This mineral is an important component of the bone mineral complex. In fact, about 85 percent of the phosphorus in the body is found in the bone. It appears that both too little dietary phosphorus and too much can result in bone loss. A high level in the blood causes the release of parathyroid hormone (PTH). And, if you recall, PTH instructs your osteoclasts to release calcium into your bloodstream. Scientists believe that a long-standing imbalance of phosphorus and calcium, caused by too much dietary phosphorus and too little dietary calcium, may contribute to bone breakdown.

On the other hand, if your diet lacks phosphorus and your blood levels become low, your body will release the mineral from your bones in an effort to keep your blood level constant (the same way that calcium blood levels remain stable at the expense of your bone). One of the symptoms of a phosphorus deficiency is bone pain. A low blood phosphorus level can result from poor eating habits, intestinal malabsorption, and excessive use of antacids that bind to phosphorus, such as Maalox, Diovol, Gelusil, and Amphogel.

The daily recommended intake for phosphorus is 700 milligrams. Most of the phosphorus in our diet comes from additives in cheese, bakery products, processed meats, and soft drinks. Other food sources include wheat bran, milk, fish, eggs, poultry, beef, and pork. As you can probably guess, most people don't have a problem getting enough phosphorus. Perhaps vegans who use no commercial bread or other commercial products are at risk of a phosphorus deficiency. Everyone else, just make sure you meet your calcium requirements so that you keep these two minerals in balance.

Magnesium

One-half of the body's magnesium stores are in the bone. Before I continue, I'd like to clear up one piece of misinformation. Magnesium does not help your body absorb calcium! I can't begin to count the number of times I have heard this said. On occasion, I've even seen it written in books. Without magnesium, you'll absorb calcium just fine; however, you won't form healthy bones. Your body needs magnesium to make parathyroid hormone, an important regulator of bone building. Animal studies show that a lack of dietary magnesium causes increased bone breakdown and decreased bone synthesis.

It's difficult to say to what extent magnesium plays a role in the development of osteoporosis since few studies have actually looked at the effect of dietary magnesium intake on bone loss. Most of the studies supporting the use of magnesium supplements have found that osteoporosis is more common in people who have other health problems that cause a magnesium deficiency, such as alcoholism or hyperthyroidism.

Scientists have found that magnesium levels in bone are actually higher, not lower, than normal in people with osteoporosis.

Nonetheless, magnesium is an important nutrient for bone health and is also required for the smooth functioning of many other processes in the body. The recommended daily intake for women is 320 milligrams. The best food sources are wheat bran, whole-grain breads, cereals and pasta, legumes, nuts, seeds, and leafy green vegetables. There's no question in my mind that most people need to step up their magnesium intake. If you stop eating refined starches like white bread and white pasta and switch to whole-grain products, you'll be making a good start. The fact that so many of my clients lack magnesium in their diets is why I recommend buying a calcium supplement that includes magnesium. But too much supplemental magnesium can cause diarrhea. For this reason, I suggest you buy a calcium-magnesium supplement that offers these two nutrients in a two-to-one (2:1) ratio: two parts calcium to one part magnesium.

Boron

While there's no daily recommended intake for boron, studies suggest that higher intakes of this trace mineral may slow down loss of calcium, magnesium, and phosphorus from the urine. And that's not all. Boosting your boron intake may also increase your blood estrogen level. Scientists aren't exactly sure how boron keeps calcium in balance, but they think that boron is needed for activation of vitamin D.

A daily intake of 1.5 to 3 milligrams is probably more than adequate to meet your requirements for bone growth and development. Fruits and vegetables are the main food sources of boron, but their boron content will depend on how much of the mineral is in the soil they were grown in. If you want to take a supplement, 3 to 9 milligrams per day is a very safe amount. Intakes greater than 500 milligrams a day can cause nausea, vomiting, and diarrhea. Your best bet is to strive for at least five servings of fruits and vegetables each day. Boron supplements are available in the United States but not in Canada.

Manganese, zinc, and copper

Your body uses these minerals to synthesize enzymes that are essential in making bone tissue. The impact of these nutrients on bone loss has been studied in postmenopausal women. In one two-year study, women who received a daily supplement of calcium, manganese, copper, and zinc had not experienced any bone loss of the spine by the end of the study. The placebo group, on the other hand, lost 3.5 percent of their bone mass.[25] Manganese is widely available in foods, and deficiencies have not been seen in humans. You may want to check, however, that your diet is supplying 5 milligrams daily, the amount used in this study (see Appendix 4 to assess your manganese intake). Meat and tap water are your best bets for copper. When it comes to zinc, reach for wheat bran, wheat germ, oysters, seafood, lean red meat, and milk.

Other lifestyle factors

THE IMPORTANCE OF EXERCISE

Regular exercise before the age of 30 helps women get a head start on building peak bone mass. Studies have found that children who spend the most amount of time being physically active have stronger bones than those who are sedentary. But the effect of exercise doesn't stop once you've achieved your peak mass. Bone cells are constantly active, tearing up old bone and laying down new bone. Participating in weight-bearing activities stimulates bones to increase in strength and density during the pre- and postmenopausal years. Weight-bearing exercise is any exercise that forces you to support your own body weight and/or additional weight (as in weight training). Swimming and cycling are not considered weight-bearing exercise: in swimming, your weight is supported by the water, and in cycling, by the bike. Brisk walking, jogging, stair climbing, and strength training are all good examples of weight-bearing activities. One study found that postmenopausal women who worked out three times a week for nine months actually increased their bone mass by 5.2 percent.

If your exercise routine includes weight training, that's fabulous. If it doesn't, consider adding this form of exercise to your routine. Researchers have learned that weight training also has a protective effect on bone density in women. Compared with women who didn't exercise, women who worked out with weights for one hour three times a week gained bone mass, to the tune of 1.6 percent. The nonexercisers actually lost 3.6 percent of the bone mass in their spine over the course of the study.[26]

If you have osteoporosis, a safe exercise program can help you slow bone loss, improve posture and balance, and build muscle strength and tone. The benefits of exercise can reduce your risk of falling and fracturing a bone. Your best bet is to incorporate a mix of activities into your week. Aim to enjoy four sessions of weight-bearing activities each week, and two or three workouts with weights. If you have never used weights before, be sure to consult a certified personal trainer to design a safe and effective program for you. Personal trainers work in fitness clubs, and many will come to your home. And don't worry, you won't need a basement full of exercise equipment. Some of the best trainers I know teach women creative ways of building muscle strength without having to purchase weights. Doing push-ups or sit-ups, or working against the resistance of a Dyna-band (available in sporting goods stores), can all be part of such an exercise program.

THE bottom LINE...

Leslie's recommendations for reducing your risk of osteoporosis and bone fracture

1   If you're approaching menopause, get your bone density measured to help you and your doctor determine if you need to take medication to prevent osteoporosis.

2   If you're already a fan of soy foods, consider boosting your intake so that your diet provides you with at least 50 milligrams daily of isoflavones, the natural plant estrogens found in soybeans. Soy's isoflavones bind to estrogen receptors on the bone and may slow down bone loss.

3   To strengthen your bones, make sure you're eating enough protein-rich foods such as fish, poultry, lean meat, legumes, tofu, and dairy products. But don't go overboard. Some studies suggest that very high intakes of protein cause your kidneys to excrete calcium.

4   If you drink alcohol, keep your intake at a moderate level of no more than two drinks daily.

5   To prevent too much calcium loss from your body, keep your caffeine intake to a daily maximum of 450 milligrams (that's no more than three small cups of coffee). If you have osteoporosis, aim for a daily maximum of 200 milligrams, but preferably none.

6 Go easy on the salt shaker and processed foods with high sodium. For every 500 milligrams (1/5 teaspoon) of sodium you consume, you'll need to consume 40 milligrams of calcium to minimize sodium-related calcium loss.

7 Depending on your age and risk of osteoporosis, get 1000 or 1500 milligrams of calcium each day from food, and if necessary, supplements.

8 To help you absorb the calcium in your diet, make sure you get 400 international units (IU) (perimenopausal women) or 800 IU (postmenopausal women) of vitamin D each day. The best food sources are fluid milk (not yogurt or cheese), fortified soy or rice beverages, oily fish, and whole eggs. Make a real effort to boost your vitamin D intake in the winter, when your body's natural production of the vitamin is reduced by a lack of sunlight.

9 Other nutrients that help build bone density include vitamin A, vitamin K, magnesium, phosphorus, boron, manganese, zinc, and copper. With the exceptions of vitamin K and phosphorus, you'll also find most of these vitamins and minerals in a multivitamin and mineral formula. Vitamin K is made in the body, and phosphorus is widespread in commercial foods.

10 If you don't already work out, begin adding regular exercise to your life. Weight-bearing activities such as brisk walking, jogging, stair climbing, tennis, soccer, and basketball, as well as strength training with weights, can stimulate an increase in bone density. If you have health problems or you take certain medications, check with your physician before embarking on a regular exercise program.

Reducing your risk of heart disease

"When I turned 50, the farthest thing from my mind was having a heart attack. I guess I should have paid more attention. It took a long time to accept the fact that at the age of 59 I suffered my first (and hopefully last) heart attack. Today I eat well, exercise, take vitamins, and feel better than ever before."

12

We tend to view heart disease as a health problem faced by middle-aged men. It's true that clogged arteries and heart attacks generally afflict men 10 to 15 years earlier than they do women. This built-in "protection" from heart disease has led many women to believe they are immune to heart attacks. But the physiological factors that protect women end when the menstruating years are over (or are absent if you have diabetes; see page 181 for more on this). In the postmenopausal years, the possibility of heart disease needs to be taken very seriously. With the loss of estrogen that accompanies menopause, a woman's risk of getting heart disease increases four-fold and continues to rise with age. If you're a woman older than 50, it's important to realize that your risk of dying from heart disease has increased significantly from when you were younger. In fact, heart disease and stroke are the top two killers among adult Canadian women, accounting for 38 percent of all deaths. Today, almost 40,000 Canadian women suffer from heart disease.

As women enter menopause, they tend to be more concerned about cancer, especially breast cancer. When asked, many of my clients say that breast cancer is the leading cause of death among women. In truth, a woman has only one-quarter the risk of dying from breast cancer as she does from heart disease. Women are more anxious about breast cancer because it strikes at a younger age and it kills a greater number of perimenopausal women than does heart disease. But clearly, heart disease takes a larger toll on Canadian women.

I can't emphasize enough how important it is for women to pay attention to their heart health and learn how to protect themselves from heart disease. Both women and their doctors tend to ignore or overlook symptoms such as chest pain, often attributing this and others to indigestion, stress, or gallbladder problems. As well, women tend to get to a hospital much later after having a heart attack than do men, and they also tend to receive less aggressive therapy. Studies have shown that compared with men, women are more likely to die in the year following their heart attack.[1] This is largely because women are older and have more advanced heart disease by the time they are diagnosed.

If you're a postmenopausal woman, do not underestimate any chest pain. If heart disease is responsible for your symptoms, the sooner you seek medical attention, the greater your chances of preventing a heart attack. Or, if you experience the warning signs of a heart attack, the sooner you get yourself to an emergency room, the better your recovery will be.

Warning signs of a heart attack

If you experience any of these symptoms, seek medical help immediately:

- Heavy feeling or pressure in the chest area that lasts more than a few minutes, or goes away and comes back
- Chest discomfort with light-headedness, fainting, sweating, nausea, or shortness of breath
- Pain that moves to your neck, arms, back, jaw

For women in particular, there are other, less common, warning signs:

- Atypical chest pain, stomach or abdominal pain
- Nausea or dizziness
- Shortness of breath and difficulty breathing
- Unexplained anxiety, weakness, or fatigue
- Palpitations, cold sweats, or paleness

Heart disease defined

"Heart disease" is a general term that includes coronary heart disease, congenital heart disease (heart disease one is born with), congestive heart failure, and malfunctioning heart valves. I will focus here on coronary heart disease, a disease affecting the blood vessels that feed the heart. Coronary heart disease is the most common type of heart disease and, at the same time, the most easily preventable through dietary and lifestyle adjustments. Coronary heart disease is caused by atherosclerosis, a gradual process of the narrowing of the heart's arteries that leads to a heart attack. To keep things simple, I will use the term *heart disease* here to refer to coronary heart disease.

THE PROCESS OF HEART DISEASE

Believe it or not, atherosclerosis can actually begin in childhood or adolescence. Even in youth, fatty streaks, which may one day cause heart disease, can appear on the lining of the arteries, the vessels through which the heart pumps blood to the body. The fatty streaks are areas where cholesterol is sticking to the artery lining. As cholesterol accumulates, fatty streaks can begin to infiltrate the artery wall. As adults, the question is not whether we have these fatty areas on our artery walls, but rather, what we can do to prevent them from progressing.

Atherosclerosis starts with an injury to the lining of an artery. An infection or virus, high blood pressure, cigarette smoke, or diabetes may cause this damage. Your body then attempts to heal itself, just as it would with any wound. The injured area becomes covered with plaque, which contains cholesterol, white blood cells, and smooth muscle cells. This plaque eventually becomes covered with a layer of muscle cells and calcium, stiffening arteries and narrowing the passage through them. Most people have well-developed plaque by the time they're 30.

Atherosclerosis is dangerous because it can restrict blood flow to the heart. Healthy arteries expand with each heartbeat to allow blood to flow easily through them. Once arteries become stiff and narrow from a buildup of plaque, they cannot expand and so blood pressure rises. High blood pressure damages the vessel walls further, and more plaque forms. As less blood flows through narrowed arteries, your kidneys respond by causing your body to hold on to sodium, which increases your blood pressure further.

HOW A HEART ATTACK HAPPENS

Blood cells called platelets respond to damaged spots on blood vessels by forming clots. Your body uses the same process to form a scab on a cut. Normally, clots dissolve in the blood. But when atherosclerosis is severe enough, clots form faster than they can disappear. A clot may stick to plaque and gradually enlarge, until it blocks blood flow to an area of the heart. That portion of the heart may die slowly and form scar tissue. But a clot may also break loose, and circulate in the blood until it reaches an artery too small to pass through. When a clot that's wedged in a vessel cuts off the supply of oxygen and nutrients to a part of the heart muscle, a heart attack results (a stroke occurs when a clot blocks an artery that leads to the brain and kills an area of brain tissue).

Risk factors for heart disease

Knowing your risk factors for heart disease is an important first step in reducing your risk. At least half of all heart attacks are the result of known risk factors. The checklist below gives the most important risk factors for heart disease. As you can see, risk factors are classified as either modifiable or nonmodifiable. Nonmodifiable factors—like your age or having a family history of early heart attacks—are risk factors that you can't change. Where you exert your control over heart disease is with modifiable risk factors. You can eliminate culprits such as poor diet, lack of exercise, or tobacco use. And you can control others, such as high blood pressure or diabetes.

ARE YOU AT RISK OF HEART DISEASE?

Assess your heart health by reviewing the risk factors below. If one or more modifiable risk factor applies to you, take action to change it and lower your odds of heart disease.

Nonmodifiable risk factors

- You're older than 40.
- You're at or past menopause.
- You have a family history of heart attack before age 60.

Modifiable risk factors

- You have high blood cholesterol—or you don't know your blood cholesterol levels.
- You have high blood triglycerides—or you don't know your triglyceride levels.
- You have low HDL cholesterol—or you don't know your HDL levels.
- You have high blood pressure—or you don't know what your blood pressure is.
- You smoke cigarettes.
- You have a poor diet (for example, you eat higher-fat foods often or your diet is lacking in fruits and vegetables).
- You don't exercise regularly.
- You have diabetes.
- Your BMI is greater than 25 (see page 181).

The more heart disease risk factors you have, the higher your risk of developing it. While 62 percent of Canadian women have at least one risk factor for heart disease, 19 percent have at least two, including regular smoking, high blood pressure, or high blood cholesterol. Women between the ages of 65 and 74 are most likely to have multiple risk factors. Even small increases in more than one factor can have an impact on your chances of getting the disease. Here's a closer look at the risk factors and how they speed up heart disease.

ADVANCING AGE

As you get older, your chances of having heart disease increase. With age, your body becomes less efficient at clearing cholesterol from the bloodstream. The cells in the lining of your blood vessels contain receptors for low density lipoprotein (LDL), a substance that carries cholesterol particles (see page 176). These receptors attach to LDL and remove the cholesterol it carries from the blood. As the adult years pass, your body produces fewer of these receptors, and the ones you do have become sluggish. Most of the age-related rise in blood cholesterol occurs between the ages of 20 and 50. This is also a time when many people gain weight, accounting for some of the rise in blood cholesterol that occurs during adulthood. With advancing age, many women develop high blood pressure and diabetes, two other important risk factors for heart disease.

ONSET OF MENOPAUSE

I mentioned earlier that women get heart disease 10 to 15 years later than men, something often referred to as "gender protection." Sometime between the ages of 50 and 55, a woman's estrogen levels decline, and her heart disease risk begins to rise. In men, by contrast, the risk of heart disease increases around the age of 40. Both natural menopause and surgical menopause (a complete hysterectomy) is associated with an increased risk. Before menopause, estrogen protects the heart by keeping cholesterol levels in check. It does this by stimulating the production of LDL receptors on cell surfaces. The more LDL receptors you have, the more cholesterol can leave the blood and enter the cells, where it will be broken down. With a loss of estrogen, LDL receptor activity declines and blood cholesterol levels rise. Before menopause, estrogen may also help keep blood vessels more flexible.

FAMILY HISTORY

If you have a first-degree relative with heart disease, you carry a higher risk than otherwise of getting the disease yourself. As a woman, your risk is even greater if you have a female relative who suffered from heart disease. Genes can make you more prone to having high cholesterol, to having LDL cholesterol that's susceptible to free-radical damage, or to sustaining an injury to your artery lining. (For more on free radicals, see Antioxidants: Disease Fighters of the New Millennium on pages 177–178). Scientists have yet to sort out how your genetic makeup contributes to heart disease. But having a family history of heart disease doesn't mean you'll get the disease. It means only that your chances of getting it are greater. As you'll see below, there are plenty of positive things you can do so that heart disease has less chance of becoming your destiny.

HIGH BLOOD LIPID LEVELS

By now I'm sure you've heard plenty about high cholesterol levels and heart disease. The strong link between the two is certainly the reason we jumped on the low-fat bandwagon in the 1980s. Back then, it was clear that a 1 percent lowering of blood cholesterol translated into a 2 percent reduction in heart disease (and as you'll read later, one of the key strategies for lowering high cholesterol levels is to cut back on animal fat).

Nevertheless, many people are still confused about cholesterol. Let me begin by telling you there are two kinds of cholesterol. Dietary cholesterol is found in foods, and blood cholesterol is made by your liver. For most people, the two are unrelated. This means that dietary cholesterol intake has little or no effect on the amount of cholesterol in the bloodstream.

Cholesterol and triglycerides, another type of blood fat made in your liver, don't dissolve in your blood. Instead, they are transported in the blood, piggyback style, on protein carriers (lipoproteins) to their cellular destinations. The lipoproteins that have received the most attention are low density lipoproteins (LDLs) and high density lipoproteins (HDLs). Here's a primer on blood fats for those of you who have heard these terms but were never sure what they meant.

LDL cholesterol

This cholesterol is transported to the arteries on low density lipoproteins (lipid, or fat-carrying proteins). LDL cholesterol is the type that contributes to the process of the hardening and narrowing of arteries. LDL receptor sites on blood vessel walls degrade this type of cholesterol, taking it out of the blood. The potential problems caused by LDL increase when, as explained above, LDL receptor sites decline in number with age. LDL is also more likely to stick to artery walls if it has been damaged by free radicals. The higher your LDL cholesterol levels, the greater your risk of developing heart disease. LDL levels are strongly influenced by what you eat.

HDL cholesterol

High density lipoproteins carry cholesterol away from the arteries toward the liver for degradation. HDLs, therefore, help prevent the accumulation of cholesterol on your artery walls. The higher your HDL levels, the lower your risk of developing heart disease. HDL levels are influenced by genetics, exercise, and, to some extent, diet.

Triglycerides

These fat particles are made in the liver from the food you eat and are transported in your blood on very low density lipoproteins (VLDLs). Although they have not received as much media attention as cholesterol, high levels of triglycerides are also associated with a greater risk of heart disease, especially in women over 50. Triglyceride levels are affected by diet, exercise, and body weight.

If you know your cholesterol and triglyceride levels, use the following reference guide to determine whether your levels are healthy or whether they put you at higher risk of heart disease. (Blood lipids are measured in millimoles per litre.)

BLOOD LIPID LEVELS: UNDERSTANDING YOUR RISK

Blood lipid	Desirable	Borderline risk	At risk
Total cholesterol	5.2	5.2–6.2	6.2
LDL cholesterol	2.0–3.4		3.4
HDL cholesterol	0.9–2.4		0.9
Triglycerides	0.6–2.3		2.3

Circulating cholesterol contributes to heart disease by becoming part of the fatty plaques that build up on artery walls. The more LDL cholesterol there is in the blood, the more LDL cholesterol is available to be attached to artery walls. (As I mentioned above, HDL cholesterol, on the other hand, is transported to the liver for excretion.) The longer you have high LDL levels, the greater the chance more cholesterol has built up in your arteries. While high LDL cholesterol levels stress your arteries, oxidized LDL cholesterol creates even worse problems. Once LDL cholesterol becomes oxidized, that is, damaged by harmful free-radical molecules, it is much more likely to accumulate in artery linings. You'll see that my recommendations to prevent heart disease include not only dietary strategies to lower cholesterol but also ways to protect your LDL cholesterol from oxidation (and you probably can guess that that's where antioxidants play a role!).

Antioxidants: disease fighters of the new millennium

The role dietary antioxidants play in disease prevention has been one of the most important discoveries made in the field of nutrition. Current knowledge indicates that many degenerative diseases (such as heart disease, cancer, and Alzheimer, to name just a few) have their origins in free-radical damage.

Free radicals are highly reactive oxygen molecules produced by normal body processes. They come into the body from the environment. What makes them so reactive is that they are missing an electron. Most molecules have equal numbers of protons (positively charged particles) and electrons (negatively charged particles). In an effort to restore their balance, free radicals seek out electrons from molecules found in body cells, destroying those cells in the process. Although the body produces substances that keep free-radical activity in check, those levels decline with age. As well, large numbers of environmental free radicals from pollution, cigarette smoke, and the like can overwhelm our natural defences.

Unchecked free-radical activity can damage many components of cells, including DNA, lipids (fats), and proteins. Free-radical damage (oxidation) to LDL cholesterol is one contributing factor to heart disease. Once oxidized, LDL cholesterol is more likely to be deposited on artery walls, where it causes hardening and narrowing of the arteries.

As I mentioned above, our bodies are equipped with built-in antioxidant enzymes that search out and neutralize free radicals. Over the past decade, we have also learned that a continual supply of dietary antioxidants is necessary for disease prevention. Dietary antioxidants include vitamins C and E, beta-carotene, and selenium. And as you'll read in this chapter and the next, there are other protective antioxidant compounds in plant foods as well. You'll learn that eating plenty of fruit, vegetables, and whole grains and adding certain antioxidant supplements to your diet are smart health protection strategies.

Blood cholesterol levels rise quickly in women after menopause. According to Canadian surveys, by the age of 55, women have higher cholesterol levels than men. In fact, 43 percent of Canadian women have a total cholesterol level above 5.2 millimoles per litre, and almost one-third have high LDL levels. It seems that having high total cholesterol does not pose as much risk for women as it does for men. What's worse, according to specialists, is having both a low HDL cholesterol level and a high triglyceride level. This combination increases a woman's risk of heart disease by a factor of ten.[2]

To get a more accurate picture of your risk of heart disease, then, it's important to get *all* types of your cholesterol measured, not just the total number. If your total cholesterol is 6.5 but your HDL is high, your risk of heart disease is lessened. If, on the other hand, your doctor determines that a high LDL level accounts for most of your total value of 6.5 and at the same time your HDL is low, this would be cause for concern. You'd want to make some lifestyle changes to change the numbers for the better.

Recent research also suggests that your risk ratio—your ratio of total cholesterol to HDL cholesterol—is a better predictor of heart disease risk than LDL or HDL values alone.[3] Following is a guide to this ratio as it applies to women:

RISK RATIO* (TOTAL CHOLESTEROL:HDL CHOLESTEROL)

Below-average risk	<3.5
Average risk	3.5–5.0
Above-average risk	5–10
Greatly above-average risk	>10

*To determine your risk ratio, divide your total cholesterol value by your HDL cholesterol value.

HIGH BLOOD PRESSURE

Elevated blood pressure, or hypertension, is considered one of the "big three" risk factors for heart disease, along with high cholesterol and cigarette smoking. The higher blood pressure is above normal, the greater the risk. Arteries stiff from atherosclerosis strain as blood pulses through them. Add high blood pressure to the equation, and arteries are put under much greater stress. Stressed and strained arteries develop more lesions, and fatty plaque grows more frequently. As I explained earlier, if you already have hypertension, atherosclerosis makes your high blood pressure worse. If hardened arteries can't expand when the heart beats, blood pressure rises. This in turn leads to further damage to the arteries. And when blood flow to the kidneys slows down, and blood pressure becomes too low for these organs to function efficiently, they respond by retaining sodium to raise the pressure. Atherosclerosis and high blood pressure can be a deadly combination.

Blood pressure is created by the pressure generated by your heart as it pushes blood through your arteries. When your heart beats, the blood pressure in your arteries rises. When the heart relaxes between beats, blood pressure falls. Your blood pressure is taken with two measures: systolic pressure (the blood pressure when the heart is contracting)

EVALUATION OF BLOOD PRESSURE (mm Hg)

Blood Pressure	Systolic Blood Pressure	Diastolic
Normal	<130	<85
High-normal	130–139	80–89
Mild hypertension	140–159	90–99
Moderate hypertension	160–179	100–109
Severe hypertension	180–209	110–119
Very severe hypertension	210 or higher	120 or higher

and diastolic pressure (the blood pressure when the heart is relaxing). The higher the blood pressure levels, the harder your heart is working. If your resting blood pressure is consistently 140/90 or higher, you have high blood pressure. Doctors use the guide on page 179 to evaluate blood pressure.

More than one-third of postmenopausal women in Canada have high blood pressure. After the age of 55, hypertension is more common in women than it is in men. High blood pressure has no symptoms. The only way to determine if you have high blood pressure is to have your blood pressure checked regularly. You can then take steps to manage it and minimize the damage it can do to your heart. Have your blood pressure taken when you are relaxed, not stressed: Many of my clients have gone to their doctor, had their blood pressure measured, and come out with a high reading. Yet, two days later, when they are retested, their blood pressure is normal. This phenomenon is known as "white coat syndrome." When you're anxious (as many of us are at medical checkups), your blood pressure rises. When you relax, it returns to normal. This is why it's a good idea to have your doctor take a few readings in a row: Instead of testing just once, test three consecutive times. Chances are, you'll begin to relax after the first two tests, allowing your doctor to obtain a more accurate reading.

High blood pressure is treated by weight loss, dietary modifications, and often medication. Later in this chapter, you'll find the latest dietary strategies to help lower high blood pressure.

CIGARETTE SMOKING

It's been estimated that smoking triples a person's risk of developing heart disease. Smoking damages the lining of the arteries, increasing the likelihood of plaque formation. Inhaling cigarette smoke also produces free radicals in the body, which then damage LDL cholesterol, making it stick to the artery walls. If this weren't enough, smoking also increases blood pressure and makes blood clot formation more likely.

Among women, smoking is the number-one preventable risk factor for heart disease. Interestingly, smoking is a more important predictor of heart attack in middle-aged women than it is in men. And the longer you smoke, the greater your chances of heart disease. The Nurses' Health Study, done by Harvard researchers, found that women who started smoking before the age of 15 had a nine-fold higher risk of heart disease than women who had never smoked. The same study found that your risk of dying from heart disease decreases to the risk level of a nonsmoker 10 to 14 years after you quit.[4] So, if you smoke, the sooner you quit the better.

Women who use estrogen and smoke cigarettes have an even higher risk, as this combination increases the possibility of blood clots forming. If you take birth control pills or hormone replacement therapy and you smoke, seriously consider quitting.

DIABETES

Diabetes, a disease in which blood sugar levels persist at high levels, increases women's risk of dying from heart disease more than it does men's. A woman with diabetes is three times more likely to experience heart disease than a nondiabetic woman.[5] In fact, if a woman develops diabetes before menopause, her built-in gender protection is gone. This is because the development of fatty plaque progresses much more rapidly in diabetes. Women with diabetes also tend to have abnormal blood lipids (high LDL, low HDL, and high triglyceride levels) and high blood pressure. These three risk factors—elevated blood glucose (sugar), abnormal blood lipid levels, and high blood pressure—act synergistically, in what is known as Syndrome X, to increase heart disease risk.

BODY WEIGHT

As your body mass index (BMI) increases, so does your risk of heart disease. (To determine your BMI, see pages 105–106.) Carrying extra weight puts stress on your heart and circulatory system, as your heart works harder to pump blood throughout your body. Being overweight can also lead to high blood pressure and elevated blood cholesterol. Today, 37 percent of Canadian women aged 16 to 64 are overweight. Even worse, one-half of all women aged 55 to 64 are overweight, and 36 percent of those overweight are considered obese.[6]

Carrying excess weight around the waist is much more dangerous to your heart than having chunky thighs. The Nurses' Health Study found that women with a waist-to-hip ratio (WHR) of 0.74 or higher had a two-fold increase in heart disease risk.[7] (To determine your WHR, see pages 106–107.) According to the Nurses' Health Study, the ideal WHR is less than 0.72. Abdominal fat appears to be more active than lower body fat: when fat stores in this area are mobilized, they go directly to the liver, where they are packed into LDL molecules. Researchers are also learning that fat around the middle interferes with blood sugar and insulin levels and can increase the risk of diabetes.

HOMOCYSTEINE LEVELS

Scientists are now turning their attention to a compound called homocysteine. A high blood level of homocysteine is present in 47 percent of people who have early heart disease unexplainable by other risk factors. Evidence for the role of homocysteine in heart disease has been mounting since 1985, when a paper in the *New England Journal of Medicine* reported that 30 percent of people with premature heart attack had high blood levels of homocysteine. Since then, a number of studies have discovered that people with high homocysteine levels have a much higher risk of developing heart disease than those with normal levels. American researchers from Boston found that among 28,263 postmenopausal women, those with the highest levels of homocysteine had more than double the risk of heart attack or stroke than women with the lowest levels.[8]

Homocysteine is an amino acid our body produces naturally in the course of daily biochemical activities. Normally we convert homocysteine to other harmless amino acids with the help of B vitamins. When this conversion doesn't occur, homocysteine can accumulate in the blood and damage vessel walls, promoting the buildup of cholesterol. Homocysteine levels can accumulate as the result of either an inherited genetic defect or a B vitamin deficiency.

Doctors do not routinely measure blood homocysteine levels—not yet anyway. According to some experts in the field of heart disease, a blood test for homocysteine levels may be standard in the near future. Although it is not routinely done, the test is readily available, so you may want to discuss having one with your doctor. If you're wondering what to do, keep reading to learn what nutrition tips can keep your homocysteine level healthy.

INACTIVITY

A sedentary lifestyle is considered an independent risk factor for heart disease, meaning that even if you are free of all the other risk factors, if you don't exercise regularly, you're at a higher risk of heart disease. Sadly, 59 percent of Canadian women are sedentary. In fact, more women are inactive than men. I'm sure you've heard health professionals promote the many benefits of exercise. For starters, regular exercise helps you maintain a healthy weight. Regular aerobic exercise can lower LDL cholesterol levels and raise those of HDL cholesterol. It also strengthens the heart and blood vessels. And there's no doubt in my mind that when people exercise regularly, they tend to make healthier food choices.

I am sure it is apparent by now that you can alter or eliminate many of the risk factors discussed above. Clearly, changing your lifestyle can have a significant impact on your risk of heart disease. According to a survey done by the Heart and Stroke Foundation, Canadian women are getting a failing grade when it comes to protecting their future heart health. Up to two-thirds of women are making lifestyle choices that put them at risk—only 30 percent maintain a healthy weight, 36 percent are physically inactive, and only about one-half have talked to their doctors about their risk of heart disease.[9]

The good news is that each one of us has the ability to do something about this situation. Many of the risk factors we've been considering are influenced by what you eat. I think doctors often forget this. I can't tell you how many clients come to see me to avoid going on cholesterol-lowering medication their doctor has recommended. These women's blood tests come back high, and the physician hands them a prescription instead of sending them to a nutritionist. Luckily, I work with a number of wonderful physicians who always send their patients my way before resorting to cholesterol-lowering drugs.

It's time to take a look at what you can do to reduce your odds for heart disease. The strategies I list in the remainder of the chapter will help in a number of ways. My nutrition and herbal recommendations will help keep your blood lipids at a healthy level, prevent damage or oxidation to your LDL cholesterol, lower blood pressure, and promote a little weight loss. So let's get started!

Dietary approaches

DIETARY FAT

One of the most important strategies for eating heart healthy is to reduce your fat intake to less than 30 percent of your total calorie intake. A 2000-calorie diet, for example, translates into no more than 65 grams of fat per day. If you're following a

1200-calorie weight-loss diet, you should be consuming no more than 40 grams of fat per day. You also need to remember that when it comes to heart health, not all fats are created equal. Some fats have a strong impact on your risk, whereas others are neutral and don't affect your heart. Other fats, as you'll read below, have a beneficial effect on heart health. If your fat intake comes mainly from these healthy fats, getting 35 percent of daily calories from fat is considered healthy. There's no question that nutrition recommendations on types and amounts of dietary fat can be confusing. To clear up this confusion once and for all, here's what you need to know about fat to reduce your risk of heart disease.

Saturated fat

This type of fat is found in animal foods—meat, poultry, eggs, and all dairy products. Without a doubt, diets containing a lot of saturated fat raise your risk of heart disease. Many studies have shown that high intakes of saturated fat are linked with high levels of blood cholesterol. Saturated fat seems to inhibit the activity of LDL receptors on cells, resulting in cholesterol accumulating in the bloodstream.[10]

Foods contain many types of saturated fats, and researchers are learning that they don't all influence our blood cholesterol to the same degree. For instance, the saturated fat in dairy products raises cholesterol more than does the saturated fat in meat. And you might be pleased to know that the type of saturated fat found in chocolate (stearic acid) does not raise blood cholesterol levels. However, I don't expect you to know the types of saturated fats in foods. What's most important is to eat less saturated fat. Saturated fat should account for less than 10 percent of your daily calories. To achieve that goal, choose foods that appear on the list on page 185.

So, what does the number accompanying the statement "% MF" (percent milk fat) on dairy products mean? It refers to the amount of fat present in a certain volume of milk or weight of cheese. For example, on a package of cheddar cheese, "31% MF" indicates that there are 31 grams of fat in 100 grams of that cheese. In other words, you're getting 9 grams of fat in a 30-gram (1-oz.) serving. Feta cheese labelled "22% MF" has 6.5 grams of fat per 30-gram (1-oz.) serving. Fat in fluid milk is measured per 100 ml of milk. For example, 1% milk contains 1 gram of fat per 100 ml of milk. That translates into 2.5 grams (less than a teaspoon) in one 8-ounce (250-ml) glass.

To eat less saturated fat, look for cheese made with part skim milk (15 to 20 per-

LOWER-FAT SUBSTITUTES FOR COMMON FOODS

Food	Lower fat choices or substitutes
Milk	Skim, 1% milk fat (MF)
Yogurt	Products with 1.5% MF or less
Cheese	Products with 20% MF or less
Cottage Cheese	Products with 1% MF
Cream	Evaporated 2% or evaporated skim milk
Sour Cream	Products with 7% MF or less
Red meat	Flank steak, inside round, sirloin, eye of round, extra-lean ground beef, venison
Pork	Centre-cut pork chops, pork tenderloin, pork leg (inside round, roast), baked ham, deli ham, back bacon
Poultry	Skinless chicken breast, turkey breast, ground turkey
Egg, whole	Two egg whites (these can usually be found in your grocery store next to the fresh eggs. (See my comment on eggs in the section on dietary cholesterol, pages 189–190.)

cent MF) or skim milk (7 percent MF). Or buy naturally lower-fat cheeses such as feta and goat's cheese. Or, use smaller portions of strong-tasting cheeses. Making lower fat choices will help you eat less saturated fat. But it's also important to watch your portion sizes of these foods. When you do eat lean meat, be sure your portion size doesn't exceed 3 ounces (90 g)—the size of a deck of cards. This way you'll also stay within the serving recommendations for the entire day (see Appendix 1 for the recommended number of daily servings of each food group).

You might be wondering about butter. It *is* a concentrated source of saturated fat, but if your blood cholesterol levels are normal, there is no reason you can't include butter in your diet. Just use it sparingly. Even if your blood cholesterol levels are high, you can still use a little butter (if you're doing everything else right to lower your cholesterol, it shouldn't make a difference). Many people have made the switch to margarine because, unlike butter, it is made from vegetable oils that don't raise cholesterol. But before you spread margarine on your toast, there's something you should know about another type of fat.

Trans fat

Chances are you've heard of trans fat; if you haven't, you might have heard about "hydrogenated fat." Trans fats are formed when vegetable oils are processed into margarine or shortening. The chemical process, called hydrogenation, adds hydrogen atoms to liquid vegetable oils, making them more solid and useful to food manufacturers. Cookies, crackers, pastries, and muffins made with hydrogenated vegetable oils are more palatable and have a longer shelf life. A margarine that's made by hydrogenating a vegetable oil is firmer, like butter.

Sounds okay so far. The bad news is that, aside from destroying essential fatty acids that we need to obtain from the vegetable oils we eat, hydrogenation makes a fat become saturated *and* it forms significant amounts of *trans fat.* Consuming too much trans fat can increase your risk of heart disease by raising LDL cholesterol, lowering HDL cholesterol, and impairing blood vessel function. Remember that for a healthy heart, we want lower LDL and higher HDL levels.

Many experts believe that trans fat is worse for our cholesterol levels than saturated fat. Harvard researchers have estimated that replacing 2 percent of daily calories from trans fat with a monounsaturated fat like olive oil can reduce the risk of heart disease in women by 53 percent. The Nurses' Health Study revealed that women who had the highest intake of trans fat had a 50 percent higher risk of heart disease than women who ate the least. Foods that contributed to trans fat intake were margarine, cookies, cake, and white bread. An Italian study found similar results. Women with a medium or high intake of margarine had a 50 percent higher risk of heart attack than those who had a low intake.[11]

The first, easy step in reducing your intake of trans fat is to start reading food labels and ingredient lists.

- Look for the words "partially hydrogenated vegetable oil" and "shortening." Eat less often foods that contain them. Trans fat accounts for as much as 40 percent of the fat in foods such as French fries, fast food, doughnuts, pastries, potato chips, snack foods, and commercial cookies.
- If you eat margarine, choose one made with "nonhydrogenated" fat. Many brands state this right on the label. If it's not, add the values for polyunsaturated and monounsaturated fats listed on the package's nutrition information panel. These values should add up to at least 6 grams per 2-teaspoon (10-ml) serving for a regular margarine, 3 grams for a light margarine. If they don't, saturated and trans fats are present in high levels.

- You won't find grams of trans fat listed on nutrition labels—yet. In the meantime, look at the nutrition information panel and add up the grams of saturated, polyunsaturated, and monounsaturated fat. Compare this number with the total grams of fat cited. You may find that these numbers don't match—the total fat grams listed may be more than the total of the individual types of fats listed. The number of the missing fat grams is the value for the trans fat in the product!

New requirements for food labels became law on January 1, 2003. Among the changes to nutrition labels is that all prepackaged foods will be required to list the grams of trans fat on the nutrition facts panel. But you won't see revised labels overnight. Food manufacturers will be granted three years to phase in their new labels (small food companies will be given five years to comply). However, it's expected that some manufacturers will start putting the new labels on their products immediately. In the meantime, continue to check ingredient lists for the terms "hydrogenated," "partially hydrogenated," and "shortening."

Polyunsaturated fat

These fats are classified by scientists according to their chemical structure. Omega-6 polyunsaturated fats are found in all vegetable oils, including canola, sunflower, safflower, corn, and sesame. Omega-3 polyunsaturates are found in fish and seafood, as well as flaxseed and walnut oil. Replacing saturated fat in your diet with polyunsaturated fats will have a cholesterol-lowering effect. For instance, using a nonhydrogenated margarine made from sunflower oil instead of butter, or eating fish instead of steak, are two ways to help your reduce high blood cholesterol levels. Most of this effect is because you are eating less saturated fat, not because the polyunsaturated fats have magical properties. In fact, animal studies have found that adding polyunsaturated fat to the diet while keeping the amount of saturated fat constant does not result in cholesterol reduction.[12]

Fish and heart health   It does seem, however, that there is something special about the polyunsaturated fat in fish. Many studies have found that populations that consume fish a few times each week have lower rates of heart disease.[13] Omega-3 fats in fish can lower high levels of triglycerides, a certain type of blood fat, as well as reduce the stickiness of platelets, the cells that form blood clots in arteries. Aim to eat fish three times each week. If you already have heart disease, consider eating fish even more often than this. The American Heart Association guidelines recommend eating one fatty fish meal per day (or alternatively a fish oil supplement) to achieve an intake of omega-3 fats beneficial for people with heart disease.

For the best sources of omega-3 fats, choose oilier fish; salmon, albacore tuna, lake trout, sardines, anchovies, herring, and mackerel are good choices. If you plan to rely on tuna sandwiches to get your omega-3s, think twice. Canned tuna has very little heart-healthy oil.

Flaxseed, canola, and walnut oils   These oils are an excellent source of another type of omega-3 fat, alpha linolenic acid (ALA). Not only is this fatty acid essential to your health, it might also ward off a heart attack. In a study of almost 77,000 women, those who consumed the most ALA had a 45 percent lower risk of dying from heart disease.[14] When investigators looked at what these women were eating, they found that a higher intake of oil-and-vinegar salad dressing accounted for the ALA in their diet. The women who used vinaigrette salad dressings at least five or six times a week reduced their risk of dying from heart disease by 54 percent. The message here: A little fat is necessary for heart health. So don't be tempted to avoid oils altogether. If you choose the right ones, and use them sparingly, you just might ward off heart disease.

Monounsaturated fat

Monounsaturated fats found in olive oil, canola oil, peanut oil, avocado, and nuts can help lower elevated blood cholesterol levels. Some studies suggest that extra-virgin olive oil also helps prevent blood clots from forming and has antioxidant effects that help protect its users from heart disease.[15] If you do use olive oil, be sure to buy extra-virgin, which is darker in colour than regular olive oil. It's more expensive, but it has been processed the least and contains more protective compounds. But don't overdo it. Whether it's olive oil, margarine, or butter, the fat still has 9 calories per gram. Too much of any type of fat can cause weight gain, and this in turn can increase your blood cholesterol levels. To follow a low-fat diet, aim to consume no more than 1 or 2 table-spoons (15 to 25 ml) of added fat each day.

The Mediterranean diet and heart health

If Greek or Italian foods are your favourite fare, you might be interested to know that these cuisines can protect your heart. Recently, researchers compared the effects of the Mediterranean diet with those of the typical Western diet in 423 people who had experienced one heart attack. After 27 months, the Mediterranean diet showed striking protective effects. Heart disease–related death rates and heart attack recurrences were much lower in those who followed the Mediterranean diet rich in fruit, vegetables, grains, beans, olive oil, and fish.[16]

Follow the guidelines below to save the airfare to Italy and reap the health benefits of this diet!

Daily foods
- Rice, pasta, couscous, breads, polenta, other grains
- Fruits and vegetables
- Legumes (lentils, kidney beans, chickpeas)
- Extra-virgin olive oil
- Yogurt and cheese

A few times a week
- Fish, chicken, eggs
- Sweets

A few times a month
- Red meat, in small amounts

DIETARY CHOLESTEROL

This wax-like fatty substance is found in meat, poultry, eggs, dairy products, fish, and seafood. It's particularly plentiful in shrimp, liver, and egg yolks. While high-cholesterol diets cause high blood cholesterol in animals, this effect is not seen in humans. In fact, dietary cholesterol has little or no effect on most people's blood cholesterol. One reason for this is that our intestines absorb roughly one-half of the cholesterol we eat. The rest is excreted in the stool. Our bodies are also efficient at secreting the cholesterol we do absorb from food into bile that's stored in the gallbladder. This means that very little dietary cholesterol becomes available for transport on LDL particles. So if you're worried about eating eggs, you need not be. A recent study done at Harvard University did not find any significant association between egg intake and risk of heart disease or stroke in healthy men and women.[17] Most experts agree that eating five or six eggs a week will not negatively affect your heart health.

In spite of these built-in protective mechanisms, too much dietary cholesterol can raise LDL cholesterol levels in some people, especially people with a hereditary predisposition to high cholesterol. Health Canada recommends that we consume no more than 300 milligrams of cholesterol each day. Choosing animal foods that are low in saturated fat also helps cut down on dietary cholesterol. Here's how foods stack up when it comes to cholesterol content:

CHOLESTEROL CONTENT OF COMMON FOODS (MILLIGRAMS)

1 egg, whole	190
1 egg, white only	0
Beef sirloin, lean only, 3 oz. (90 g)	64
Calf's liver, fried, 3 oz. (90 g)	416
Chicken breast, no skin, 3 oz. (90 g)	73
Pork loin, lean only, 3 oz. (90 g)	71
Salmon, 3 oz. (90 g)	54
Shrimp, 3 oz. (90 g)	135
Butter, 2 tsp. (10 ml)	10
Milk, skim, 1 cup (250 ml)	5
Milk, 2% MF, 1 cup (250 ml)	19
Cheese, cheddar, 31% MF, 1 oz. (30 g)	31
Cheese, mozzarella, part skim, 1 oz. (30 g)	18
Cream, half and half, 12% MF, 2 tbsp. (25 ml)	12
Yogurt, 1.5% MF, 3/4 cup (175 ml)	11

Source: *Nutrient Value of Some Common Foods*. Health Canada, 1999. Adapted and reproduced with the permission of the Minister of Public Works and Government Services Canada, 2003.

SOY PROTEIN

It's clear that a daily dose of soy lowers blood cholesterol. So clear, in fact, that in October 1999 the U.S. Food and Drug Administration passed a regulation allowing manufacturers of soy foods to add a health claim to the label. Cartons of tofu, soy beverages, and veggie burgers now tell American shoppers that eating a low-fat diet containing 25 grams of soy protein daily lowers the risk of heart disease.

The soy and heart disease link became popular knowledge back in 1995, when researchers from Lexington, Kentucky, published a report in the *New England Journal of Medicine* that analyzed 38 studies on soy and cholesterol. The analysis determined that eating soy protein instead of animal protein significantly lowered high levels of LDL cholesterol and triglycerides. Since then, other studies have confirmed soy's cholesterol-lowering power. One study showed that 20 grams of soy protein taken daily significantly lowered cholesterol levels in 53 perimenopausal women who had *normal* cholesterol levels to begin with. Another study found that a high soy diet lowered LDL cholesterol by 4 percent in people with mildly elevated cholesterol levels. This same study found the effect of soy to be even more pronounced in participants with higher cholesterol levels. In these people, LDL cholesterol levels dropped by 10 percent. More recently, American researchers gave 80 women, 45 to 55 years of age, either 33 milligrams of soy isoflavones or a placebo three times daily. After four months of treatment, the women taking the isoflavones had a significant reduction in total and LDL cholesterol levels (not to mention hot flashes!).

Soy can keep your heart healthy in other ways, too. Studies show that soy raises HDL cholesterol levels, lowers blood pressure, and keeps blood vessels healthy. Soy also prevents oxidation or damage to LDL cholesterol. As I discussed above, when LDL becomes damaged by free radicals, it sticks to artery walls much more easily. In one study, American researchers found that postmenopausal women who consumed three glasses of soy beverage each day experienced a significant delay in oxidation of LDL cholesterol.[18]

The heart-protective effects of soy foods are attributed to the proteins and isoflavones (phytoestrogens) found in soybeans. When it comes to lowering cholesterol levels, it seems that you need both components. This is why studies using purified soy isoflavone supplements don't show a cholesterol-lowering effect. A daily dose of 25 grams of soy protein is routinely recommended to lower high blood cholesterol levels. But research conducted at the University of Toronto suggests that if your daily diet contains soluble fibre (see following page) and vegetable protein foods, 14 grams might be enough to lower your cholesterol.[19] And if you just want the antioxidant benefits of soy foods, experts suggest consuming 10 grams of soy protein per day. Make your meal plans armed with the following information.

SOY PROTEIN CONTENT OF SOY FOODS (GRAMS)

Soy beverage, 1 cup (250 ml)	9
Soybeans, canned, 1/2 cup (125 ml)	14
Soy nuts, 1/4 cup (50 ml)	14
Soy flour, defatted, 1/4 cup (50 ml)	13
Soy protein powder, isolate, 1 scoop (30 g)	25
Tempeh, 1/2 cup (125 ml)	16
Tofu, firm, 1/2 cup (125 ml)	19
Tofu, regular, 1/2 cup (125 ml)	10
Veggie burger, Yves Veggie Cuisine, 1	17
Veggie dog, small, Yves Veggie Cuisine, 1	11

SOLUBLE FIBRE

Plant foods contain a mixture of two types of fibre: soluble and insoluble. While both are important to your health, it's soluble fibre that can help keep your heart healthy. (Insoluble fibre found in wheat bran and other plant foods helps keep your bowels healthy.) Soluble fibre consists of plant components that either dissolve or swell in water. In plants, soluble fibres help "glue" cells together. The best food sources of these fibres include oats and oat bran, psyllium, legumes or beans, fruits, and vegetables.

Strong evidence exists to support the idea that adding soluble fibre from oats and beans to your low-fat diet significantly lowers total and LDL cholesterol levels. American researchers from Chicago studied 146 adults with high LDL cholesterol and found that adding oatmeal and oat bran to a low-fat diet lowered LDL cholesterol levels by 10 and 16 percent respectively.

Psyllium is another type of soluble fibre with cholesterol-lowering effects. An analysis of 12 studies conducted among 404 adults with high cholesterol levels revealed that a psyllium-enriched breakfast cereal, eaten as part of a low-fat diet, lowered total cholesterol levels by 5 percent and LDL cholesterol levels by 9 percent.[20]

Based on years of research showing the protective effects of oat fibre (beta glucan) and psyllium, the U.S. Food and Drug Administration now allows foods rich in these fibres to carry a health claim on their labels. Breakfast cereals and other foods that meet specific criteria (high in fibre, low in saturated fat and cholesterol) may, like foods rich in soy protein, state that they help reduce the risk of heart disease in conjunction with a low-fat diet.

Soluble fibre exerts its cholesterol-lowering effect in your intestinal tract. When these fibres reach your intestines, they attach themselves to bile acids, causing these to be excreted in the stool. Bile is a digestive aid that's released from your gallbladder after you eat. Your liver makes bile from cholesterol and sends it to your gallbladder to be stored until it's needed. This means that if a high-fibre diet is causing you to excrete more bile, your liver has to make more of it from cholesterol. The result? Lower blood cholesterol levels. But soluble fibre probably works another way, too. When unabsorbed fibre reaches your colon, intestinal bacteria degrade it; short chain fatty acids are by-products of this bacterial activity. These fatty acids then make their way to the liver, where they are able to hamper cholesterol production.

To boost your intake of soluble fibre, here are the foods you'll want to add to your diet:

FOODS HIGH IN SOLUBLE FIBRE

Breakfast cereals	Legumes	Fruits	Vegetables
All Bran Buds	Black beans	Apples	Carrots
Oat bran	Chickpeas	Cantaloupe	Green peas
Oatmeal	Kidney beans	Grapefruit	Potatoes
Psyllium-enriched cereals	Lentils	Orange	Sweet potatoes
	Navy beans	Pears	
	Soybeans	Strawberries	

If you decide to try a pysllium-rich breakfast cereal, start slowly. These cereals are a great way to get a hefty dose of soluble fibre, and I often encourage my clients with high cholesterol to add them to their breakfast routine. However, they can cause gastrointestinal upset if you're not used to them. As a rule, it takes about two weeks for the bacteria that reside in your intestine to adjust to a higher fibre intake. In the meantime, you may experience bloating and gas. So start by adding 1/4 to 1/2 cup (50 to 125 ml) of All Bran Buds to your usual cereal. Over the course of two or three weeks, work up to 1 cup (250 ml). Be sure to drink more water as you increase your fibre intake: soluble fibre needs fluid in order to do its job.

WHOLE GRAINS

When you think of whole grains, you probably think of fibre. While it's true that foods such as whole-wheat bread, whole-grain breakfast cereals, and brown rice are higher in fibre than their white counterparts, they also have other protective ingredients that might help lower the risk of heart disease.

Harvard researchers learned from the Nurses' Health Study that women who had the highest intake of whole grains had a 33 percent lower risk of heart disease than women who consumed the least. Once the researchers accounted for other risk factors such as body weight, alcohol intake, and physical activity, whole grains still reduced the risk by 25 percent. Interestingly, whole grains offered the most protection for women who had never smoked—these women had a 52 percent lower risk than smokers. The Iowa Women's Health Study also found a link between whole-grain intake and heart health. In this study of almost 35,000 postmenopausal women, those who ate two servings of whole grains each day had the lowest rates of heart disease.[21]

Experts attribute the heart protective effects of whole grains to a number of natural compounds. Whole grains are important sources of vitamin E; minerals such as zinc, selenium, copper, iron, and manganese; and phenolic compounds. All these natural compounds have antioxidant properties and may offer protection from heart disease. Antioxidants protect your LDL cholesterol from oxidation caused by free radicals. I mentioned earlier that when your LDL cholesterol becomes oxidized, it sticks to artery walls, causing a buildup of fatty plaque.

Eating foods made from whole grains means you're getting *all* parts of the grain—the outer bran layer where nearly all the fibre is, the germ layer that's rich in nutrients like vitamin E, and the endosperm that contains the starch. When whole grains are milled, scraped, refined, and heat processed into flakes, puffs, or white flour, all that's left is the starchy endosperm. This means these products offer significantly less vitamin E, B6, magnesium, potassium, zinc, fibre, the list goes on. Use the guide on page 195—a list of common whole grains and whole-grain products, and where applicable, their refined counterparts—to help you get more nutritious whole grains into your diet.

Need a change from pasta? Bored of rice with your chicken? Maybe it's time to add a little adventure—and nutrition—to your meals with these tasty whole grains.

Buckwheat   Probably familiar to many of you as a grain used in pancakes, buckwheat is the main ingredient in Japanese soba noodles. Kasha, sometimes called roasted buckwheat groats, cooks quickly and is very versatile. Try it in soups, stews, stuffing, and stir-fries. It has a nutty taste that boosts the flavour of any meal.

Bulgur   If you've eaten Middle Eastern cuisine, chances are you've encountered bulgur, or cracked whole wheat, in tabouli salad. High in iron, calcium, and fibre, it's great in pilafs, soups, and stuffings. It's another quick-cooking grain.

Kamut   This grain is related to wheat but is less likely to cause an allergic reaction. Kamut grains are about two or three times the size of wheat berries and have more fibre and protein than most grains. Kamut's chewy texture and buttery flavour make it a great addition to salads. Commercial food processors grind it into flour for use in baked goods, cereals, and pasta.

Quinoa   Sacred to the Incas, this fluffy grain is sold as a whole grain or in pasta form. It's lower in carbohydrate and higher in protein than most grains. Try it in pilafs, salads, casseroles, and stir-fries.

Spelt   Touted, like kamut, as a grain well tolerated by people with wheat allergies,

WHOLE AND REFINED GRAINS

Whole grain	Refined grain
Hulled barley	Pearled barley
Brown rice	White rice
Bulgur	Couscous, semolina, Cream of Wheat
Coarse corn meal or grits	Cornmeal
Flaxseed	
Kamut	
Oat Bran	
Oatmeal	
Quinoa	
Whole-wheat bread*	White bread
Whole-grain pasta (brown rice, kamut, quinoa, spelt, whole wheat)	Durum semolina or wheat pasta
Whole rye bread	Light rye bread
Spelt	

*When buying bread, look for the words "whole wheat flour" or "whole rye flour" on the list of ingredients. The terms "wheat flour" and "unbleached wheat flour" mean that refined wheat flour has been used.

spelt is sold as a whole grain or a flour. You can also buy spelt bread, breakfast cereal, and pasta. Try using the flour in baking and cooking. It adds a delicious nutty taste to pizza crusts and multigrain breads.

NUTS

It seems that adding a handful of nuts to your diet on a regular basis may also help keep your heart in shape. Populations that include nuts as a regular part of their diet have lower rates of heart disease. The diets of vegetarians, Seventh-Day Adventists, Mediterranean, and Asian cultures all include nuts. The Nurses' Health Study discovered that women who ate 5 ounces (150 g) of nuts each week had a 35 percent lower risk of heart attack and death from heart disease than women who never ate nuts or ate them less than once a month.

Nuts are a good source of monounsaturated fat, which can help to lower cholesterol levels when added to a healthy diet. Toronto researchers recently learned that adding 1/2 cup (125 ml) of plain almonds to the diets of men and women with high blood cholesterol resulted in a 9.4 percent reduction of LDL cholesterol levels. The protective effect of nuts may also be due to ingredients similar to those found in whole grains. Nuts and seeds are also rich sources of the potent antioxidant vitamin E and many important minerals. And, of course, nuts are good sources of essential fatty acids (alpha-linolenic acid and linoleic acid), as well as of dietary fibre. A French study found that a high level of HDL cholesterol was associated with a diet rich in walnuts.[22]

While researchers continue to try to determine exactly how nuts work to reduce the risk of heart disease, it makes sense to add them to your diet. Go easy though; eating too many nuts each day can lead to weight gain—consider that 1 cup (250 ml) of nuts packs about 850 calories and 18 teaspoons (90 ml) of oil! Keep your serving size to one ounce (30 g)—about 1/4 cup (50 ml). Aim to get nuts into your diet five times a week. Here's how you might do that:

- Toss a handful of peanuts into an Asian-style stir-fry.
- Nuts are great with greens. Stir-fry collard greens with cashews and 1 teaspoon (5 ml) of sesame oil; add walnuts to your green or spinach salad; try a little walnut oil in your next salad dressing (use half olive oil and half walnut oil).
- Mix sunflower or pumpkin seeds into a bowl of hot cereal or yogurt.
- Snack on a small handful of almonds with a few dried apricots.
- Serve your casserole with a sprinkling of mixed nuts.

TEA AND FLAVONOIDS

You've probably never thought of your afternoon cup of orange pekoe as a source of antioxidants that can protect your heart. Well, according to researchers, it's true—green and black teas may lower the risk of heart attack. One recent study investigated the effects of tea, coffee, and decaffeinated coffee on heart attack risk. Compared with non–tea drinkers, those who enjoyed at least one cup a day had a 44 percent lower risk of heart attack. In this study, coffee showed no protective (or harmful) effects.

Another study from the Netherlands looked at tea intake in men and women over 55 years old. The researchers found that tea had significant protective effects. The more tea consumed, the lower the risk of atherosclerosis. Drinking one to two cups of tea each day was associated with a 46 percent lower risk of severe atherosclerosis, and drinking more than four cups a day lowered the risk by 60 percent. This study found the protective effect of tea to be stronger in women than men.[23]

Tea leaves contain dietary compounds called flavonoids. Hundreds of different flavonoids have been identified in plants; the ones in tea are called catechins. You'll find catechins in green tea, black tea, and oolong tea, but not herbal teas. This is because herbal teas are not made from the leaves of the tea plant but from the roots, leaves, stems, flowers, and fruits of other plants that do not contain catechins.

A daily cup or two of tea can do more than keep your arteries healthy. You'll read in Chapter 13 about how tea might help reduce your risk of breast cancer too. The following suggestions will help you incorporate tea into your daily diet:

- Replace that afternoon coffee with a mug of tea.
- Instead of drinking soft drinks, try iced tea. Make your own to avoid the large amounts of sugar found in commercial brands.
- Try flavoured black tea—Earl Grey, orange spice, apricot, raspberry, and black currant are a few of my favourites.
- Try a chai latte at your local coffee shop. It's a hot drink made with tea, milk, and spices. Again, these drinks tend to be sweet. Ask that less syrup or sugar than usual be added.

Other ways to boost your flavonoid intake

If you've starting drinking more tea to get heart protective flavonoids, that's great. But don't stop there. Research suggests you should also be reaching for other foods rich in flavonoids. A study done in the Netherlands found that the risk of dying from heart disease was 48 percent lower in men who had the highest intake of dietary flavonoids (I'm afraid this study didn't look at women). Tea, onions, and apples were the flavonoid-rich foods that appeared to offer these men protection. The Iowa Women's Health Study also found a protective effect from a flavonoid-rich diet. Among these 34,000 post-menopausal women, those who consumed the most flavonoids from food had a 38 per-cent lower risk of dying from heart disease. In this study, broccoli was strongly linked to a reduced risk.[24] It seems you can't go wrong with plenty of vegetables!

ALCOHOL

Those of you who enjoy a glass of wine with dinner might be doing your heart a favour. Many studies have found that a moderate intake of alcohol reduces the risk of heart disease. The Nurses' Health Study determined that, compared with nondrinkers, women who consumed one to six drinks a week had a 12 to 17 percent lower risk of dying from heart disease. Women who drank more than six drinks a week had a slightly higher risk of death from heart disease.

Scientists believe that alcohol may work in three ways to protect the heart. First, drinking alcohol, whether it's wine, beer, or liquor, raises the level of HDL cholesterol. A Boston study found that men and women who regularly consumed a few alcoholic drinks had higher levels of HDL cholesterol and a lower risk of heart attack.[25] Second, alcohol may also reduce blood clotting; excessive clotting, as discussed, is part of the process of heart disease. Before you get too excited, though, you should know that the protective effects of alcohol are most apparent in people over the age of 50 and in those with more than one risk factor for heart disease. If you're a healthy, premenopausal woman, a daily drink probably won't do much for your heart.

Third, some evidence exists to support the theory that antioxidants in wine, especially red wine, may help keep LDL cholesterol healthy and reduce blood clotting. This is one explanation for the French Paradox—that people living in France have much lower rates of heart disease than North Americans, even though they have the same risk factors we do. Some believe that the French are protected by their daily intake of red wine.

Despite the positive research findings, I'm not advising you to consume a couple of glasses of wine a day. There are too many negative health effects associated with a mod-erate alcohol intake (one to two drinks daily). For starters, light to moderate drinking increases the risk of breast cancer (Chapter 13 tells you more about this). And if you're suffering through perimenopausal symptoms such as hot flashes, mood swings, and insomnia, alcohol will only make you feel worse. Here are my recommendations regarding alcohol:

- If you drink now, keep your intake to no more than two drinks a day, preferably one.

- If you are a nondrinker, don't start now. I believe it's a healthier way to go and, as you can see by now, there are plenty of other nutrition strategies you can put in place to reduce the odds of heart disease.

DASH FOR HEALTH

I promised you earlier that I'd give you strategies for lowering high blood pressure. Many of the recommendations already mentioned in this chapter will help lower elevated blood pressure at the same time as they work to keep your cholesterol levels healthy—eating a low-fat diet, drinking alcohol in moderation, and maintaining a healthy weight are all important strategies for keeping blood pressure normal. In addition, there are some other modifications you should consider making to your diet and lifestyle if you want to keep your blood pressure healthy and your risk of heart disease down.

Much of this advice comes from the Dietary Approaches to Stop Hypertension research study—DASH for short—an eight-week trial that measured the effects of diet on blood pressure in 459 adults. Researchers gave participants one of three diets: 1) a control diet that contained low amounts of fruit and vegetables (3.6 servings a day) and dairy products (0.5 servings a day); 2) a diet high in fruits and vegetables (8 to 10 servings a day) and; 3) a combination diet high in fruits and vegetables with added low-fat dairy products (2 servings a day). All diets provided the same amounts of sodium and a maximum of two alcoholic drinks per day.

When it came to lowering blood pressure, the combination diet gave the best results. People on this diet who had mild hypertension achieved a reduction in blood pressure similar to that obtained by drug treatment.[26] What's more, a second study revealed that reducing the salt content of the DASH diet lowered blood pressure even more.

If you have high blood pressure and would like to follow the DASH diet, use the following as your guide:

EATING TO LOWER BLOOD PRESSURE

Food group	Number of servings* per day
Whole-grain foods	7–8
Vegetables	4–5
Fruits	4–5
Low-fat/nonfat dairy products	2
Meat, poultry, fish	4–6 oz. (120–180 g) or less
Legumes, nuts, seeds	4–5 servings per week
Added fats	3
Sweets	1 serving per week

*For serving size information, refer to Appendix 2

Here are a few more strategies that will help you maintain healthy blood pressure:

- Don't smoke. Every cigarette you smoke raises your blood pressure.
- Limit your alcohol intake to no more than two drinks daily.
- Limit sodium intake. To see where we get most of our sodium, refer to pages 147–149.
- Get regular exercise. A fitness program of brisk walking can help lower blood pressure.

Vitamins and minerals

B VITAMINS

The B vitamins won't lower your cholesterol, but they will help keep your homocysteine level down. I told you earlier that a high level of homocysteine is associated with a higher risk of heart attack. To prevent homocysteine from accumulating and damaging blood vessels, the body uses three B vitamins to convert it into other harmless compounds. Folate, vitamin B6, and vitamin B12 are needed for normal homocysteine metabolism; without them, homocysteine levels rise.

One of the simplest strategies for lowering elevated homocysteine levels, then, is to boost your intake of B vitamins. Harvard researchers proved this point when they studied 80,000 women for 14 years and found that those who consumed the most folate and vitamin B6 had a 45 percent lower risk of heart disease than those women who consumed the least.[27] Among those women who got plenty of B vitamins in their diet, the risk of heart disease was also lower if they regularly took a multivitamin and mineral supplement, a major source of folate and B6. Here's how to get more Bs into your daily diet.

FOOD SOURCES OF THE B VITAMINS

B vitamin	Recommended dietary allowance (RDA)	Best food sources
Folate	400 micrograms (0.4 mg)	Spinach, orange juice, lentils, wheat germ, asparagus, broccoli, leafy greens, whole grains
Vitamin B6	1.3–1.5 milligrams	Whole grains, bananas, potatoes, legumes, fish, meat, poultry
Vitamin B12	2.4 micrograms	Meat, poultry, fish, dairy products, eggs, fortified soy and rice milk

What about a B vitamin supplement?

I just told you that a daily multiple vitamin offered women in the Nurses' Health Study a little more protection. It's also true that meeting the daily requirement for folate (called folic acid when it's in a supplement) is a challenge for many people. The top three food sources are spinach (262 micrograms per cup [250 ml] cooked), lentils (357 micrograms per cup [250 ml] cooked), and orange juice (109 micrograms per cup [250 ml]). If you don't eat these foods every day, be sure to eat plenty of other folate-rich foods.

For those of you who have difficulty eating a varied diet, I recommend taking a good-quality multivitamin and mineral supplement to ensure you're getting your daily B vitamins. It will provide 100 percent or more of the recommended daily amount of each B vitamin. If you're over 50, you should be getting your B12 from a supplement anyway. This is because, as I mentioned earlier, as we age, we become less efficient at producing stomach acid, which is necessary for B12 to be absorbed from food. If you're a vegan and don't consume animal foods or fortified beverages, you won't be getting any vitamin B12 from your diet—yet another reason to take a supplement. Use the following criteria when choosing a multivitamin:

- It offers 0.4 to 1.0 milligrams of folic acid (folate).
- It offers enough iron. Premenopausal women should choose a product with 15–18 milligrams. Postmenopausal women have lower iron requirements and can choose a multi containing 8 milligrams or less.
- It contains beta carotene, vitamin A, and vitamins D, B1, B2, B6, B12. Biotin and pantothenic acid aren't important since they're easily found in food.
- It contains iron, copper, zinc, magnesium, iodine, selenium, and chromium. Don't worry if it doesn't contain phosphorus or potassium, as these minerals are easily obtained through the diet. As for calcium, you can't get enough from a multivitamin. If you need supplemental calcium, you'll have to take that separately.
- If you're looking for more B vitamins than a regular multi gives you, choose a high-potency formula that contains from 30 to 75 milligrams of most of the B vitamins. One word of caution: The B vitamin niacin may cause flushing of the face and chest when it's taken in doses greater than 35 milligrams (this reaction is easily avoided by taking your supplement just after a meal). While this symptom is harmless and goes away within 20 minutes, some people find it uncomfortable. If you want to avoid the flushing response, look for a formula that contains no more than 35 milligrams of niacin. Or choose one containing *niacinamide*, a form of niacin that doesn't cause flushing.

  To boost your B intake, have your multivitamin with a glass of orange juice each morning, order a spinach salad with your whole-grain sandwich at lunch, or throw some canned lentils into your pasta sauce at dinner. That doesn't sound so bad does it?

Take your supplement with food to allow for better breakdown and absorption of the pill. Plan to take your supplement at the meal you are most likely to remember it.

VITAMIN C

Chances are, you're familiar with this vitamin's role in treating the common cold. But you might be surprised to learn that vitamin C could help reduce your risk of a heart attack. Many studies have reported links between high dietary intakes of this vitamin, high blood levels of vitamin C, and a lower risk of heart disease. Finnish scientists measured 13 risk factors for heart attack in a large group of men and found that low blood levels of vitamin C were the strongest predictor of heart disease. Back home in North America, researchers observed an 11 percent reduction in rates of heart disease with every 0.5 milligram per decilitre rise in blood vitamin C among 6624 men and women. In fact, in the men and women with the highest blood vitamin C levels, rates of heart disease were 27 percent lower than in those study participants with the lowest vitamin C levels.

It is well accepted that the level of vitamin C in your bloodstream is a good indicator of the amount of vitamin C in your diet. A Portuguese study of 194 adults determined that, compared with those individuals with marginal vitamin C intakes, those who consumed the most vitamin C had an 80 percent lower risk of heart attack.[28]

Vitamin C's claim to fame lies in its ability to act as an antioxidant. The vitamin is able to neutralize harmful free-radical molecules that damage your LDL cholesterol (for a more detailed explanation of what free radicals are and how they affect you, read "Antioxidants: Disease Fighters of the New Millennium" on pages 177–178). As a result, LDL cholesterol is less likely to accumulate on artery walls. But vitamin C may

VITAMIN C CONTENT OF FOODS (MILLIGRAMS)

Cantaloupe, 1/4 medium	56
Orange, 1 medium	70
Orange juice, fresh, 1 cup (250 ml)	131
Grapefruit, red or pink, 1/2	47
Kiwi, 1 large	68
Mango, 1	49
Strawberries, raw, 1 cup (250 ml)	89
Broccoli, raw, 1 spear	141
Brussels sprouts, cooked, 1/2 cup (125 ml)	50
Cauliflower, raw, 1/2 cup (125 ml)	38
Potato, baked with skin, 1	27
Red pepper, raw, 1/2 cup (125 ml)	95
Tomato juice, 1 cup (250 ml)	47

Source: *Nutrient Value of Some Common Foods*. Health Canada, 1999. Adapted and reproduced with the permission of the Minister of Public Works and Government Services Canada, 2003.

protect your heart in other ways as well. It may raise levels of HDL cholesterol and, at the same time, lower LDL cholesterol. And studies suggest the vitamin may also help to inhibit the formation of blood clots by reducing the stickiness of platelets.[29]

The daily recommended vitamin C intake for adult women is 75 milligrams (smokers need an additional 35 milligrams). This amount is easy to get from your diet. If your diet needs an infusion of vitamin C, the foods listed on page 203 are your best bets.

What about a vitamin C supplement?

For those of you who don't eat at least two foods rich in vitamin C each day, taking a supplement is a good idea. Keep in mind, though, that fruits and vegetables contain many other natural chemicals that may work together with vitamin C to keep you healthy. So even if you do take a vitamin C pill each day, I recommend that you also try to add foods rich in vitamin C to your diet. Here's what you need to know about vitamin C supplements:

- If you're looking for the most C for your money, choose a supplement labelled "Ester-C." Lab studies have found this form of vitamin C to be more available to the body.
- If you don't like to swallow pills and prefer a chewable supplement, make sure it contains calcium ascorbate or sodium ascorbate. These forms of vitamin C are less acidic and corrode your tooth enamel less.
- Take a 500-milligram supplement once or twice a day. There's little point in swallowing much more at one time since your body can only use about 200 milligrams at one time. If you want to take more, split your dose over the day.

VITAMIN E

Data showing that vitamin E protects against coronary heart disease date back to the 1970s. As scientists began to understand the antioxidant effects of the vitamin, more and more reports emerged suggesting a beneficial cardiovascular effect. Most of the evidence indicates that vitamin E is more effective at preventing heart disease from establishing itself in the first place than it is at treating it. A number of studies have shown that vitamin E supplements prevent heart attacks in men and women. The relationship between vitamin E and the heart was made famous in 1993 by two reports in the *New England Journal of Medicine.* In one of these, a large study of American nurses, women who took 100 international units (IU) of supplemental vitamin E for two years had a 41 percent lower risk of heart attack than nonsupplement users. In 1996, a Canadian study reported that the use of vitamin supplements, especially of vitamin E, was associated with a reduced risk of heart attack among 2313 French-Canadian men.

Whether vitamin E can help prevent a heart attack if you already have heart disease remains to be seen. The Cambridge Heart Antioxidant Study gave people with heart disease 800 IU or 400 IU of vitamin E daily for one year. The researchers determined that vitamin E use lowered the risk of fatal and nonfatal heart attacks by 47 percent.[30] However, other studies have found no benefit.

Recently, a report in the November 2002 issue of the *Journal of the American Medical Association* suggested that vitamin E (and vitamin C) does more harm than good in women taking hormone replacement therapy. This study looked at the effects of vitamin E and C, either alone or in combination with HRT, in 423 postmenopausal women with existing heart disease. The researchers measured narrowing of the arteries and found that, compared with women taking the placebo pills, artery narrowing was the same or slightly worse for women taking HRT and also for women taking the vitamin therapy. Rates of death and nonfatal heart attacks were also higher for both groups of women, compared with women taking the placebo pills.[31]

While these results suggest that antioxidant vitamins do not improve the course of heart disease and may be slightly harmful, it is important to know that none of these findings was statistically significant. This means that the findings could have occurred by chance alone. Based on the evidence to date, we certainly can't say that a vitamin E supplement is beneficial for people with heart disease. On the other hand, research does suggest that vitamin E—from foods and supplements—reduces the risk of developing heart disease in the first place.

Vitamin E is often referred to as a lipid antioxidant. Once consumed, vitamin E makes its way to the liver, where it is incorporated into cell membranes and carrier molecules, such as the lipoproteins that transport cholesterol. It is in these carrier molecules that vitamin E works to protect the lipids (fats) from damage by free radicals. Vitamin E may also inhibit blood clot formation and preserve the health of the blood vessels that feed the heart.

The current recommended daily intake of vitamin E is 22 IU (15 mg) per day. Wheat germ, nuts, seeds, vegetable oils, whole grains, and kale are all good sources. These foods contain vitamin E along with alpha-linolenic acid, an essential fatty acid which, as I mentioned earlier, might help reduce your risk of heart disease.

What about a vitamin E supplement?

Even if you boost your daily intake of foods rich in vitamin E, you still won't come close to getting 100 IU, the amount deemed to offer protection in the study of nurses mentioned above. For this reason, you must rely on a supplement. To help you choose the right vitamin E supplement, consider these suggestions:

- Start with a dosage of 400 IU per day. If you're healthy, there's not much evidence that supports taking more than this. If you have heart disease, some evidence suggests that 800 IU per day is beneficial.
- Buy a "natural source" vitamin E supplement. Although the body absorbs both synthetic and natural vitamin E equally well, your liver prefers the natural form. It incorporates more natural vitamin E into lipoprotein carrier molecules.
- If you're on blood-thinning medication such as warfarin (Coumadin), don't take vitamin E without first consulting your doctor, as the vitamin has slight anticlotting properties.

LYCOPENE

If you want to add another dietary antioxidant to your dinner plate, consider lycopene. Scientists are only now discovering this compound's role in disease prevention. You might be interested to know that not only is lycopene being studied for its role in heart disease prevention but also for its potential as an anticancer agent (lycopene may help fight cancers of the prostate, lung, and cervix).

Lycopene is a cousin of beta-carotene, the antioxidant nutrient found in carrots. It turns out that, compared with beta-carotene, lycopene is twice as potent an antioxidant. Lycopene is found in red-coloured fruits and vegetables. It's the pigment that gives these foods their bright colour. It also protects these plants from disease. Tomatoes are the richest source of lycopene, but it's found in pink grapefruit, watermelon, guava, and apricots, too.

Researchers have observed a relationship between the amount of lycopene in a person's blood and body fat stores and that person's risk of developing heart disease. A study looking at participants from 10 European countries reported that men with marginal lycopene stores had a 52 percent increased risk of heart attack compared with those individuals with the highest body stores.[32]

As an antioxidant, lycopene provides yet another dietary defence mechanism against free-radical damage to LDL cholesterol. Toronto researchers studied the effect of dietary lycopene in 19 healthy adults. A diet supplemented with tomato products doubled lycopene blood levels and significantly reduced free-radical damage to LDL cholesterol. Lycopene may also lower the level of LDL cholesterol by hampering its production in the liver. One small study found that a 60-milligram lycopene supplement taken for three months was able to lower LDL levels by 14 percent.[33]

While more work needs to be done to unravel the precise role lycopene plays in heart health, there's no reason to wait for the research to be completed before taking steps to get a good supply in your daily diet—foods containing lycopene are healthy for all sorts of other reasons, anyway. Based on the research that has been conducted, it appears than an intake of 5 to 7 milligrams daily offers protection. And that's easy to get if you eat heat-processed tomato products.

LYCOPENE CONTENT OF FOODS (MILLIGRAMS)

Tomato, raw, 1 small	0.8–3.8
Tomatoes, cooked, 1 cup (250 ml)	9.25
Tomato sauce, 1/2 cup (125 ml)	3.1
Tomato paste, 2 tbsp. (25 ml)	8.0
Tomato juice, 1 cup (250 ml)	12.5–29.0
Ketchup, 2 tbsp. (25 ml)	3.1–4.2
Apricots, dried, 10 halves	0.3
Grapefruit, pink, 1/2	4.2
Papaya, 1 whole	6.2–16.5
Watermelon, 1 slice, 10 in. (25 cm) × 3/4 in. (2 cm)	8.5–26.4

As you can easily see from the list above, heat-processed tomato products are the best source of lycopene. It's also easier for your body to absorb lycopene from these foods. Even though one fresh tomato packs up to 4 milligrams of lycopene, your body doesn't absorb it all. Eat the equivalent amount of canned tomato and you'll absorb more lycopene. Here's another tip to help you increase the amount of lycopene your body absorbs: Add a little olive oil to your pasta sauce. Lycopene is a fat-soluble compound and so it's better absorbed in the presence of a little fat.

What about a lycopene supplement?

If you're looking for a lycopene boost, all you really have to do is add a glass of low-sodium tomato juice to your lunch. However, lycopene supplements are available in health food stores and drug stores. If you opt for a supplement, I recommend that you choose a brand made with either Lyc-O-Mato or LycoRed extract. These extracts, produced in Israel, are derived from whole tomatoes. They are also the extracts that have been used in clinical studies. Most supplements offer 5 milligrams of lycopene per tablet, so one a day is all you need.

COENZYME Q10

Here's an antioxidant that you may not have heard about. Coenzyme Q10 (CoQ10) was discovered back in 1957 at the University of Wisconsin. Today, believe it or not, it's one of the six top-selling pharmacological agents in Japan. Coenzyme Q10 is also known as ubiquinone, a name derived from the word "ubiquitous"—because it's found in all plant and animal cells.

If you haven't heard about CoQ10, it's probably because it is not considered a nutrient; there's no daily recommended intake for this substance. Our cells form CoQ10 with the help of vitamin B6 and an amino acid called tyrosine (amino acids are the building blocks of proteins). As we age, our CoQ10 levels decline.

You should be familiar with this compound for two reasons. First, it is an antioxidant and may prevent free-radical damage to LDL cholesterol. In the liver, CoQ10 is packaged into LDL cholesterol molecules and, from there, transported on LDL carriers to other parts of the body. As a part of the LDL particle, CoQ10 is able to neutralize harmful free radicals that attack LDL cholesterol. In fact, CoQ10 levels in your blood may represent the amount of oxidative stress your body is regularly faced with. One study found that, compared with healthy individuals, CoQ10 levels were lower in patients with high cholesterol and in those who smoked. CoQ10 levels were the highest in younger people.[34]

If you're taking medication for high blood cholesterol, you might also consider taking a CoQ10 supplement. This is because the so-called "statin" drugs (such as Mevacor,

Zocor, Pravachol, Lescol, and Lipitor) have been shown to cause a significant reduction in blood CoQ10 levels. The higher the drug dose taken, the lower CoQ10 levels fall.[35]

If you have heart disease, CoQ10 may help keep your LDL and HDL cholesterol levels within the normal range. In studies in India, patients were given 60 milligrams of CoQ10 twice daily. Not only did cholesterol levels improve but there was also a reduction in complications during the first 28 days after a heart attack.[36]

Studies have used anywhere from 60 to 120 milligrams of CoQ10 per day. The supplement is well tolerated and no serious side effects have ever been reported with long-term use. Laboratory studies do indicate that supplements containing CoQ10 in an oil base are more available to the body.

Herbal remedies

GARLIC (ALLIUM SATIVUM)
Garlic contains many different sulphur compounds. One in particular, S-allyl cysteine (SAC), appears to lower total cholesterol, LDL cholesterol, and triglycerides, and raise levels of HDL cholesterol. SAC is present in small amounts in raw garlic, but its concentration increases when garlic is aged. The scientific studies that show a positive effect have used an aged garlic extract (Kyolic brand) to achieve a cholesterol reduction. Aged garlic extract contains many different sulphur compounds, but research points to SAC as the compound with the most biological activity.

One American study from Brown University School of Medicine gave 41 men with high cholesterol nine aged garlic capsules (for a total of 7.2 grams) or placebo pills daily for six months. Those taking the garlic tended to show a 7 percent lowering of total cholesterol levels, a 4.6 percent lowering of LDL levels, and a 5.5 percent reduction in blood pressure. Other studies have found 900 milligrams of dried garlic powder in capsule form to be effective at reducing levels of blood cholesterol.[37]

While the findings on other forms of garlic have been less consistent, some studies have shown positive results with garlic powder capsules and fresh garlic.

Garlic may reduce the risk of heart disease in a number of ways:
- It inhibits cholesterol production in the liver.
- It lowers blood triglyceride levels.

- It thins the blood and reduces the stickiness of platelets.
- It acts as an antioxidant and prevents damage or oxidation to LDL cholesterol (many studies have found SAC in aged garlic extract to significantly inhibit free-radical damage to LDL cholesterol).
- It lowers blood pressure.

When it comes to fresh garlic, we don't yet know the optimal intake needed for heart health. Many scientists agree that as little as one-half clove each day will offer health benefits. Most people can take one or two cloves a day (about 3 to 6 grams raw garlic) without any problems. Some people, however, are sensitive to garlic. The oil soluble compounds in fresh garlic account for its potential to upset the stomach and to cause that wonderful garlic smell.

I encourage you to use more garlic in your cooking. Add it to sauces, soups, casseroles, and raw to salad dressings. By using raw, cooked, and, if you choose, an aged garlic supplement, you get a variety of protective sulphur compounds. You should also know that although raw garlic contains very little SAC, a recent study from Penn State University found that if you let crushed garlic sit at room temperature for 10 minutes before cooking with it, more beneficial allyl sulphur compounds will be formed.[38]

What about a garlic supplement?

Scientific research points to aged garlic extract as the supplement of choice because of its higher concentration of SAC. (Another plus: aged garlic extract supplements will not cause an odour.) Generally, experts recommend taking from one to nine capsules daily (take one to three at a time, with a meal). Because garlic can thin the blood, it should not be used if you are taking blood-thinning medications such as warfarin (Coumadin). If you're taking an aspirin a day, make sure you inform your physician that you have started taking garlic.

GUGGUL

Although not technically an herbal remedy, this plant-based product has a long tradition of use in Ayurvedic medicine, a traditional medicine of India. Only recently has it made its way to the Western world. Today you'll find supplements of guggul, or guggulipid, in health food stores. These products are made of myrrh, a resin from the bark of the *Commiphora mukul* plant.

Guggul's claim to fame is its cholesterol- and triglyceride-lowering ability. Studies conducted in India have demonstrated that guggul can significantly lower these blood fats. One study measured the effect of adding 50 milligrams of guggulipid twice daily to a low-fat, high-fibre diet in 61 patients with high cholesterol levels. All participants followed a cholesterol-lowering diet for 12 weeks, during which time LDL cholesterol and triglycerides fell. For the next 12 weeks, participants continued their diet, but half of them were given guggul and the remaining participants were given a placebo capsule. At the end of the study, those taking guggul were doing significantly better than the participants on placebo. The addition of the resin reduced both LDL cholesterol and triglycerides another 12 percent.[39]

If you have high blood cholesterol and you want to add guggul to your cholesterol-lowering regime, you should be aware that it has not been well studied. We know very little about its safety or long-term efficacy (in fact, I had difficulty finding much information at all about the product). For this reason, many herbalists don't recommend its use. I have included it in my book only because it is becoming widely available in health food stores and I've recently had a number of clients ask me about the product. If you do decide to try guggul, buy a product that states the amount of guggulsterone on the label. According to some experts, 25 milligrams of guggulsterone taken three times daily is the effective dose.

THE bottom LINE...

Leslie's recommendations for reducing your risk of heart disease

1 To keep your cholesterol levels in the healthy range, reduce your intake of saturated fat. Buy low-fat milk products: skim or 1 percent milk fat (MF) milk, yogurt with 1.5 percent MF or less, and cheese with 20 percent MF or less. Choose lean cuts of meat and poultry such as inside round, flank steak, sirloin, pork tenderloin, and chicken or turkey breast. And use butter sparingly.
2 To eat less trans fat, avoid as much as possible foods that contain partially hydrogenated vegetable oils and shortening. If you use margarine, choose one labelled "nonhydrogenated" or make sure that grams of polyunsaturated and monounsaturated fats add up to 6 grams or more per 2-teaspoon (10-ml) serving.

3   Be sure to include the heart healthy omega-3 fats (a type of polyunsaturated fat) in your diet. Aim to eat oily fish, such as salmon, lake trout, sardines, anchovies, herring, and mackerel, three times a week.

4   To increase your intake of alpha-linolenic acid, a member of the omega-3 family, use flaxseed oil, walnut oil, and canola oil. Also aim to include a 1/4 cup (50 ml) of nuts in your diet up to five times a week.

5   If you use olive oil, buy extra-virgin. It's been processed the least and contains the most antioxidant compounds.

6   If your cholesterol levels are in the normal range, feel free to eat an egg up to six times a week.

7   If your cholesterol levels are high, add 14 to 25 grams of soy protein to your diet each day.

8   Every day, include a source of soluble fibre in your diet. Foods like psyllium-enriched breakfast cereals, oatmeal, and oat bran do lower elevated cholesterol in conjunction with a low-fat diet, and they also help sustain your energy levels for a longer period of time.

9   When it comes to buying breads, cereals, rice, and pasta, always choose whole-grain products.

10 Drink a cup (or more) of tea as part of your daily diet. Tea contains catechins, antioxidant compounds that protect LDL cholesterol.

11 If you drink alcohol, limit your intake to no more than one alcoholic beverage per day.

12 Boost your intake of B vitamins to help keep your homocysteine levels down. Food sources of B12, B6, and folate can be found on page 201 and in earlier chapters. To ensure you are meeting your needs, take a daily multivitamin and mineral supplement or try a B-complex supplement.

13 Eat at least one food rich in vitamin C each day. As an important dietary antioxidant, vitamin C protects your LDL cholesterol from damage caused by free-radical molecules. If you're concerned that you are not getting enough vitamin C, add 500 or 600 milligrams of Ester-C to your supplement regime.

14 For even more antioxidant protection, add vitamin E to your daily diet. Wheat germ, nuts and seeds, and kale are good food sources. To get the amount of vitamin E found protective in the research, take a daily vitamin E supplement (400 or 800 IU).

15 Each day include a source of lycopene, a cousin of beta-carotene. Just like vitamins C and E, lycopene is an antioxidant and may even help lower high blood cholesterol. Heat-processed tomato products are the best food sources; see page 207 for a list of others. If you want to take a lycopene supplement, buy a brand containing Lyc-O-Mato or LycoRed extract.

16 If you're currently taking "statin" drugs to lower your cholesterol (see page 208), take 60 to 120 milligrams of coenzyme Q10 (CoQ10) daily. These drugs lower your body's CoQ10 levels, and CoQ10 is yet another important antioxidant.

17 To get more heart protective sulphur compounds, increase your intake of garlic, both raw and cooked. Use one-half to one clove each day in cooking. If your cholesterol levels are high, consider taking aged garlic extract (it's odourless, too!).Take one to two capsules (300 to 600 mg) up to three times daily with meals. If you are on blood-thinning medication, be sure to check with your physician or pharmacist for possible side effects or interactions.

18 If you have a high cholesterol level and you're wondering whether you should take guggul, or guggulipid, be wary. Few studies have been done to assess this product's safety or long-term efficacy. Based on what is known, the effective dose may be 25 milligrams of guggulsterone three times daily.

Reducing your risk of breast cancer

"There are only two types of women today: women who have breast cancer and women who are afraid they are going to get breast cancer."

13

The thought of breast cancer probably scares women more than the spectre of any other type of cancer. With menopause the fear often becomes magnified. Most of us know that the risk of developing cancer increases with age, and we are also concerned about hormone replacement therapy and its possible effect on our breasts. As with any other disease, some things encourage cancer and other things discourage it, and our knowledge of factors influencing cancer in general, and breast cancer in particular, is growing steadily. I hope that after you read this chapter you will feel ready to take a proactive approach to reducing your cancer risk. As you will see, there is plenty of action you can take.

Breast cancer statistics

Breast cancer is the most common type of cancer among Canadian women. The Canadian Cancer Society estimated that 20,500 new cases of breast cancer would develop in 2002, representing 30 percent of all cancers (official figures won't be released until later in the year 2003). Breast cancer deaths in Canada in 2002 were estimated at 5400, accounting for 17 percent of all cancer deaths in the country (lung cancer tops the list, followed by breast, then colon, cancer). Sadly, 15 Canadian women die every day from breast cancer. But the good news is that the death rate from breast cancer has decreased by 10 percent since 1986. This is largely because more and more women are having mammograms, allowing for earlier detection (more on mammograms later in this chapter).

Most women want to know what their risk of developing this disease is, and what they can do to prevent it. The following table shows you the risk of developing breast cancer by a certain age.

LIFETIME BREAST CANCER RISK

Age	Risk
25 years	less than 1 in 1000
50 years	1 in 63
75 years	1 in 15
90 years	1 in 9

These numbers mean that by the age of 50, 1 in every 63 women (1.5 percent) will get breast cancer. By the age of 90, 1 in every 9 women will get the disease (11 percent). As you read these numbers, keep in mind that statistical risks can't be applied to you as an individual. They represent the average risk of the entire population of Canadian women. If you have certain risk factors for breast cancer, such as a family history of breast cancer or a poor diet, these numbers underestimate your risk. Conversely, if you have no risk factors at all for the disease, the numbers overestimate your chances of getting breast cancer.

At this point, you're probably wondering what factors can increase your odds of getting breast cancer. But before we get to that, I want take you through a short pathology (the study of diseases) course. If you understand the cancer process, it might help ease your worry that cancer is an inevitable disease.

Cancer 101

Simply put, cancer is a disease in which abnormal cells grow out of control. When enough of these cells accumulate, a tumour forms. If the cancer cells are able to break away from the tumour, they can circulate throughout the body and take up residence in another organ, a process called metastasis. But let's go back to the earliest steps in cancer development.

Cancer begins at the cellular level. When we are healthy, our body cells divide every day in order to repair damaged tissues, replace old cells, and grow new tissue. Normal cell growth and division is regulated by internal controls. For instance, if you cut yourself, your body will release messenger chemicals to tell cells in the wounded area to quickly divide and make new cells. Certain receptors on your cells receive the messenger chemicals and then trigger specific enzymes to speed up cellular division. When your wound has healed, the delivery of these messenger chemicals is shut off and cellular life returns to normal. Besides the types of controls that take care of healing, healthy cells are also programmed to die at a certain age so that cellular death will be in balance with new cell growth. But sometimes the process can go awry. Cells don't stop dividing even though your body tells them to. They take on a life of their own and grow in an unregulated fashion. These cells don't die when they are programmed to. This is what happens in cancer.

WHAT MAKES A CELL CANCEROUS?

Every cell has a genetic blueprint, called deoxyribonucleic acid (DNA). The DNA of cells contains genes that program cell reproduction, growth, and repair of all body tissues. Sometimes genes can become damaged, and this damage can result in cancer. In essence, there are three ways in which your genes can become faulty:

- A mutation can occur during normal cell division such that the newly formed cell contains an abnormal gene. This can happen randomly or if the cell is exposed to some other agent.
- Cells might be exposed to an environmental agent, called a carcinogen, that harms the DNA. For instance, cigarette smoking is a carcinogen that promotes the development of lung cancer.
- Flawed genes can be inherited from your parents. However, very few types of cancer are the result of inherited genes.

Just because you have one damaged gene does not mean you are destined to get cancer. Many processes must take place before a cancer develops. Your body has what are called tumour suppressor genes, which keep an eye out for damaged DNA and halt it in its tracks. But if these tumour suppressor genes become mutated, cells with abnormal genes can multiply at an uncontrolled rate. It is estimated that in 20 to 40 percent of breast cancer cases, a particular tumour suppressor gene (called p53) is mutated.

Several genetic mutations are probably needed for breast cancer to develop. Genes that go on to cause cancer are called oncogenes.

Cancer is not explained by genetics alone. Some people who have a family history of a certain cancer never get that cancer. Experts agree that cancer is the result of an *interaction* between genes and environmental factors, such as diet. For instance, you might have a mutated gene that predisposes you to breast cancer, but because you eat a low-fat diet high in antioxidant-rich fruits and vegetables, you may never get cancer. On the other hand, if you are regularly exposed to pollutants and eat a poor diet, the risk that any faulty genes you carry will catalyze a cancerous growth is increased.

How breast cancer develops

The breast consists mainly of fatty tissue, which gives it its size and shape. Within this fatty tissue are milk glands. Lobules are groups of individual milk-forming glands, and each lobule empties into a duct, a small passageway that carries milk to the nipple. It's in the lobules and ducts that most breast cancer begins. Within the breast is also a network of lymphatic vessels, which connect to lymph nodes under the arm, under the collarbone, and near the breastbone. The lymphatic system drains fluid and particles (called lymph) from the breast into the lymph nodes. The lymph then enters the bloodstream and is eventually removed from the body.

Breast cancer begins with a single cell that runs amok, usually in the lobule or duct. Cancers probably start here because these are two areas where cells divide rapidly during the normal menstrual cycle. Estrogen and progesterone stimulate the breast cells to begin dividing each month, preparing the body for pregnancy. If conception does not occur, breast cell receptors receive a message to stop cell division. The process begins again the following month, and every month in which menstruation occurs, until menopause. Because fairly rapid cell division occurs regularly in the breast for such a span of years, there is a greater chance for a genetic mutation to occur. While most breast cancers are not detected until after menopause, it is believed that the majority actually begin to develop in the premenopausal years.

BREAST CANCER GENES

Some cases of breast cancer are caused by inherited mutations in the genes BRCA1 and BRCA2. The gene BRCA1 was identified in 1994 and, in its mutated form, is now believed to cause inherited early-onset breast cancer; this disease accounts for 5 percent of breast cancers. BRCA1 is actually a tumour suppressor gene, the type of gene that's supposed to work to keep DNA healthy. Families carrying a faulty BRCA1 gene experience a high incidence of both breast and ovarian cancers occurring at a young age. However, 80 percent of breast cancers occur in older women who don't have the flawed BRCA1 gene. Genetic testing that screens for faulty BRCA1 and BRCA2 genes is available across Canada. Testing is done at what are usually called familial breast cancer clinics, often connected to a cancer treatment centre. Eligibility for the test will vary depending on the province in which you live. Usually you will be eligible if you have two or more close relatives with breast cancer and a referral from your physician. At the clinic, a woman will be counselled as to the pros and cons of having such a test. If she decides to take it, she will be counselled as to how to deal with the ramifications of the results.

Genetic tests, I am sure, will add a great deal of worry to many women's lives. It will become important to remember that not all mutated genes go on to catalyze a cancer. And in the case of those who find they have the mutated BRCA1 or BRCA2 gene, this information will no doubt be used to spur important preventative decisions in response to a higher breast cancer risk.

RISK FACTORS FOR BREAST CANCER

While we don't yet know all the causes of breast cancer, ongoing research is rapidly adding to our knowledge base. Studies of large numbers of women have been able to identify risk factors that increase a woman's chance of developing breast cancer. To date, the clearest risk factors for the disease are associated with hormonal and reproductive factors. Exactly how hormones play a role is not yet fully understood. However, researchers do believe that estrogen can promote the growth and development of mutated breast cells. As you will see below, a common thread in many of the identified risk factors is the length of time your breast tissue has been exposed to your body's circulating estrogen via the menstrual cycle. The longer the exposure, the greater the risk of breast cancer.

Age

As you saw in the risk chart on page 215, breast cancer is more common in women over 50. In fact, more than 75 percent of breast cancers occur in postmenopausal women. While it is possible to develop breast cancer at a younger age, most women don't. Keep in mind also that increasing age makes other risk factors discussed below more likely to occur. When two or more risk factors are combined, your risk becomes greater than when you have been exposed to one risk factor alone.

Previous breast cancer

A history of breast cancer increases the odds that a woman will get breast cancer again, in both the same and the opposite breast.

Family history

If you have a first-degree relative (a mother or a sister) with breast cancer, your risk of developing the disease is approximately doubled. You run an even greater risk if more than one close relative is affected, or if the cancer has occurred at a young age in a first-degree family member. But while it is true that a history of breast cancer in the family increases risk, the additional risk may not be as great as you think. If you have a breast cancer gene, there is a 50 percent chance you will pass it on to your daughter. If she, in turn, gets the gene, there is a 50 percent chance that she will pass it on to her child, and so on. Purely hereditary breast cancer accounts for about 10 percent of all cases. And remember, even if you are unlucky enough to inherit a breast cancer–causing gene, you are not fated to get the disease. You can take preventive action.

Age at first pregnancy

Women who have children before 30 years of age have a lower risk of developing breast cancer. Women who have their first child after 30 have a higher risk, and women who never have children are at an even greater risk. Many experts believe that the important factor here is the amount of time that lapses between menarche (the onset of menstruation) and first pregnancy. The theory is that the developing breast tissue is most sensitive to cancer-causing agents (carcinogens) during this time. Hormones produced only during pregnancy mature the breast cells and make them more resistant to carcinogens. It may be that these same pregnancy hormones stimulate mutated breast cells in a woman who has her first baby after 30 years of age.

Age at first period

If your period began before you were 12 years of age, you have, statistically, a slightly higher risk of developing breast cancer. In fact, each year that puberty is delayed may offer as much as a 20 percent reduction in risk. Many of the changes that occur at puberty are because of higher levels of endogenous estrogen (estrogen that's made in your body). It is believed that the longer breast tissue is exposed to higher levels of endogenous estrogen, the greater the chance for cells to become cancerous.

Late menopause
Women who menstruate for longer than 40 years have a slightly higher risk of breast cancer. Like early menarche, late menopause influences the amount of time breast cells are exposed to estrogen.

The list above describes the stronger risk factors for the disease. In addition, however, the following factors may play a role, though they are less well understood.

Exposure to radiation
Radiation from X-rays taken during a woman's younger years may increase the risk of breast cancer later in life. It appears that this factor is more significant if exposure occurs before the age of 40. Despite this, experts feel exposure to radiation is probably a minor contribution to overall risk.

Use of hormones
In animal studies, estrogen intake is associated with an increased occurrence of breast cancer. Recently, the Women's Health Initiative (WHI), in a large trial sponsored by the National Institutes of Health, linked the use of combined hormone replacement therapy (HRT) to breast cancer. In July 2002, the trial was halted after 5.2 years, when the researchers reported that the risk of breast cancer was 26 percent higher in the group of women taking estrogen plus progestin. On average there were about 38 cases of invasive breast cancer per 10,000 women, compared with 30 cases among women taking the placebo pills. This translates into an increased risk of less than one-tenth of 1 percent a year. Despite this small increase in risk, the study revealed that the longer a woman stayed on HRT, the more her breast cancer risk increased.[1]

Clearly, the pros and cons of combined HRT need to be discussed with your physician. Factors to consider include your other risk factors for breast cancer, heart disease, osteoporosis, and the severity of menopausal symptoms.

Diet

More and more studies are determining that certain dietary factors increase the risk of developing breast cancer. Diet affects breast cancer development by either initiating cancer growth through causing a genetic mutation or by promoting the growth of cancerous cells. This chapter includes an extensive discussion of the many dietary and nutritional factors that have been studied in relation to breast cancer risk.

SCREENING FOR BREAST CANCER

The larger and better established a breast cancer tumour is, the more difficult it is to treat. This is especially true if the tumour metastasizes before treatment begins. Experts agree that your best protection against breast cancer is prevention, and that's what I'll discuss in much of the rest of this chapter. If you do develop a tumour, the earliest possible detection makes successful treatment more likely. For this reason, it's also important to use the methods currently available for early detection.

Mammograms

You should be thinking about getting your first mammogram around the time of menopause. Doctors recommend that all Canadian women between the ages of 50 and 69 have a mammogram every two years in combination with a physical exam of the breasts by a trained health professional. Guidelines for women under 50 or over 70 will vary by province. A mammogram is a special X-ray of the breast that will reveal the location of a breast lump, its size, and certain characteristics that may be suggestive of cancer. If a lump looks suspicious to your physician, he or she will order further tests to determine if it's malignant. Mammograms use very low doses of radiation and do not cause breast cancer; nor do they make an existing cancer worse. Rather, a mammogram is a very important screening tool that can catch breast cancer early.

However, not all lumps are seen on a mammogram. Younger women have denser breasts, which make detection more difficult. This is one of the reasons women under 50 are not encouraged to have regular mammograms. (Another reason is that breast cancer is less common in premenopausal women.)

While it is generally accepted that mammograms save the lives of women who are over 50 years of age and have breast cancer, there is debate about whether women in the premenopausal transitional years between 40 and 49 should start having routine mammograms. Currently, because of the results of the Canadian National Breast Screening Study, health authorities do not recommend routine mammograms for this age group. In this 10-year study of 25,000 women 40 to 49 years old, there was no difference in breast cancer death rates between women who were screened and women who were not.[2]

Breast self-exam

Although less reliable at detecting cancer than a mammogram combined with a physical examination by your doctor, the breast self-exam is an important way to detect physical changes in your breasts. By the age of 40, all Canadian women should be performing monthly breast self-exams. Use the pads of your fingers to examine the tissue in your breasts and in your armpits. Breast self-exams should be done at the same point during each menstrual cycle. Be sure to also look carefully at your breasts in the mirror. Any of the following changes, whether detected manually or visually, should prompt a visit to your family doctor:

- A lump or thick area in the breast or underarm area
- Unusual swelling of the breast
- Change in colour or texture of the skin on the breast
- Blood leakage from the nipple or areola (the dark ring surrounding the nipple)
- Inversion of the nipple (the nipple puckers inward, rather than pointing outward)

PREVENTING BREAST CANCER

Changing your lifestyle

Factors such as lifestyle and diet definitely make a difference to your risk of developing many types of cancer. In 1997, an international expert panel of the World Cancer Research Fund and the American Institute for Cancer Research released a 653-page report outlining dietary advice to prevent cancer. The report stated that between 30 and 40 percent of all cancer cases are preventable by a healthy diet, regular exercise, and maintaining a healthy weight. The report went on to say that diets high in fruits and vegetables could alone prevent at least 20 percent of all cancer cases.[3]

When it comes to breast cancer, dietary factors such as fat, alcohol, fibre, fruits, and vegetables have all been well studied. Below are my nutrition recommendations based on current scientific knowledge. While some of these strategies have strong research to support their adoption, others do not have such strong evidence backing them. However, evidence does exist to suggest that they *may* be helpful. And certainly when it comes to eating a low-fat diet packed with fibre and antioxidant nutrients, I really don't think you can go wrong. While we are still learning about breast cancer, making the dietary changes I list below will help you improve your overall well-being. And they just might lower your odds of getting breast cancer.

Dietary strategies

DIETARY FAT

When most women think of diet and breast cancer, they think of fat. The main hypothesis among nutrition researchers has long been that a high-fat diet increases the risk of getting the disease. And certainly no other nutrient has been studied so in depth in terms of breast cancer. Throughout the 1980s and 1990s, however, the fat hypothesis has come under debate. It seems the link between a high-fat diet and breast cancer is not as clear-cut as we had thought.

Scientists became interested in the link between fat intake and breast cancer when they noticed that women in countries with low-fat intakes had much lower rates of breast cancer as compared with women in countries with higher-fat diets. It has been hypothesized that dietary fat may increase breast cancer risk by increasing estrogen production (you'll recall I told you earlier that a woman's circulating estrogen is thought to be related to breast cancer risk by stimulating the growth of breast tissue). Studies do show that vegetarian women with low-fat, high-fibre diets have lower levels of estrogen and, among them, there are fewer incidences of breast cancer.[4] Another way high-fat diets may cause breast cancer is through weight gain and body fat accumulation, which in turn increases the risk of breast cancer. This is because fat cells produce estrogen.

Theory aside, does the amount of fat you eat make a difference to your risk? In animal studies, very high-fat diets stimulate breast cancer growth, but this effect has not been seen in human studies. Most large studies have failed to show a strong relationship between total fat intake and breast cancer risk. Toronto researchers summarized 23 studies done up until 1993 and concluded that a high-fat diet increased the risk of breast cancer by about 12 percent. A recent 14-year study of 89,000 women found no evidence that a high-fat diet promoted breast cancer or that a low-fat diet protected against it. Many experts, however, believe that the women in these studies didn't reduce their fat intake enough to see a benefit.[5] The no more than 30 percent of daily calories from fat that Health Canada recommends might be too high to offer protection from breast cancer.

A large Toronto study is currently underway to determine if a very low-fat diet can prevent breast cancer. So far the results look promising. One report found that women who ate a low-fat (21 percent), high-carbohydrate (61 percent) diet for two years had significantly reduced dense breast areas as seen by mammogram (dense breast areas are a risk factor for cancer), as compared with women on a 30 percent–fat diet. Another report from this research group revealed that women who followed a 15 percent–fat diet for two years had lower levels of circulating estrogen, which could offer protection.[6] We won't know whether these two findings will translate into a lower rate of breast cancer in the women in these studies consuming a low-fat diet until more time has passed. But based on these initial reports, I certainly believe that following a low-fat diet is a wise precautionary measure.

In addition to studying how much fat a woman eats, researchers have been busy looking at the different types of fat and their effects on breast cancer. But before we look at what they've found, it's important that you understand the differences between the various fats found in food.

Saturated fat   Saturated fat is solid at room temperature. Animal fat is saturated—a block of butter or the marbled fat in meat and poultry, for example. The fat in cheese, milk, and eggs is also saturated. Certain oils, called hydrogenated vegetable oils, can be saturated, too. Hydrogenation is a chemical process that adds hydrogen atoms to liquid vegetable oils, making them more solid and useful to food manufacturers. Cookies, crackers, pastries, and muffins made with hydrogenated vegetable oils are more palatable and have a longer shelf life. A margarine made by hydrogenating a vegetable oil is firmer, like butter.

Polyunsaturated fat   This term refers to fats that are liquid at room temperature. An example is vegetable oil, be it corn, sunflower, safflower, or sesame. There are two types of polyunsaturated fats in foods: omega-6s and omega-3s. Omega-6 polyunsaturated fats are found in all vegetable oils. Omega-3 polyunsaturated fats are found in fish. The oilier the fish, the more polyunsaturated fat it contains. Omega-3 fats are also found in flaxseed oil, canola oil, walnut oil, and, of course, omega-3 eggs.

Monounsaturated fat   This fat is slightly different from saturated and polyunsaturated fat. If you refrigerate a monounsaturated fat, it becomes semisolid. If you take it out of the fridge and store it at room temperature, it will return to a liquid form. Olive oil, canola oil, and peanut oil are the best sources of monounsaturated fat. (And if you're wondering why canola oil doesn't get as hard as olive oil does when refrigerated, it's because canola contains both monounsaturated and polyunsaturated fat.) Nuts and avocado are also rich in monounsaturated fats.

Saturated fat, meat, and milk

Several studies have looked at the relationship between foods high in saturated fat—meat and dairy products—and breast cancer. When it comes to meat, the findings are mixed. Some studies show that higher meat intakes are linked with a greater risk, whereas others don't show any effect. Based on a review of the research, the international panel of experts from the World Cancer Research Fund and the American Institute for Cancer Research recently concluded that meat might possibly increase a woman's risk.

The harmful effect of meat may be due to its saturated fat content, or it may be due to the way it's prepared. Cooking meat at high temperatures forms compounds called heterocyclic amines, which have been shown to cause breast tumours in animals. It appears that well-cooked meat may not be that healthy for women either. Researchers at the University of Minnesota have learned that women who eat their hamburger, steak, and bacon well done are more than four times as likely to have breast cancer than women who enjoy their meat rare or medium done.[7] Until we know more about the effects of cooked meat, breast cancer experts advise that we consume no more than 3 ounces (90 g) of meat each day.

Not all the studies looking at the relationship between dairy products and breast cancer have reported a higher risk from dairy consumption. In fact, a Finnish study suggests that drinking a glass of whole milk might offer protection against breast cancer. Researchers in Helsinki studied 4697 women for 25 years and discovered that those participants who had the highest intake of milk had a 48 percent lower risk of developing breast cancer than the women who drank the least milk.

Scientists speculate that a special fat might be responsible for milk's protective effect. Conjugated linoleic acid (CLA) occurs naturally in milk (and meat) and has been shown in a number of animal studies to inhibit breast cancer growth. Scientists believe that CLA protects cells from becoming cancerous when breast cells are dividing.[8]

Polyunsaturated fat and fish

In animals, very high intakes of polyunsaturated vegetable oils can promote breast tumour growth. But keep in mind that the studies that came to these conclusions were looking at animals fed 45 percent of their calories from fat. That's pretty high. The average Canadian eats less fat than that, getting more like 32 percent of daily calories in the form of fat. The data on humans show that vegetable oils have no effect on breast cancer risk, at least in the amounts we typically consume. So there's no need to throw away your bottle of sunflower seed oil!

You may want to start eating more fish. In studied populations, women who eat plenty of fish for many years have a lower incidence of breast cancer. And while no trials have been done on women, one experimental study did find that omega-3 fats from fish oil actually suppressed human breast cancer cell growth and metastatic cancer in female mice (scientists inject human breast cancer cells into mice to study the effects of different carcinogens).[9] Although there is not a lot of evidence for fish's protective effect, results of the existing studies do suggest that you get more omega-3 fats into your diet. My recommendation is to eat fish three times a week. Here are a few of my ways to cook tasty fish:

Lemon dill salmon   Place a salmon filet or salmon steak on a piece of aluminum foil. Squeeze the juice of 1/2 lemon over the fish and top with fresh chopped dill and black pepper. Wrap in foil and bake at 450° Fahrenheit (220° Celsius) for 20 to 25 minutes.

Hoisin salmon   Mix hoisin sauce with a touch of hot chili paste, chopped fresh ginger, and a little roasted sesame oil. Brush over fish. Bake at 450° Fahrenheit (220° Celsius) for approximately 15 minutes or until done to your liking.

Asian-style marinated fish   Marinate a filet or steak of white fish (halibut, swordfish, sea bass) in a Ziploc bag for 30 minutes with Mo's Authentic Japanese dressing. (Mo's is my favourite brand, but you can use any dressing you like.) If you don't have time to marinate the fish, drizzle about 1/4 cup (50 ml) of the dressing over the fish just before baking. Bake at 450° Fahrenheit (220° Celsius) for approximately 15 minutes or until done to your liking. For a different flavour, use oyster sauce.

Monounsaturated fat and olive oil

No doubt you've read that olive oil is good for your heart. But can it help you reduce your odds of developing breast cancer too? It's true that breast cancer is less common in Mediterranean countries where olive oil is the main source of fat. A few studies have even found that women with breast cancer use significantly less olive oil compared with women free of the disease.[10] I've already told you that olive oil is a rich source of monounsaturated fat. Could this be the protective factor? Or perhaps the secret ingredients are olive oil's natural antioxidants, such as vitamin E? Researchers don't think so. At this time there appears to be no relationship between monounsaturated fat or vitamin E and breast cancer risk. It may be that if you consume more olive oil, you eat less of other fats that might increase your risk (such as saturated fat).

SOY FOODS

We're back to soy again. You can't escape the health benefits of this humble bean. Populations (including Japanese people and vegetarians) that consume the largest amounts of soy have the lowest rates of breast cancer. Researchers attribute soy's possible protective effect to naturally occurring compounds called isoflavones. When we consume soy foods, bacteria in our intestinal tract convert isoflavones to compounds that act like a weak estrogen hormone in the body. This is why isoflavones are called phytoestrogens (plant estrogens). Two soy isoflavones, genistein and daidzein, have been studied extensively.

Acting as weak estrogen compounds, isoflavones are able to attach to estrogen receptors in the body. In fact, genistein has a much stronger pull to certain estrogen receptors than does estradiol, one of your body's own estrogen hormones. Researchers believe that if genistein can bind to estrogen receptors in the breast, it blocks a woman's own estrogen from taking those spots. And that's good news because it means that breast cells have less contact with estrogen.

A regular intake of soy isoflavones may also alter hormone production and lower levels of circulating hormones in the bloodstream. A small study done at the University of Texas found that premenopausal women who drank three 12-ounce (375-ml) glasses of soy beverage each day had lower blood levels of estrogen than women on a soy-free diet. The lower estrogen levels lasted up to three menstrual cycles after the women stopped taking the soy. A Tufts University study also found that a high-soy diet lowered blood estrogen by 20 percent in menopausal women.

A high-soy diet can also influence how much estrogen your breast cells come in contact with by lengthening the menstrual cycle slightly. One study showed that a daily intake of soy products containing 45 milligrams of isoflavones lengthened the menstrual cycle of premenopausal women.[11] Over a lifetime, longer menstrual cycles mean fewer menstrual cycles; this in turn means the breasts have less exposure to estrogen.

Before you get too excited about soy's protective breast cancer effects, I should tell you that most experts believe soy exerts its benefits with respect to protecting from breast cancer during puberty, when breast cells are most sensitive to carcinogens. In other words, you need to be consuming soy as a young girl to get protection from breast cancer later in life. Two recent studies lend support to this notion. One measured soy food intake among Asian-Americans during adolescence and found a much lower risk of breast cancer later in life among the women who consumed the most soy in their teen years. American researchers found similar results when they studied a large group of Chinese women.[12]

Should you eat soy if you're a breast cancer survivor?

The estrogen-like properties of isoflavones have led some experts to be concerned about the use of soy in women with breast cancer because estrogen may increase this risk. Some preliminary studies show that soy has protective effects for breast cancer while others suggest soy might increase breast cell growth.[13] Laboratory research has also found that genistein inhibits the growth of estrogen-positive and estrogen-negative human breast cancer cells. Let me briefly explain these terms. Postmenopausal women tend to get *estrogen-positive* tumours. The cells in an estrogen-positive tumour have estrogen receptors and will respond to estrogen. In general, these tumours have a better prognosis than estrogen-negative tumours because they are slower growing and they respond to hormone treatments. Premenopausal women are more likely to get an *estrogen-negative* tumour, which rarely responds to hormonal treatments, since the cells in it do not have estrogen receptors.

While the studies show that soy has an anti-estrogen effect and prevents breast cancer cells from growing, a few laboratory studies suggest that *high intakes* of genistein might enhance breast tissue growth. British researchers studied the effect of a 60-gram soy supplement (containing 45 milligrams isoflavones) in 48 premenopausal women with benign breast disease or breast cancer. Soy supplementation for two weeks did stimulate growth of normal breast cells.[14] This finding does not mean, however, that short-term soy consumption increases the chance of breast cancer. Rather, it means we need more research in this area to understand how soy works in women with breast cancer.

Because we lack sufficient reliable information about the effect of soy foods in women with breast cancer, a history of breast cancer, or a family history of breast cancer, women should use soy cautiously. Unfortunately, there are no specific recommendations for women with estrogen-positive breast cancer. Until more is known, avoid consuming large amounts of soy each day. Absolutely avoid using soy protein powders and isoflavone supplements. While most experts feel that consuming soy foods three times a week as part of a plant-based diet is considered safe, there are some who feel isoflavones from any source pose a risk. Clearly the decision to eat soy foods is a personal one.

If you want to start eating soy foods because they *might* help reduce your risk of breast cancer *and* because they have many other health benefits (if you haven't already, read Chapter 12 on soy's cholesterol-lowering power), try adding one soy food to your diet each day. Chapter 4 outlines different types of soy foods and how to enjoy them.

FLAXSEED

The tiny brown or golden seeds of flax are now being studied for their possible role in preventing breast cancer. Flaxseed contains natural compounds called lignans. (You might also be interested to know that flax seeds are rich in soluble fibre and alpha-linolenic acid, an essential fatty acid.) When we eat flaxseed, bacteria in our gut convert the plant lignans into human lignans, which act very much like estrogen in the body. Once in the body, phytoestrogens from flaxseed have a weak estrogen-like action and are able to bind to estrogen receptors. In so doing, they can, like other phytoestrogens, help block the action of our body's own potent estrogen on breast cells.

Two studies conducted at the University of Toronto found that lignans from flaxseed reduced the size of breast tumours in rats.[15] Whether flaxseed can do this in humans is another question. And it's a question that's being addressed now by Dr. Lillian Anderson and her team at the University of Toronto. In their study, women with breast cancer are being given 25 grams (about 2 tablespoons) of flaxseed daily, in the form of a muffin, to see if the flaxseed lignans have any beneficial effect on tumour size between diagnosis and surgery. Preliminary findings suggest that flaxseed can slow the growth of breast tumours.

In the meantime, should you be eating flax? It's too early to say that eating flaxseed will reduce breast cancer risk, but you can still make it part of your regular diet, just in case. It certainly won't do you any harm. If nothing else, you'll add a source of fibre and essential fat to your diet. Aim to get 1 to 2 tablespoons (15 to 25 ml) of ground flaxseed each day. It is very important that you grind your flaxseed to release the lignans. Otherwise all you'll be getting is a source of fibre. Grind flaxseed in a clean coffee grinder or with a mortle and pestle. You can also buy it pre-ground at health food stores, though it is more expensive (Omega Nutrition makes a good product).

Now the real question: What do you do with it? Plenty! Here are just a few ideas that will add crunch and a great nutty flavour to your meals:

- Add ground flaxseed to hot cereals, pancakes, muffin batters, and cookie mixes. I have clients who even add it to cold breakfast cereal.
- Mix ground flaxseed into yogurt and applesauce.
- Sprinkle flax on salads and soup.
- Add flaxseed to casseroles.
- Try a loaf of flaxseed bread. Check your local bakery, health food store, or super-market.
- Try Red River cereal, another good source of flaxseed.

Once you grind flaxseed, store it (along with any whole seeds you have remaining) in an airtight container in the fridge. The natural fats in flaxseed go rancid quickly if exposed to air and heat.

What about flax oil?

I've had many clients tell me they add flaxseed oil to their foods or take flaxseed oil capsules with their morning juice. When I ask them why, many reply, "To protect myself from breast cancer." I then explain to them what I'm about to tell you. Flaxseed oil is a great source of alpha-linolenic acid (ALA), an essential fatty acid belonging to the omega-3 family that our body needs to get from food. But it is not a good source of lignans—the phytoestrogens that may protect the breast. Lignans are found in the seed, along with ALA and fibre. So if you're looking to add to your arsenal of breast cancer–fighting foods, choose ground flaxseed, not flax oil.

FRUITS AND VEGETABLES

Looks like Mom was right when she told you to finish your vegetables. Over 200 studies from around the world have shown that a diet high in fruits and vegetables lowers the risk of developing many cancers, including breast cancer. American researchers from Harvard University studied over 89,000 women and found that those who ate more than 2.2 servings of vegetables daily had a 20 percent lower risk of breast cancer than those who ate less than one serving. Another study of premenopausal women found that high total vegetable intake lowered the risk of breast cancer by 54 percent.[16]

It appears that dark green vegetables, which contain beta-carotene, other carotenoid compounds, and folate (a B vitamin) are most protective. Beta-carotene is an antioxidant nutrient, which means it is able to protect cells from damage caused by harmful free-radical molecules. Our bodies form free radicals from oxygen every day as a consequence of normal metabolism. Pollution and cigarette smoke increase free radical levels in our bodies. Free radicals roam the body and damage the genetic material of cells, which may lead to cancer development. They can also damage protein and fat molecules in our cells. Every cell in our body has defence mechanisms against free radicals, including a system of enzymes and antioxidants that act as scavengers, mopping up free radicals before they cause harm. Without continuous antioxidant protection, our cells would not survive. Dietary antioxidants like beta-carotene (and vitamins E and C) provide the body with extra ammunition against free radicals. You'll read more about the effect of beta-carotene in the "Vitamins and Minerals" section that starts on page 241.

The protective effects of fruits and vegetables have not been replicated, however, in studies focusing on isolated antioxidants such as beta-carotene or vitamin C supplements. We are learning that there's more to fruits and vegetables than vitamins, minerals, and fibre. Plant foods also contain thousands of phytochemicals, naturally occurring compounds that act as antioxidants and natural antibiotics, and inhibit cancer development. Experts believe that phytochemicals play a unique role in health and that they probably work together with vitamins and minerals in the food. This is probably why we don't see the same disease prevention in studies using supplements—it's the *whole food* that seems to be important.

Despite our knowledge that these foods are good for us, many of us still don't manage to get our recommended daily 5 to 10 servings. We say we don't have time. We grab a bagel instead of an apple. Or we throw together pasta with pesto instead of eating a salad with a baked potato. Some people just don't like vegetables. Maybe some of us think that a strawberry cereal bar counts as a fruit serving. Or, when it comes right down to it, we'd rather have French fries than a bowl of steamed spinach.

Well, it's time to make sure you get at least 5 to 10 servings of fruits and vegetables each day. Aim to eat at least three different-coloured fruits and three different-coloured vegetables daily. Try these tricks to sneak them into your diet:

- Buy pre-chopped and washed vegetables at the supermarket. Try baby carrots, broccoli and cauliflower florets, or "salad in a bag." These veggies are ready to be thrown into the microwave, steamer, or your salad bowl.
- Pick up fresh fruit or raw veggies from the salad bar at your local supermarket.
- Grab a can of vegetable juice instead of Diet Coke at lunch.
- Order a green or spinach salad at lunch (ask for the dressing on the side).
- For a nutrient boost, use romaine and other dark green lettuces when making salad (I've always referred to iceberg as the "polyester of lettuces"!).
- When ordering a sandwich, ask for tomatoes, cucumbers, and lettuce. When making a sandwich, try spinach leaves as a change from lettuce.
- Add quick-cooking greens such as spinach, kale, rapini, or Swiss chard to soups and pasta sauces.
- Fortify soups, pasta sauces, and casseroles with grated zucchini and grated carrot.
- Bake (or microwave) a sweet potato for a change from rice or pasta.
- Add slices of lemon, lime, or orange to water for flavour and a little vitamin C boost.
- Enjoy chocolate cake? Top it with a few spoonfuls of strawberries.
- Replace that cereal bar with two pieces of fruit.

Antioxidant all-stars

An American research team has measured the ability of fresh produce to provide antioxidant protection, that is, to protect cells from harmful free-radical molecules. They compared fruits and vegetables with vitamin C and E supplements. Guess what? Most fruits and vegetables outperformed the supplements by a long shot. Here are the winners, ranked according to antioxidant performance:

Vegetables		Fruits	
1	kale	1	blueberries
2	beets	2	strawberries
3	red peppers	3	plums
4	broccoli	4	oranges
5	spinach	5	red grapes
6	red grapes	6	kiwi
7	potato	7	white grapes
8	sweet potato	8	apples, tomatoes, bananas, pears
9	corn		

FIBRE AND WHEAT BRAN

Although the research is preliminary, there is evidence to suggest that a high-fibre intake may offer protection from breast cancer. When Toronto researchers looked at the findings from 12 controlled studies, they found that 20 grams of fibre per day was associated with a modest, but significant, lower risk of developing breast cancer.

One way fibre may help is by binding to estrogen in the intestine and causing it to be excreted in the stool. Every day our intestines reabsorb estrogen from bile, a compound that your liver manufactures and that your gallbladder releases into your intestines. Bile is needed to digest fat. If dietary fibre can attach itself to estrogen and facilitate its removal from the body, your body has to take estrogen out of the bloodstream to make more bile. The net result—a lower level of circulating estrogen. If you eat a high-fibre diet for many years, then, you could possibly lower your risk of breast cancer.

Diets high in wheat bran and low in fat do lower blood estrogen levels in premenopausal women. A study from the UCLA School of Medicine found that women who ate a 10 percent–fat diet with 25 to 35 grams of fibre each day for two months had significantly lower serum estrogen levels than when they ate their regular diets. A more recent study showed that adding 20 grams of wheat bran to the diet had a significant estrogen-lowering effect after one month. Women in this study ate 10 grams of wheat bran daily and achieved a significant reduction in estrogen levels after two months.[17]

High-fibre diets, because they are high in plant foods, tend to be higher in antioxidant vitamins and lower in fat, both factors that might protect against breast cancer. And people who eat plenty of fibre tend to maintain a healthy weight. There are many explanations for fibre's protective effect, all of which may be true. The studies do suggest, however, that dietary fibre works best if you follow a low-fat diet. So adding a little wheat bran to a diet that's high in fat and low in fruits and vegetables probably won't do you much good. More and more we are learning that health protection comes from a *combination of factors* in the diet—the ideal diet includes many low-fat foods, high-fibre foods, soy foods, and foods rich in antioxidant nutrients and phytochemicals.

Dietary fibre defined

Dietary fibre is the structural material in plants—fruits, vegetables, grains, and legumes—that cannot be broken down by the human digestive tract (although bacteria in our colon are able to digest some of these fibres). Thanks to heavy advertising campaigns, fibre is, to many people, synonymous with certain brands of breakfast cereal. But you're shortchanging yourself if you rely on a single food to get your fibre. That's because dietary fibre comes in two varieties, *soluble* and *insoluble*. Both are present in varying proportions in plant foods, but some foods may be rich in one or the other. And both types of fibre function differently in your body to promote health.

As their name suggests, soluble fibres dissolve in water. Dried peas, beans, lentils, oats, barley, psyllium husks, apples, and citrus fruits are good sources of soluble fibre. After you've consumed these foods, the soluble fibres form a gel in your stomach and slow the rate of digestion and absorption. Foods such as wheat bran, whole grains, and some vegetables contain mainly insoluble fibres. Although these fibres do not dissolve in water, they do have a significant capacity for retaining water. In this way they act to increase stool bulk and promote regularity. It's wheat bran (containing mostly insoluble fibre) that's been studied the most in relation to breast cancer risk.

How much fibre do you need?

It's estimated that North Americans are getting 11 to 14 grams of fibre each day, only one-half of the daily intake recommended. Experts recommend that women get 25 grams (men need 38 grams) of dietary fibre each day to reap its health benefits. The list of high-fibre foods that follows will give you some ideas of which foods to choose to sneak more fibre into your diet. And, for those of you who are not sure how many grams of fibre you're getting each day, I've also listed the fibre content of various foods.

Note that it's important to *gradually* build up to consuming 25 grams of fibre daily.

Too much too soon can cause bloating, gas, and possibly diarrhea. When adding fibre to your diet, spread it out over the course of the day. Getting all your fibre at once may reduce the benefits and increase the discomfort. And don't forget that fibre needs water if it's going to do its job. Aim to consume a minimum of 1 cup (250 ml) of water with each high-fibre meal and snack.

FIBRE CONTENT OF HIGH-FIBRE FOODS (GRAMS)

To reach the recommended 25 grams of fibre each day, slowly add high-fibre foods to your diet, replacing lower-fibre foods you're eating now. All measurements given below refer to amounts after cooking, unless otherwise specified.

LEGUMES

Black beans, 1 cup (250 ml)	12.0
Chickpeas, 1 cup (250 ml)	6.1
Kidney beans, 1 cup (250 ml)	6.7
Lentils, 1 cup (250 ml)	8.4
Pinto beans, 1 cup (250 ml)	14.0

NUTS

Almonds, 1/2 cup (125 ml)	5.0
Peanuts, 1/2 cup (125 ml)	6.0

CEREALS

100% bran cereals, 1/2 cup (125 ml)	10.0
Bran Flakes, 1 cup (250 ml)	5.0
Bran Buds, 1/3 cup (75 ml)	13.0
Corn Bran, 1 cup (250 ml)	7.6
Red River Cereal, 1 cup (250 ml)	5.0
Shreddies, 1 cup (250 ml)	4.0

BREAD AND GRAINS

Bran muffin, 1 medium	2.5
Flaxseed, ground, 1 tbsp. (15 ml)	1.2
Pasta, whole wheat, 1 cup (250 ml)	6.0
Pita pocket, whole-wheat, 1	4.5
Rice, brown, 1 cup (250 ml)	2.5
Wheat bran, 1 tbsp. (15 ml)	1.2
Whole-wheat bread, 100%, 2 slices	3.0

FRUITS (RAW UNLESS OTHERWISE SPECIFIED)

Apple, 1 medium with skin	3.5
Apricots, dried, 1/2 cup (125 ml)	6.0
Blackberries, 1/2 cup (125 ml)	3.5
Figs, 3 dried	5.0
Orange, 1 medium	2.6
Pear, 1 medium with skin	4.7
Prunes, 3 dried	4.0
Raisins, 1/2 cup (125 ml)	7.5

VEGETABLES

Broccoli, 1/2 cup (125 ml)	2.0
Brussels sprouts, 1/2 cup (125 ml)	2.5
Carrots, 1/2 cup (125 ml)	2.5
Green peas, 1/2 cup (125 ml)	4.0
Lima beans, 1/2 cup (125 ml)	4.8
Sweet potato, mashed, 1/2 cup (125 ml)	4.0

Source: *Nutrient Value of Some Common Foods.* Health Canada, 1999. Adapted and reproduced with the permission of the Minister of Public Works and Government Services Canada, 2003.

PROBIOTICS (FERMENTED MILK PRODUCTS)

The last time you sat down to a bowl of yogurt, you probably didn't think you might be staving off breast cancer. One Dutch study in which researchers compared the diets of women who had breast cancer with the diets of women free of the disease showed that women who ate a low-fat diet with plenty of fibre and fermented milk products (the equivalent of 1.5 glasses daily) had a 50 percent lower risk of developing breast cancer than women who did not use fermented milk products regularly. Another study found that fermented milk inhibited the growth of breast cancer cells in the laboratory.[18]

The term "probiotic" means "to promote life" and refers to living organisms which, upon ingestion in certain numbers, improve the microbial balance in the intestines and exert health benefits. In this sense, yogurt is considered a probiotic food. Once in our intestinal tract, the bacteria in probiotic foods can produce active compounds that suppress the growth of other microbes that produce cancer-causing substances.

These friendly bacteria, known collectively as lactic acid bacteria, include *Lactobacillus acidophilus, Lactobacillus bulgaricus, Lactobacillus casei, Streptococcus thermophilus,* and the many strains of *Bifidobacteria.* The human digestive tract contains hundreds of strains of bacteria, making up what is called the normal intestinal flora. Among the intestinal flora are the lactic acid bacteria. They inhibit the growth of unfriendly, or disease-causing, bacteria by producing lactic acid and antibacterial substances that suppress their growth, and by preventing unfriendly bacteria from attaching themselves to the intestinal walls. Fermented milk products become even more important when you're on a course of antibiotics. When you take a broad-spectrum antibiotic, you end up killing both the disease-causing bacteria and the friendly ones.

Fermented milk products have a long history of medical use. Records show that foods such as yogurt and kefir (a drink made by adding live bacteria to milk) were used by 16th-century doctors to treat intestinal infections. Today scientists are learning that these friendly bacteria may do much more than keep our intestinal tract healthy. In addition to possible cancer prevention, lactic acid bacteria can help stimulate the immune system, lower blood cholesterol, treat candida yeast infections, and speed recovery from diarrhea.

Adding fermented milk products to your diet

Lactic acid bacteria in fermented milk products and supplements will exert their health effects only if they reach the intestines in sufficient numbers. This means you must consume adequate "doses" of live bacteria. Experts generally recommend consuming between 1 and 10 billion living, healthy bacterial cells daily. The amount of live bacteria in a 3/4-cup (175-ml) container of yogurt ranges from 175 million to 17,500 million. During storage, many of these bacteria may die. In Canada, all commercial yogurts are made using *Lactobacillus bulgaricus* and *Streptococcus thermophilus*. Some manufacturers add other strains such as some of the *Bifidobacteria, Lactobacillus acidophilus,* and *Lactobacillus casei.* To begin reaping the health benefits of probiotics, include one serving of yogurt in your daily diet. If you're a little more adventurous you might try kefir or sweet acidophilus milk, two fermented milk beverages available in many supermarkets.

What about a probiotic supplement?

If you don't eat dairy products, probiotic capsules or tablets are a good alternative. Many natural health experts believe that taking a high-quality probiotic supplement is the only way to ensure you're getting a sufficient number of friendly bacteria into your intestinal tract. Even if you do enjoy yogurt or kefir, you might still consider adding a supplement to your daily nutrition regime, as some of the bacteria in yogurt (and in a supplement, for that matter) will be killed by acid in the stomach. Here are a few considerations to keep in mind when choosing a product:

- Buy a product that offers 1 to 10 billion live cells per dose. Taking more than this may result in gastrointestinal discomfort.
- Know the types and sources of the bacteria in the supplement. Since research has shown that both *Lactobacillus acidophilus* and the various *Bifidobacteria* offer health benefits, a product that contains both types is recommended if you're looking for overall health protection. Some experts believe that human strains of bacteria are better adapted for growth in the human intestinal tract. When choosing a product, you might ask the pharmacist or retailer if the formula contains human or nonhuman strains.
- For greater convenience, choose a product that is stable at room temperature and does not require refrigeration. This allows you to continue taking the supplement while travelling or at the office.
- Always take your probiotic supplement with food, as the stomach contents become less acidic with the presence of food. This allows more live bacteria to withstand stomach acid and reach their final destination in the intestinal tract.

GREEN AND BLACK TEA

As you learned in Chapter 12, tea and its flavonoids have been shown to protect the heart. A growing body of evidence suggests that tea also protects us from certain cancers, including breast cancer. While not all studies that investigate a woman's tea intake have found a protective effect against breast cancer, some do. The famous Nurses' Health Study from Harvard found that drinking four or more cups of tea per day (versus one or fewer) was associated with a 30 percent lower risk of breast cancer. Animal studies also show that clear tea, tea with milk, and extracts of tea can suppress or block breast cancer development. And interestingly, a Japanese study discovered that breast cancer patients who drank more green tea before diagnosis had significantly lower recurrence rates and better prognosis than those who didn't.[19] The researchers who did this study now believe that something in green tea may somehow modify the cancer and make it easier to treat.

Tea is harvested from the *Camellia sinensis* bush. Tea leaves contain natural chemicals that act as antioxidants. These antioxidants belong to a special class of compounds called catechins. By mopping up harmful free-radical molecules in the body, catechins in tea may protect your cells' genetic material from damage.

A study done at Tufts University in Boston compared tea's antioxidant ability with that of 22 types of vegetables (including broccoli, onions, garlic, corn, and carrots) and found that 7 ounces (230 ml) of green or black tea, brewed for five minutes, had an antioxidant power equivalent to that found in the same amount of fruit or vegetable juice.[20]

Tea

There are three main types of tea: green, black, and oolong. All three come from the same tea bush but are processed differently.

Green tea   The leaves are allowed to wilt naturally after picking.

Black tea (orange pekoe)   The leaves are rolled to break them up and allow air (and thus oxygen) to come into contact with their enzymes. This process of the contact between the tea enzymes and the oxygen is called fermentation. After fermentation, the leaves are dried.

Oolong teas   These are made of partially fermented leaves, which gives them a flavour in between that of green and black teas.

As I noted earlier, herbal teas are not made from tea leaves but from the roots, stems, leaves, and flowers of other plants. They don't have the antioxidant properties of green or black teas.

Here are a few tips to help you get tea into your diet:

- If you drink coffee in the afternoon, substitute tea.
- The next time you're at the grocery store, pick up a box of green tea bags or loose-leaf green tea. Then, the next time you're having a meal inspired by Asian cuisine at home, you'll be ready to serve it with a pot of green tea. (Of course, you don't have to wait until you're having Asian food to enjoy this delicious beverage.)
- Substitute tea for all soft drinks.
- Enjoy a cup of black or oolong tea with your midday snack. Try flavoured tea; Earl Grey, apricot, and black currant are some of my favourites.
- The next time you're at your local coffee bar, try chai, a spicy hot drink made from tea and spices. You might ask that they add only half the amount of syrup as usual—it is often very sweet.

If you're trying to cut back on caffeine *and* lower your odds of getting breast cancer, try tea instead of coffee. As you can see from the chart below, a cup of tea has one-quarter of the caffeine found in the same amount of coffee. Plus, you get all its health-protecting antioxidants. To reach Health Canada's daily upper caffeine limit of 450 milligrams, you'd have to drink 10 to 12 cups of tea a day!

CAFFEINE CONTENT OF COMMON BEVERAGES (MILLIGRAMS)

Black tea, 8 oz. (250 ml)	46
Green tea, 8 oz. (250 ml)	33
Coffee, drip, 8 oz. (250 ml)	100–175
Cola, 12 fluid oz. (355 ml)	37

ALCOHOL

So far, I've been recommending mostly that you *add* foods to your diet—foods that research shows might offer some protection against breast cancer. Although alcohol is not a food, it is a component of many women's diets that needs to be addressed. Unfortunately, that glass of red wine that keeps your heart healthy likely increases your risk of breast cancer. So likely, in fact, that diet and cancer experts recommend that women do not drink alcohol. The current recommendations state that if you consume alcoholic drinks at all, you should limit them to one per day.

In the late 1970s and early 1980s, studies began reporting that breast cancer risk increased with alcohol intake. In a review of 38 studies conducted up until 1992, researchers concluded that having one, two, or three drinks daily all increased the risk of breast cancer. The more alcohol a woman consumed, the higher her risk. Women who drink three alcoholic beverages daily increase the risk of breast cancer by 140 percent as compared with the risk carried by nondrinkers. At three drinks a day, the risk is also 20 percent higher than for women who have one drink a day.

We don't fully understand why alcohol increases breast cancer risk. It may be that alcohol weakens breast cells' defences against carcinogens, or it may be that alcohol causes the liver to activate carcinogens. Alcohol may inhibit the ability of cells to repair faulty genes. Alcohol can also influence estrogen levels in the body. In one study, postmenopausal women who consumed two drinks a day had significantly higher blood estrogen levels than women who didn't drink.[21]

Enough evidence has been accumulated for us to conclude that alcohol probably does increase the risk of breast cancer. To help lower your risk, take the following advice to heart:

- If you don't drink alcohol now, don't start.
- If you do drink, aim to consume no more than one drink daily.
- If you need to lower your daily intake, try replacing alcoholic beverages with sparkling mineral water, Clamato or tomato juice, or cranberry and soda.
- You might try cutting out alcoholic beverages on evenings you are not entertaining or out for dinner. Save your glass of wine or cocktail for social occasions.

MANAGE YOUR WEIGHT

A number of studies have determined that gaining weight after menopause is linked with a higher risk of breast cancer.[22] Obesity may influence breast cancer risk by increasing your circulating estrogen levels—this is because estrogen is produced in body fat cells. If you are overweight or you have gained some weight since menopause, I strongly advise you to read Chapter 10 on preventing weight gain. On pages 105–106 I show you how to determine your body mass index, which is a key indicator of how your current weight is affecting your health. I also give you plenty of strategies, as well as a meal plan (see Appendix 1) to help you achieve a healthy weight.

Vitamins and minerals

BETA-CAROTENE AND OTHER CAROTENOIDS

In my discussion of fruits and vegetables, I told you that vegetables high in beta-carotene appear to be more protective against cancer than other vegetables are. Beta-carotene has two roles in the body. As you read above, it has an antioxidant effect, which can help protect our genes from oxidative damage caused by free radicals. But beta-carotene is also converted to vitamin A inside the body. Vitamin A is essential for proper cell growth and development, and also enhances our immunity. Both of these functions of vitamin A may help our body keep cancer at bay.

When all the studies are considered together, beta-carotene does appear to offer some protection from breast cancer. Toronto scientists have estimated that women who get the most beta-carotene in their diets reduce their risk of breast cancer by 15 percent. A diet that is high in fruits and vegetables rich in beta-carotene might also improve breast cancer survival. Two studies on this topic found that women who consumed more than 8 milligrams of beta-carotene daily had a lower risk of dying from breast cancer than women who got less than 3.5 milligrams each day.

At this time, I am unable to tell you exactly how much beta-carotene you need each day; unfortunately, those studies haven't been done yet. But most experts believe a daily intake of 5 milligrams will offer plenty of antioxidant protection. For the record, one medium-sized carrot packs 11 milligrams! You'll get plenty of beta-carotene if you make a point to eat at least two foods from the list below. To boost your beta-carotene, think orange and green. Not sure what to do with these foods? Read on…

Go for green!

Beet greens   When you buy beets, save the greens and eat them too—the leaves of root vegetables have more vitamins and minerals than do the roots. Beet greens are also a good source of vitamins A and C, calcium, and iron. They're good in soups, stir-fries, and, if tender enough, salad.

Collard greens   In addition to plenty of vitamins and minerals, this member of the cabbage family contains sulphur compounds that may prevent certain cancers. Stir-fry collards; once cooked, add a dash of roasted sesame oil and a handful of cashews.

Kale   Just 1 cup (250 ml) of this cabbage-family green provides more than twice the daily requirements for beta-carotene and vitamin C. Kale is also high in calcium and vitamin E. Steam or stir-fry with other vegetables, or throw chopped kale into soup and allow to simmer. Kale shrinks a lot during cooking; 3 cups (750 ml) raw gives you 1 cup (250 ml) cooked.

Spinach   One-half cup (125 ml) of cooked spinach provides plenty of vitamin C, a full day's dose of vitamin A, and plenty of folate, a B vitamin important during pregnancy and for preventing heart disease (see pages 200–202). Like kale, spinach shrinks a lot during cooking: 2 cups (500 ml) of raw leaves will give you 1/2 cup (125 ml) cooked spinach; for this reason, 1/2 cup (125 ml) of cooked spinach packs more nutrition than 1 cup (250 ml) raw. As well, the body is able to break down spinach proteins more easily when the vegetable is heated. Steam, braise, or stir-fry it with a little garlic. Add a splash of balsamic vinegar at the end of cooking.

Swiss chard   Another great way to get calcium, beta-carotene, vitamin C, and some iron. Use both the leaves and stalks, but add the leaves at the end of cooking—the stalks take longer to soften. Stir-fry with a little olive oil and garlic. Or add lemon juice and Parmesan cheese to cooked Swiss chard. Steamed Swiss chard with a little olive oil and red pepper flakes is great over pasta.

There are more than 600 types of carotenoids. While beta-carotene is a plant's most plentiful carotenoid, other important carotenoids include lutein and lycopene. Researchers are investigating the link between a lutein-rich diet and breast cancer risk. The famous Harvard Nurses' Health Study found that premenopausal women who ate five or more servings of carotenoid-rich fruits and vegetables had a lower risk of breast cancer than women who ate less than two servings daily. In another study of postmenopausal women with breast cancer, researchers discovered that women with higher lutein levels in their blood were more likely to have estrogen-positive breast cancer.[23] As outlined above, breast tumours that contain estrogen receptors are associated with a better chance of survival and better response to hormone treatment.

Our bodies don't absorb dietary carotenoids well—our small intestines take in roughly 10 to 30 percent of the amount of these nutrients found in a particular food. Because they are fat-soluble molecules, you'll absorb more if you eat carotenoid-rich foods with a little fat. Try a yogurt dip with carrot sticks, a little olive oil in lycopene-rich pasta sauce, or a splash of salad dressing on your roasted red pepper.

To increase your intake of carotenoid-rich fruits and vegetables, try getting five servings (1/2 cup/125 ml each) from a variety of the following foods every day:

CAROTENOID-RICH FOODS

Beta-carotene	Lycopene	Lutein
Carrots	Tomatoes	Beet greens
Squash	Tomato juice	Collards
Sweet potato	Tomato sauce	Corn
Red pepper	Grapefruit, red and pink	Kale
Cantaloupe	Guava	Okra
Mango	Watermelon	Red pepper
Nectarine		Romaine lettuce
Papaya		Spinach
Peach		

VITAMIN C

Although the research findings on vitamin C are less consistent than those on beta-carotene, there is evidence to suggest you might need to be getting more in your diet. Nine studies comparing women with breast cancer and those free of the disease found that vitamin C was protective. Women with the most vitamin C in their diet were 27 percent less likely to have breast cancer.[24] The vitamin may keep women healthy by acting as an antioxidant, or it may work by enhancing immune system functioning. Vitamin C also plays an important role in collagen synthesis. Collagen is an important tissue found throughout the body, including in the breast—it helps bind cells together, giving the various body structures integrity.

The daily recommended intake of vitamin C for women is 75 milligrams (smokers need an additional 35 milligrams). Refer to page 203 for a list of good food sources of vitamin C and to page 204 for information about taking vitamin C supplements.

VITAMIN B12

Although preliminary, one recent study suggests that a deficiency of vitamin B12 may increase the risk of breast cancer. Harvard researchers reported that postmenopausal women with the lowest B12 levels in their blood had a higher risk of breast cancer than women with much higher levels.[25] It's thought that depleted levels of vitamin B12 can lead to DNA damage.

In the body, vitamin B12 works closely with folate, an important B vitamin that's needed to synthesize DNA in cells. Folate is needed to activate B12, and vice versa. So without enough B12, your body is unable to use folate and you will eventually develop a folate deficiency. That's why you may have heard that it's important to take extra B12 when you take folic acid supplements (folic acid is the name for folate when it's in supplement form). Taking plenty of folic acid without additional B12 can hide a B12 deficiency—everything will look normal on a blood test, even though your body is depleted of vitamin B12.

Most B12 deficiencies are caused by impaired absorption, however, rather than a poor diet. After we consume B12 in our diet, the acid in our stomach helps release the B12 from food. The vitamin then binds to something called "intrinsic factor," which enables B12 to be absorbed into our bloodstream. Vitamin B12 deficiencies can occur for two reasons:

- Inadequate hydrochloric acid in the stomach, which is common in older adults. Without enough acid, B12 can't be released from food. This means it won't be absorbed into the blood.
- An inherited defective gene for intrinsic factor. Some people don't produce this necessary factor required for B12 to enter their bloodstream. In such cases, regular B12 injections are necessary.

How to get more B12

This vitamin is found exclusively in animal foods. If you eat meat, poultry, and dairy products on a regular basis, you're probably getting enough B12. The recommended intake for adults is 2.4 micrograms per day. On page 49, you'll find a table outlining various foods and their vitamin B12 content.

For strict vegetarians who eat no animal products and don't drink a fortified soy or rice beverage, I strongly recommend a B12 supplement. For that matter, anyone over the age of 50 should be getting their B12 from supplements or fortified foods. Up to one-third of older adults produce inadequate amounts of stomach acid and have lost the ability to properly absorb B12 from food. For these cases, I recommend a good multivitamin and mineral supplement or a B-complex supplement that contains the whole family of B vitamins.

FOLATE

If you drink alcohol, you might consider getting more folate into your diet. A recent Harvard study found that among women who consumed 15 grams of alcohol per day (about a glass and a half of beer or wine), those with the highest daily intake of folic acid (600 micrograms daily) had a 45 percent lower risk of breast cancer than women with the lowest folate intake (150 to 299 micrograms daily).[26] The correlation between folate intake and breast cancer risk remained even after the researchers took into account the intake of other nutrients, such as beta-carotene or vitamin A. It's thought that alcohol interferes with the transport and metabolism of folate, and may deprive body tissues of this B vitamin, which is essential for DNA synthesis.

So while I told you earlier that drinking alcohol increases the risk of developing breast cancer, this study would suggest that by getting plenty of folate in your diet and taking a folic acid supplement, you might be able to modify that risk. To help you meet the recommended daily intake of 400 micrograms daily, put the following tips into action:

- Eat spinach, asparagus, and artichokes more often. These vegetables have the most folate, with spinach in the lead, with a whopping 278 micrograms per cup (cooked).
- Drink orange juice. One glass packs roughly 110 micrograms.
- Use lentils and other legumes in salads, pasta sauces, chilies, and tacos. One-half cup (125 ml) of cooked lentils packs about 180 micrograms of folate.
- Choose whole-grain breads and cereals; they are also good sources of folate.
- Take a multivitamin and mineral supplement or a B-complex supplement.
- If you take a folic acid supplement, be sure to use one that has added vitamin B12.

THE bottom LINE...

Leslie's recommendations for reducing breast cancer risk

1 Reduce your intake of saturated fat (animal fat and hydrogenated vegetable oils) in the following ways: Eat no more than 3 ounces (90 g) of meat each day; for protein, choose lean poultry, beans, and soy foods most often; when you do eat meat, avoid cooking it well done (unless you're using ground beef, which should be cooked well done to prevent food poisoning); choose lower-fat dairy products, including 1 percent milk fat (MF) or skim milk, yogurt with 1 percent MF or less, and cheese with 20 percent MF content or less.

2 Include monounsaturated and polyunsaturated fats and oils in your diet: to get

more omega-3 polyunsaturated fat, eat oily fish three times a week. Use olive oil and canola oil in cooking and baking, and flaxseed oil in salad dressings or as an addition to cooked foods such as pasta sauce and lentil soup.

3   Eat one soy food each day to boost your intake of soy protein and isoflavones. To get lignans (plant estrogens), add 1 or 2 tablespoons (15 to 25 ml) of ground flaxseed to your daily diet.

4   Eat at least 5 to 10 servings of fruits and vegetables every single day. Make sure 5 of these servings are of foods brimming with carotenoid compounds.

5   Gradually increase your dietary fibre intake to 25 grams each day. To help lower blood levels of your body's own estrogen, focus on foods rich in wheat bran, such as whole-grain breads, 100-percent bran cereals, and whole-wheat pasta.

6   Include one probiotic food (fermented milk product) in your diet each day to get more friendly bacteria into your intestinal tract. Eat one yogurt serving as a daily midday snack, or try kefir, a fermented milk product available in most grocery stores. If you don't eat these foods, consider taking a probiotic supplement daily with a meal.

7   Drink more green and black teas for their catechins, natural antioxidant compounds found in tea leaves.

8   Avoid alcoholic beverages. If you do drink, consume no more than one drink each day.

9   Manage your weight before and after menopause. Use my strategies in Chapter 10 to take charge of weight gain.

10 Get more B vitamins, especially folate and vitamin B12, into your diet every day. These two vitamins work closely together—folate is needed for DNA synthesis and a deficiency of B12 may increase the risk of breast cancer by leading to damage of DNA molecules. The best food sources of folate include spinach, lentils, orange juice, artichokes, asparagus, and whole-grain breads and cereals. If you drink alcoholic beverages, be sure to boost your intake of this B vitamin. Vitamin B12 is found in animal products only—meat, poultry, eggs, and dairy products. Take a multivitamin and mineral supplement daily to ensure you're getting enough B12 and folate. If your multivitamin and mineral is low in B vitamins (less than 5 milligrams of each per dose), consider adding a B-complex supplement to your regime.

Appendix 1

Leslie's total nutrition plan for the menopausal years

This daily nutrition plan focuses on foods high in fibre and calcium. Phytoestrogens are provided from daily servings of soy foods and ground flaxseed. Keep in mind that how you eat throughout the day affects how you feel. To help you boost your metabolic rate and keep energy levels up, I recommend the following:

- Eat your meals four to five hours apart.
- If meals are eaten more than five hours apart, a between-meal snack is a good idea.
- Snacks should provide some protein and carbohydrate, as well as calcium, vitamin D, and antioxidants. To achieve this kind of nutrient profile in your snacks, avoid refined starchy foods (bagels, crackers, pretzels, commercial fat-free muffins, cereal bars, and the like). These foods lack protein and calcium and provide only a short-term energy boost. You'll find my snack suggestions below.

MEAL OPTIONS AND RECOMMENDED SERVINGS

Breakfast option 1
- 1 to 2 starchy food servings (whole grain)
- 1 fruit serving (citrus fruit at breakfast to enhance iron absorption from whole grains)
- 1 milk/milk alternative serving
- Ground flaxseed, 1 to 2 tbsp. (15 to 25 ml)
- Green or black tea

Breakfast option 2

- 1 starchy food serving (whole grain)
- 2 fruit servings
- 1 milk/milk alternative serving
- Ground flaxseed, 1 to 2 tbsp. (15 to 25 ml)
- Green or black tea

Breakfast option 3

- 1 protein serving
- 1 to 2 starchy food servings (whole grain)
- 1 fruit serving
- 1 fat serving
- Green or black tea

Midmorning snack options

If breakfast and lunch are five to six hours apart, eat:

- 1 piece fruit OR 1 milk/milk alternative serving; 2 cups (500 ml) water throughout morning

If breakfast and lunch are more than six hours apart, eat:

- 1 piece fruit AND 1 milk/milk alternative serving; 2 cups (500 ml) water OR
- 1 piece fruit AND 1 protein serving; 2 cups (500 ml) water OR
- If you're on the go, 1 energy bar containing 10 to14 grams protein and 20 to 25 grams of carbohydrate (for example, Balance Bar, Zone Perfect Bar, Clif Luna Bar, SoyOne Bar, Genisoy Bar); 2 cups (500 ml) water

Lunch

- 2 starchy food servings (whole grain)
- 3 protein servings
- 1 to 2 vegetable servings
- 2 fat/oil servings
- 2 cups (500 ml) water

Midafternoon snack options

If lunch and dinner are five to six hours apart, eat:

• 1 fruit serving OR 1 milk/milk alternative serving; 2 cups (500 ml) water

If lunch and dinner are more than six hours apart, eat:

• 1 fruit serving and 1 milk/milk alternative serving; 2 cups (500 ml) water
  OR

• 1 fruit serving and 1 protein serving; 2 cups (500 ml) water
  OR

• If you're on the go, 1 energy bar with 10 to 14 grams protein and 20 to 25 grams of carbohydrate; 2 cups (500 ml) water

Dinner

• 3 to 5 protein servings
• 0 to 2 starchy food servings (whole grain)
• 1 green vegetable serving
• 2 other vegetable servings
• 2 fat/oil servings
• 2 cups (500 ml) water

Evening snack (optional)

• 1 milk/milk alternative serving

MEAL IDEAS

Breakfast ideas

• 1 cup (250 ml) 100% bran cereal OR 1 1/2 cups (375 ml) whole-grain flake cereal. (Choose a cereal with at least 4 grams of fibre per serving.)
• 1 tbsp. (15 ml) ground flaxseed, sprinkled over cereal
• 1 cup (250 ml) skim or 1% milk or low-fat, calcium-fortified soy beverage
• 3/4 cup (175 ml) unsweetened citrus juice OR 1 cup (250 ml) strawberries
• Green or black tea
  OR
• 1 cup (250 ml) cooked oatmeal or Red River cereal, made with skim or 1% milk instead of water.

- 1 tbsp. (15 ml) ground flaxseed and 2 tbsp. (25 ml) raisins/dried cranberries, added to cereal
- 1/2 cup (125 ml) low-fat plain or vanilla-flavoured yogurt, as cereal topping
- 3/4 cup (175 ml) calcium-fortified orange or grapefruit juice
- Green or black tea

OR

- 2 whole-wheat toaster waffles
- Top with 1 cup (250 ml) fresh fruit or berries, 3/4 cup (175 ml) low-fat vanilla-flavoured yogurt, and a drizzling of maple syrup
- 3/4 cup (175 ml) calcium-fortified orange or grapefruit juice
- Green or black tea

OR

- Blender smoothie: 3/4 to 1 cup (175 to 250 ml) low-fat, calcium-fortified soy beverage, 1 small banana, 1/2 cup (125 ml) orange juice or handful of frozen berries, and 1 tbsp. (15 ml) ground flaxseed
- 1 slice whole-grain or rye toast with 1 tbsp. (15 ml) sugar-reduced jam or honey
- Green or black tea

OR

- 1 hard-boiled or poached egg OR 1 oz. (30 g) low-fat cheese OR 1/4 cup (50 ml) 1% cottage cheese
- 2 slices whole-grain or rye toast
- 1–2 tbsp. (15–25 ml) sugar-reduced jam or honey
- 1 cup fruit salad or 1 piece fruit
- 1 cup (250 ml) water
- Green or black tea

Midmorning snack
- 1 apple and/or 3/4 cup (175 ml) low-fat yogurt
- 2 glasses (500 ml) water

Lunch ideas
- Sandwich on two slices of whole-grain bread, with 3 oz. (90 g) turkey or chicken breast, 2 tsp. (10 ml) light mayonnaise, romaine lettuce or spinach leaves, and sliced tomato

- Handful of baby carrots or side salad with seasoned rice vinegar
- 2 glasses (500 ml) water
  OR
- 1 1/2 cups (375 ml) hearty bean soup
- 4 whole-wheat or whole-rye crackers OR 1/2 whole-wheat pita
- Green or spinach salad with 1 tbsp. (15 ml) mixed nuts
- 4 tsp. (20 ml) salad dressing
- 2 glasses (500 ml) water
  OR
- Large green or spinach salad
- 4 oz. (120 g) or 1 can tuna or salmon packed in water
- 4 tsp. (20 ml) salad dressing
- 1 whole-grain or rye roll
- 2 glasses (500 ml) water
  OR
- 1 cup (250 ml) vegetable soup
- Add 1/2 cup (125 ml) cubed firm tofu when heating soup
- Toasted vegetable sandwich on 2 slices whole-grain bread (tomato, cucumber, fresh basil leaves, spread with goat cheese)
- 2 glasses (500 ml) water
  OR
- 1 cup (250 ml) canned beans (try kidney or black beans) heated with 2 tbsp. (25 ml) water, chili powder, and other spices as desired. Place on one 8-inch (20-cm) whole-wheat tortilla and top with chopped green pepper, tomato, lettuce, grated cheese, salsa
- 2 glasses (500 ml) water

Midafternoon snack ideas
- Blender smoothie: 1 cup (250 ml) low-fat, calcium-fortified soy beverage, 1/2 small banana, and handful of frozen strawberries or blueberries
- 2 glasses (500 ml) water
  OR
- 1 piece fruit and 2 tbsp. (25 ml) roasted soy nuts or other nuts
- 2 glasses (500 ml) water

Dinner ideas

- 5 oz. (150 g) grilled or baked salmon filet, baked in foil with lemon juice, garlic, and chopped fresh dill
- 1/2 to 1 cup (125 to 250 ml) cooked brown rice
- Stir-fried broccoli, red pepper, mushrooms, and slivered almonds, stir-fried in chicken or vegetable broth to prevent sticking
- 2 glasses (500 ml) water

OR

- Omelette made with 1 whole egg and 4 egg whites (these can be Pure Egg Whites, available at grocery stores)
- Add fresh basil leaves and crumbled goat cheese, or try grated cheddar, chopped green onion, and salsa
- 1 whole-grain roll or slice of toast
- Green salad
- 4 tsp. (20 ml) salad dressing
- 2 glasses (500 ml) water

OR

- 3 oz. (90 g) roasted pork tenderloin, brushed with hoisin sauce, or, if you have more time, marinate in soy sauce, garlic, and chopped ginger, then bake at 375° Fahrenheit (190° Celsius) for 25–30 minutes
- 1/2 cup (125 ml) roasted new potatoes with 1 tsp. (5 ml) olive oil, salt, and herbs
- Steamed vegetables (1 orange and 1 green)
- 2 glasses (500 ml) water

OR

- 1 to 1 1/2 cups (250 to 375 ml) vegetarian chili (homemade with assorted canned beans tastes great. I also add veggie ground round.)
- 1 small whole-wheat tortilla
- 2 cups (500 ml) green salad
- 4 tsp. (20 ml) salad dressing
- 2 glasses (500 ml) water

OR

- 5 oz. (150 g) baked white fish, such as halibut, grouper, or sea bass (marinate for 30 minutes with a Japanese-style dressing or brush with hoisin sauce and bake at 450° Fahrenheit/220° Celsius for approximately 15 minutes or until done)
- Stir-fried collard greens; at the end of cooking, add 1 tsp. (5 ml) roasted sesame oil and some cashew nuts
- 1/2 to 1 cup (125 to 250 ml) cooked yam or sweet potato mashed with 2 tbsp. (25 ml) orange juice
- 2 glasses (500 ml) water

  OR

- 1 cup (250 ml) cooked whole-wheat pasta
- 3/4 cup (175 ml) tomato-based pasta sauce
- Add 2/3 cup (150 ml) veggie ground round or white kidney beans to sauce (I recommend Yves Cuisine soy products, such as veggie ground round; they are sold in the produce section of the grocery store.)
- Green salad
- 4 tsp. (20 ml) salad dressing
- 2 glasses (500 ml) water

Dessert or evening snack
- 3/4 cup (175 ml) low-fat yogurt with fruit added
- 1 tbsp. (15 ml) ground flaxseed, mixed into yogurt

Daily and weekly super-nutrition-plan checklists

Post this list somewhere easily visible in your kitchen. After a few weeks of meeting these requirements, you'll find you've developed a new and healthier set of eating habits.

DAILY CHECKLIST

Foods
- ☐ 1 soy food serving
- ☐ 2 to 3 milk/milk alternative servings
- ☐ 1 calcium-rich vegetable

☐ 1 dark green vegetable

☐ 1 citrus fruit

☐ 1 to 2 tbsp. (15 to 25 ml) ground flaxseed

☐ Flaxseed oil, walnut oil, or nuts

Beverages

☐ 8 or more glasses of water

☐ 1 cup (250 ml) or more green or black tea

☐ No more than 1 alcoholic drink

Supplements

☐ Multivitamin/mineral

☐ Vitamin E, 400 or 800 IU

☐ Vitamin C, 500 mg

☐ Calcium citrate with vitamin D and magnesium, 300 to 350 mg once or twice daily

WEEKLY CHECKLIST

Foods

☐ Fish, 3 times weekly

☐ Nuts, 3 to 5 times weekly

☐ Dessert or other "treat," once weekly

Beverages

☐ Alcoholic drinks, no more than 7 weekly

Leslie's meal plan for healthy weight loss

BREAKFAST

Every morning, choose among the following breakfast menus:

Breakfast option 1

- 1/2 cup (125 ml) 100% bran cereal OR 1 cup (250 ml) whole-grain cereal (Choose a cereal with at least 4 grams of fibre per serving.)

- 1 cup (250 ml) skim or 1% milk or calcium-fortified soy beverage
- 3/4 cup (175 ml) calcium-fortified orange juice OR 1 whole citrus fruit
- Water; tea
- Vitamin supplements

Breakfast option 2

- 1–2 slices whole-wheat toast with 1 tbsp. (15 ml) sugar-reduced jam or honey
- 3/4 cup (175 ml) low-fat yogurt (fruit bottom okay) OR 1 medium-sized skim milk latte
- 3/4 cup (175 ml) calcium-fortified orange juice OR 1 piece fruit
- Water; tea
- Vitamin supplements

Breakfast option 3

- 1 cup (250 ml) cooked oatmeal, Red River, or Cream of Wheat cereal
  (To boost the nutritional content of your hot cereal, add ground flaxseed, wheat germ, or 2 tbsp. (25 ml) dried fruit—cherries, cranberries, raisins.)
- 3/4 cup (175 ml) low-fat plain or vanilla-flavoured yogurt OR 1 cup (250 ml) calcium-fortified soy beverage (or milk)
- 3/4 cup (175 ml) calcium-fortified orange juice
- Vitamin supplements; water; tea

Breakfast option 4

- Soy breakfast smoothie (see recipe, page 263)
- Water, tea, and vitamin supplements

MIDMORNING SNACK

Have a midmorning snack if you eat lunch more than five hours after breakfast. Choose one of the following:

- 3/4 cup (175 ml) 1% yogurt
- 1/4 cup (50 ml) soy nuts or other nuts
- 1 piece fruit (for example, 1 medium apple)

LUNCH

Your lunch options are as follows:

Lunch option 1

- Sandwich on rye, pumpernickel, whole wheat, or pita pocket filled with 2 to 3 oz. (60 to 90 g) lean protein: turkey, chicken breast, roast beef, ham, salmon, or tuna with low-fat mayonnaise
- 2 tsp. (10 ml) mayonnaise OR 4 tsp. (20 ml) salad dressing if desired
- 1 vegetable serving (baby carrots, vegetable soup, green salad, vegetable juice)
- Water

Lunch option 2

- 3 oz. (90 g) grilled chicken breast OR 3 oz. (90 g) salmon OR 3/4 cup (175 ml) 1% cottage cheese
- Large green salad
- 4 tsp. (20 ml) salad dressing OR 2 tsp. (10 ml) olive or flaxseed oil
- 1 whole-grain roll
- Water

Lunch option 3

- Veggie burger made with soy protein (not a "grain" burger)
- Whole-wheat roll OR 1/2 whole-wheat pita pocket
- Mustard, relish, plenty of sliced vegetables
- Green salad with 4 tsp. (20 ml) salad dressing
- Water

Lunch option 4

- 1 cup (250 ml) cooked whole-wheat or brown rice pasta with tomato sauce and 3 oz. (90 g) seafood or chicken or ground soy
- Large green salad
- 4 tsp. (20 ml) salad dressing
- Water

MIDAFTERNOON SNACK

Have a midafternoon snack if you eat dinner more than five hours after lunch. Choose one of the following:

- 1 piece of fruit and 3/4 cup (175 ml) low-fat yogurt
- 1 piece of fruit and 2 tbsp. (25 ml) roasted soy nuts or other nuts
- 1 energy bar (look for a bar containing 10 to 14 grams of protein and no more than 200 calories; try Balance Bar, Zone Perfect Bar or Clif Luna Bar)
- 1 medium-size skim milk or soy milk decaf latte

DINNER

I've handled the dinner section a little differently than the others. I'll start by outlining your basic dinner and then go on to give you a few menu options that fit the basic pattern.

Your basic dinner

- 4 to 5 oz. (120 to 150 g) baked or grilled poultry, lean meat, fish, or seafood
- No starchy foods*
- 1 to 2 cups (250 to 500 ml) vegetables: aim for at least two types of vegetables
- 2 tsp. (10 ml) oil OR 4 tsp. (20 ml) salad dressing
- Water

*If you want to add whole-grain starch at dinner, such as 2/3 cup (150 ml) brown rice or 1 cup (250 ml) of cooked pasta, reduce your protein servings to 3.

Dinner option I

- Large green salad
- 1 can salmon or tuna (packed in water, drained) OR 1 grilled chicken breast
- 4 tsp. (20 ml) salad dressing
- Water

Dinner option 2

- Omelette made with 2 whole eggs* OR omelette made with 1 whole egg and 2 egg whites; add vegetables, 2 tbsp. (25 ml) grated low-fat cheese, salsa
- Steamed vegetables and/or large green salad

- 4 tsp. (20 ml) salad dressing OR 1 tsp. (5 ml) oil/margarine

*Try omega-3 eggs, available in most grocery stores

Dinner option 3

- 5 oz. (150 g) baked salmon fillet (wrap in foil with lemon juice and fresh chopped dill; bake at 450° Fahrenheit/220° Celsius for approximately 25 minutes)
- Plenty of steamed vegetables and/or green salad
- 4 tsp. (20 ml) salad dressing
- Water

Dinner option 4

- 4 oz. (120 g) roasted pork tenderloin (brush with hoisin sauce; bake at 375° Fahrenheit/190° Celsius for 25 to 30 minutes)
- Plenty of steamed vegetables and/or salad
- 4 tsp. (20 ml) salad dressing OR 1 tsp. (5 ml) oil
- Water

Dinner option 5

- 4 oz. (120 g) grilled lean beef or chicken breast
- Large green salad and/or steamed vegetables
- 4 tsp. (20 ml) salad dressing OR 1 tsp. (5 ml) oil
- Water

Dinner option 6

- 5 oz. (150 g) white fish, such as halibut, grouper, or sea bass (marinate in your favourite dressing or brush with hoisin sauce; bake at 450° Fahrenheit/220° Celsius for approximately 15 minutes)
- Plenty of steamed or stir-fried vegetables or salad
- Water

Daily food intake targets for weight loss

If you follow the meal plan outlined here, you will meet the daily food intake targets given below. In my opinion, maintaining your daily food intake at these target levels is essential for maintaining your health while losing weight. These targets are also your guide to lifelong healthy eating patterns. Remember: Everything you do to lose weight has to be everything you do to keep it off. The only reason you may need to increase your food intake is if you step up your exercise level. Refer to Appendix 2 for a detailed list of serving sizes.

- Protein foods, daily intake target: 6 to 8 servings
- Starchy foods, daily intake target: 3 to 4 servings
- Vegetables, daily target intake: 3 or more servings
- Fruit, daily intake target: 2 or 3 servings
- Milk products and milk alternatives, daily target intake: 2 to 3 servings
- Fats and oils, daily target intake: 3 to 4 servings

Appendix 2

What's a serving?

What constitutes a serving of a particular food? Here's a list of serving sizes for the foods we commonly eat. Use it to help you keep on track with your daily portions. Unless noted otherwise (and where not applicable), all serving sizes refer to measures *after* cooking.

PROTEIN FOODS	I SERVING
Fish, lean meat, poultry	1 oz. (30 g)
Egg, whole	1
Egg whites	2
Legumes (beans, chickpeas, lentils)	1/3 cup (75 ml)
Soy nuts	2 tbsp. (25 ml)
Tempeh	1/4 cup (50 ml)
Tofu, firm	1/3 cup (75 ml)
Texturized vegetable protein	1/3 cup (75 ml)
Veggie dog, small	1

STARCHY FOODS*

Bagel, regular size	1/4
Bread, whole-grain	1 slice
Pita pocket	1/2
Roll, large	1/2
Tortilla, 6-inch (15-cm)	1
Cereal, flake type	3/4 cup (175 ml)
Cereal, 100% bran	1/2 cup (125 ml)
Cereal, hot	1/2 cup (125 ml)
Crackers, soda	6
Corn niblets	1/2 cup (125 ml)
Grains (e.g., millet, barley, quinoa)	1/2 cup (125 ml)
Pasta	1/2 cup (125 ml)
Popcorn, plain	3 cups (750 ml)
Rice	1/3 cup (75 ml)

Choose whole grain as often as possible.

VEGETABLES

Vegetables, cooked or raw	1/2 cup (125 ml)
Vegetables, leafy green (e.g., salad)	1 cup (250 ml)
Vegetable juice	3/4 cup (175 ml)

FRUIT

Fruit, whole	1 piece
Fruit, small (plums, prunes, apricots)	4 pieces
Fruit, cut up	1 cup (250 ml)
Berries	1 cup (250 ml)
Juice, unsweetened	1/2 to 3/4 cup (125 to 175 ml)

MILK PRODUCTS AND MILK ALTERNATIVES

Cheese	1.5 oz. (45 g)
Milk	1 cup (250 ml)
Rice beverage, fortified	1 cup (250 ml)
Soy beverage, fortified	1 cup (250 ml)
Yogurt	3/4 cup (175 ml)

FATS AND OILS

Avocado, medium	1/8
Butter	1 tsp. (5 ml)
Margarine, nonhydrogenated	1 tsp. (5 ml)
Nuts, seeds	1 tbsp. (15 ml)
Olives	10 small or 5 large
Peanut and nut butters	1 1/2 tsp. (7 ml)
Salad dressing	2 tsp. (10 ml)
Salad dressing, fat-reduced	4 tsp. (20 ml)
Vegetable oil	1 tsp. (5 ml)

Appendix 3

Soy food recipes

This collection of recipes has got my clients enjoying soy foods. I hope you enjoy them too.

BREAKFAST

Breakfast shake with tofu

From the low-fat kitchen of my friend and fellow dietitian Sandi Williams, RD
Serves 1

1 cup	calcium-enriched orange juice	250 ml
1	small ripe banana or other fruit that appeals	1
3/4 to 1 cup	soft tofu	175 to 250 ml

Blend all ingredients into a smoothie for a quick breakfast.
Optional: *For a nutty flavour, add 1 tbsp. (15 ml) ground flaxseed.*
Source: Sandi Williams, RD. Used with permission.

LUNCH AND DINNER

Minestrone soup with soybeans

Serves 8

1 tbsp.	olive oil	15 ml
1	medium onion, chopped	1
2	garlic cloves, minced	2
6 cups	vegetable stock or chicken stock	1.5 l
28 oz.	canned tomatoes, chopped (reserve the juice)	840 g
2	potatoes, cut into cubes	2
2	carrots, diced	2
2 cups	green beans, chopped	500 ml
2 cups	cauliflower, chopped	500 ml
1 cup	dried pasta, shell-shaped or fusilli	250 ml
1 can	cooked soybeans, drained and rinsed	1 can
2	zucchini, cubed	2
6-oz. can	tomato paste	180-g can
2 tbsp.	dried basil	25 ml
1 tbsp.	dried oregano	15 ml
1/2 to 1 cup	chopped fresh parsley	125 to 250 ml
1/4 tsp.	ground black pepper	2 ml

Heat the oil in a nonstick pan. Sauté onion and garlic. Cook until softened.

Add vegetable stock, canned tomatoes and juice, potatoes, carrots, green beans, and cauliflower. Bring to boil, then reduce heat and simmer for 15 minutes. Add pasta, soybeans, zucchini, and tomato paste. Simmer for 20 minutes. Add basil, oregano, parsley, and pepper. Cook for another 10 minutes.

Optional: *Add pesto to taste, either to the pot of soup or to each bowl as served; or serve with a sprinkle of Parmesan cheese if desired.*

Source: Sandi Williams, RD. Used with permission.

Sweet potato soup

Serves 6

2 tsp.	canola oil	10 ml
2	cloves garlic, crushed	2
1	medium onion, chopped	1
1 tsp.	curry powder	5 ml
2 large	sweet potatoes, peeled and chopped	2 large
2 cups	water	500 ml
1	vegetable stock cube, crumbled	1
1 1/2 cups	calcium-fortified soy beverage	375 ml

Heat oil in large saucepan. Sauté onion and garlic with curry powder until soft. Add sweet potato, water, and stock cube. Simmer covered for 15 minutes or until vegetables are tender. Cool. Blend or process sweet potato mixture until smooth. Gradually add soy beverage, blending until well combined. Return to saucepan and heat through. Do not boil. Season with salt and pepper to taste.

Serve with crusty bread.

Source: So Good Soy Beverage, Soyaworld, www.sogoodbeverage.com. Used with permission.

Veggie chili

Serves 4

2 tbsp.	canola oil	25 ml
1	large onion, diced	1
1	red or green pepper, diced	1
1	large carrot, diced	1
2	19-oz. (570-g) cans red kidney beans, drained	2
3	14-oz. (420-g) cans tomatoes	3
2 tbsp.	tomato paste	25 ml
1 tbsp.	crushed dried chilies	15 ml
1 tsp.	chili powder	5 ml
1 tsp.	cumin	5 ml
1 tbsp.	dried oregano	15 ml
1 tbsp.	dried basil	15 ml

	salt and pepper, to taste	
11-oz. pkg.	Yves Veggie Ground Round Original	340-g pkg.
	(found in the produce section of	
	grocery stores)	

Heat oil in Dutch oven until hot, then add onion, pepper, and carrot. Sauté for 6 to 8 minutes, stirring occasionally until partially cooked. Add remaining ingredients except Yves Veggie Ground Round. Mix well. Bring to a boil and reduce heat to low. Cook 1 hour. Add crumbled Yves Veggie Ground Round. Mix well. Turn off heat and let stand 5 minutes before serving.

Note from author: This recipe can also be made with texturized vegetable protein (TVP). Rehydrate 1 cup (250 ml) of TVP in an equal amount of boiling water or stock before adding to chili.

Source: Yves Veggie Cuisine. Used with permission.

Tofu cutlets

Serves 4

1 lb.	firm tofu	500 g
1/4 cup	lime juice	50 ml
2 tbsp.	soy sauce	25 ml
1 tsp.	sesame oil	5 ml
1 tbsp.	honey	15 ml
1 tbsp.	onion, minced	15 ml
1 tbsp.	garlic, minced	15 ml
1 tbsp.	fresh ginger, minced	15 ml
1/4 tsp.	black pepper	2 ml
1 tbsp.	sesame seeds	15 ml

Slice tofu into 4 pieces lengthwise. Combine all other ingredients except sesame seeds. Add tofu to the marinade and refrigerate for 2 to 4 hours, turning occasionally. Return dish to room temperature. Preheat oven to 350° Fahrenheit (175° Celsius). Sprinkle tofu with sesame seeds. Bake for 45 minutes.

Source: Recipe courtesy of Try-Foods Canada, Ltd.

Hot and sour tofu

Serves 4

1 lb.	firm tofu	500 g
2 tbsp.	canola oil	25 ml
1	leek, trimmed, cut in 1-inch (2.5-cm) pieces	1
2	cloves garlic, thinly sliced	1
1 tbsp.	chopped ginger	15 ml
1 tsp.	Asian hot sauce	5 ml
3 tbsp.	soy sauce	45 ml
2 tbsp.	balsamic vinegar	25 ml
3	green onions, slivered	3

Wipe tofu dry, then cut into 1-inch (2.5-cm) cubes. Heat oil in skillet or wok over high heat. Add leek, garlic, and ginger, and stir-fry for 30 seconds or until garlic colours slightly. Add tofu and fry 2 minutes per side or until lightly browned. Stir in hot sauce, soy sauce, and vinegar. Bring to boil, cover pan, and simmer 3 minutes. Sprinkle with green onions.

Serve with steamed rice and vegetables.

Source: Lucy Waverman, "On Cooking" column, *Globe and Mail.* Used with permission.

DESSERT

Cinnamon raisin rice pudding

Serves 4

1/3 cup	arborio rice (short-grain Italian rice)	75 ml
1/3 cup	raisins	75 ml
2 cups	calcium-fortified soy beverage	500 ml
3 tbsp.	maple syrup or honey*	45 ml
1 tsp.	vanilla	5 ml
2 tsp.	butter or margarine	10 ml
1/8 tsp.	nutmeg	1.5 ml
pinch	cinnamon	pinch

Preheat oven to 275° Fahrenheit (135° Celsius). Mix together all ingredients except cinnamon. Pour into a greased 2-quart (2-litre) baking dish. Bake for 2 hours. Sprinkle with cinnamon. Serve hot or cold.

Variations: *Add 1 tsp. (5 ml) grated orange or lemon rind or try dried cranberries instead of raisins.*

*This pudding is delicious, but the maple syrup makes it an unappealing brown colour. If you can't get past the colour, use honey instead.

Source: Sandi Williams, RD. Used with permission.

Angel food cake with chocolate orange sauce

Serves 8

Sauce

10.5-oz. pkg.	silken tofu, rinsed and drained	297-g pkg.
1/4 cup	Dutch Process cocoa	50 ml
1/4 cup	sugar	50 ml
1 tbsp.	Grand Marnier or other orange-flavoured liqueur	15 ml

Cake

1	prepared angel food cake	1
2	peaches, peeled and thinly sliced	2
1/2 pint	raspberries, washed	275 ml
3	oranges, cut in sections	3
1 tbsp.	Grand Marnier or other orange-flavoured liqueur	15 ml
8	fresh mint sprigs for garnish	8

In a blender, process tofu, cocoa, sugar, and orange liqueur. Refrigerate. Place prepared angel food cake on a serving platter and set aside. Put prepared fruit in a bowl and sprinkle with liqueur, then spoon around cake on the serving platter.

When ready to serve, pour chocolate sauce into a serving pitcher and pour over individual servings. Garnish each serving with a mint sprig.

Source: Adapted from the Ontario Soybean Growers' Marketing Board "Tofu Recipe Booklet." Used with permission.

Appendix 4

A quick reference guide to vitamins and minerals

Eat right and live well, or so the saying goes. A diet that's low in fat and chock full of vegetables, fruit, and whole grains will give you plenty of vitamins and minerals. Your body needs more than 45 nutrients to stay healthy—and you're most likely to find them in whole, unprocessed foods. Whole foods also offer many other natural compounds that help your body fight disease, such as fibre and phyto-(plant) chemicals.

Yet despite the overload of information available today on the benefits of eating what's good for you, many of us don't get enough vitamins and minerals. If you're on the go, under stress, or a haphazard eater, chances are you don't always eat right. Nutrition surveys show that many of us don't get enough of very important nutrients like calcium, iron, and zinc.

Even if you are getting the recommended dietary allowance (RDA) of all the major vitamins and minerals, there are certain vitamins you probably should get even more of. Vitamins C, E, and folate may reduce your risk of cancer, heart disease, and other age-related illness when taken in amounts greater than the RDAs.

Use the table following to choose foods that are brimming with protective vitamins and minerals. Nutrient recommendations are given for adults, aged 19 and older.

FAT SOLUBLE VITAMINS

	WHAT IT DOES	**BEST FOOD SOURCES**	**DAILY NEEDS**
Vitamin A	Needed for night and colour vision; supports cell growth and development; maintains healthy skin, hair, nails, bones, and teeth; enhances immune system; may help prevent lung cancer	*Vitamin A:* liver, oily fish, milk, cheese, butter, egg yolks *Beta-carotene:* orange and yellow fruits and vegetables; dark green vegetables	Women: 700 mcg Men: 900 mcg
Vitamin D	Regulates body calcium levels; needed for calcium absorption; maintains bones and teeth	Fluid milk, fortified soy and rice beverages, oily fish, egg yolks, butter, margarine (also made by body when exposed to sunlight)	Women and men: 19–50 years: 400 IU 51+ years: 800 IU
Vitamin E	Protects cell membranes; enhances immune system; strong antioxidant; needed for iron metabolism	Vegetable oil, margarine, nuts, seeds, whole grains, green leafy vegetables, asparagus, avocado, wheat germ	Women and men 22 IU
Vitamin K	Essential for blood clotting	Green peas, broccoli, spinach, leafy green vegetables, liver	Women: 90 mcg Men: 120 mcg

WATER SOLUBLE VITAMINS

Vitamin C	Supports collagen synthesis and wound healing; strengthens blood vessels; boosts immune system; helps body absorb iron; antioxidant	Citrus fruit, strawberries, kiwi, cantaloupe, broccoli, bell peppers, Brussels sprouts, cabbage, tomatoes, potatoes	Women: 75 mg Men: 90 mg (smokers need an additional 35 mg per day)
B1 (Thiamin)	Needed for energy metabolism; maintains normal appetite and nerve function	Pork, liver, whole grains, enriched breakfast cereals, legumes, nuts	Women: 1.1 mg Men: 1.2 mg

	WHAT IT DOES	BEST FOOD SOURCES	DAILY NEEDS
B2 (Riboflavin)	Used in energy metabolism; supports normal vision; maintains healthy skin	Milk, yogurt, cheese, fortified soy and rice beverages, meat, whole grains, enriched breakfast cereals	Women: 1.1 mg Men: 1.3 mg
B3 (Niacin)	Used in energy metabolism; maintains skin, digestive system, and nerve function	Chicken, tuna, liver, peanuts, whole grains, enriched breakfast cereals, dairy products, all high-protein foods	Women: 14 mg Men: 16 mg
B6 (Pyridoxine)	Needed for protein and fat metabolism; used to make red blood cells; supports brain serotonin production	Meat, poultry, fish, beans, nuts, seeds, whole grains, green and leafy vegetables, bananas, avocados	Women and men: 19–50 years: 1.3 mg Women, 51+ years: 1.5 mg Men, 51+ years: 1.7 mg
Folate	Supports cell division and growth; used to make DNA and red blood cells; prevents neural tube defects in newborns; may prevent heart disease	Spinach, lentils, orange juice, asparagus, avocados, whole grains, seeds, liver	Women and men: 400 mcg
B12 (Cobalamin)	Maintains nerve function; needed to make DNA and red blood cells	All animal foods, fortified soy and rice beverages	Women and men: 2.4 mcg (adults over 50 years should get B12 from a supplement or fortified foods)
Biotin	Used for energy metabolism, fat synthesis, and amino acid and carbohydrate metabolism	Kidney, liver, oatmeal, egg yolk, soybeans, brewer's yeast, clams, mushrooms, bananas	Women and men: 30 mcg
Pantothenic acid	Needed to break down fats, protein, and carbohydrate for energy; used to make bile, red blood cells, hormones, vitamin D	Widespread in foods	Women and men: 5 mg

	WHAT IT DOES	BEST FOOD SOURCES	DAILY NEEDS
Choline	Necessary for fat metabolism and cell membrane structure; building block for acetylcholine, an important chemical for brain and nerve function	Egg yolks, liver, kidney, meat, brewer's yeast, wheat germ, soybeans, peanuts, green peas	Women: 425 mg Men: 550 mg

MINERALS

Calcium	Needed for strong bones and teeth, muscle-fortified contraction and relaxation, nerve function, blood clotting; maintains blood pressure	Milk, yogurt, cheese, soy and rice beverages, tofu, canned salmon (with bones), kale, bok choy, broccoli, chard	Women and men: 19 to 50 years: 1000 mg 51+ years: 1500 mg
Chromium	Helps insulin regulate blood sugar	Brewer's yeast, molasses, mushrooms, whole grains	Women: 25 mcg Men: 35 mcg
Copper	Helps the body absorb iron; needed for nerve fibres, red blood cells, connective tissue, and many enzymes	Liver, meat, shellfish, legumes, prunes	Women and men: 900 mcg
Fluoride	Essential in formation of bones and teeth; helps prevent tooth decay	Drinking water (if fluoridated), tea, seafood	Women: 3 mg Men: 4 mg
Iodine	Used to make thyroid hormones, which regulate growth, development, and metabolism	Iodized salt, seafood, sea vegetables, plants grown in iodide-rich soil	Women and men: 150 mcg
Iron	Needed to transport oxygen to all cells; supports metabolism	Red meat, seafood, poultry, eggs, legumes, whole grains, enriched breakfast cereals	Women: 18 mg (after menopause 8 mg) Men: 8 mg
Magnesium	Involved in bone growth, protein building, muscle contraction, and transmission of nerve impulses	Nuts, legumes, whole grains, leafy green vegetables, meat, poultry, fish, eggs	Women: 320 mg Men: 420 mg

	WHAT IT DOES	BEST FOOD SOURCES	DAILY NEEDS
Manganese	Part of many enzymes; facilitates cell metabolism	Coffee, tea, legumes, nuts, wheat bran	Women: 1.8 mg Men: 2.3 mg
Molybdenum	Used for metabolism; helps the body mobilize iron stores	Hard drinking water, meat, whole grains, legumes, green leafy vegetables, organ meats	Women and men: 45 mcg
Phosphorus	Maintains strong bones and teeth; used in metabolism; part of genetic material	Dairy products, meat, poultry, fish, egg yolks, legumes	Women and men: 700 mg
Selenium	Antioxidant; works with vitamin E to prevent cell damage from free radicals	Seafood, meat, organ meats, grains, onion, garlic, mushrooms	Women and men: 55 mcg
Sulphur	Necessary for body proteins, bones, and teeth; activates enzymes; regulates blood clotting	Meat, organ meats, poultry, fish, eggs, legumes, dairy products	Not established
Zinc	Crucial for growth and reproduction; used to make genetic material, immune compounds, enzymes; helps transport vitamin A	Oysters, seafood, red meat, poultry, yogurt, whole grains, enriched breakfast cereals	Men: 11 mg Women: 8 mg

Appendix 5

Compounding pharmacists in Canada

Bio-identical hormone replacement therapy is readily available with a prescription from a compounding pharmacist. When a pharmacist compounds a prescription, he or she takes the raw form of a medication, often a powder, and prepares it to meet the patient's needs. The pharmacist decides on the best delivery route for the medication, be it tablet, capsule, cream, gel, or suppository. The compounding pharmacist works closely with the prescribing physician to arrive at the best-possible dosage for each patient.

BRITISH COLUMBIA

Clayburn Rexall Drugstore
Unit 150-3033 Immel Road
Abbotsford, BC V2S 6S2
(604) 852-9217

Northmount Pharmacy
145 East 13th Street
North Vancouver, BC V7L 2L4
(604) 985-8241
Toll-free: 1-800-816-5533
www.northmountpharmacy.com

Skaha Pharmacy
3030 Skaha Lake Road
Penticton, BC V2A 7H2
(250) 493-8155

McDonald's Prescriptions
746 West Broadway
Vancouver, BC V5Z IG8
(604) 872-2662
www.macdonaldsrx.com

Victoria Compounding Pharmacy
1089 Fort Street
Victoria, BC V8V 3K5
(877) 688-5181
www.**pbnisystems**.com/victoria_
pharm/hrt.asp

ALBERTA

Script Pharmacy
506-71 Avenue Southwest
Calgary, AB T2V 4V4
(403) 253-6773

Lemarchand Dispensary
11503-100 Avenue, Main Floor
Edmonton, AB T5K 2K7
(780) 482-3322
www.lemarchand-rx.com

Stafford Pharmacy
1475 St. Edward Boulevard North
Lethbridge, AB T1H 2P9
(403) 320-6500
Toll-free: 800-320-1260
www.staffordpharmacy.com

SASKATCHEWAN

Victoria Square Dispensary
2345-10th Avenue West
Prince Albert, SK S6V 7V6
(306) 922-5855
www.compoundingpharmacy.sk.ca

Hill Avenue Drugs
3410 Hill Avenue
Regina, SK S4S 0W9
(306) 586-6262

Saskatoon Medical Arts Pharmacy
133-750 Spadina Crescent East
Saskatoon, SK S7K 3H3
(306) 652-5252

Wall Street Pharmacy
140 Wall Street
Saskatoon, SK S7K 1N4
(306) 652-5194

MANITOBA

Dauphlin Clinic Pharmacy
622-3rd Street Southwest
Dauphlin, MB R7N 1R5
(204) 638-4602
www.dcp.ca

CD Whyte Ridge Pharmacy
123 D. Scurfield Boulevard
Winnipeg, MB R3Y 1L6
(204) 488-1819

Tache Pharmacy
400 Tache Avenue
Winnipeg, MB R2H 3C3
(204) 233-3469
www.tachepharmacy.com

ONTARIO

Pickering Village Pharmacy
59 Old Kingston Road
Ajax, ON L1T 3A5
(905) 683-9271

Dell Pharmacy (multiple locations in southern Ontario)
4057 New Street
Burlington, ON L7L 1S8
(905) 637-2880
www.dellpharmacy.com

Beveridge & Brown Clinic Pharmacy
167 Hespeler Road
Cambridge, ON N1R 3H7
(519) 623-4116

Hunter's Pharmacy
3019 Tecumseh Road
East Windsor, ON N8W 1G8
(519) 945-4333

Marchese Pharmacy
316 James Street North
Hamilton, ON L8L1H2
(905) 528-4201

Village Pharmacy and Health Food
Store
225 Lakeshore Road East
Mississauga, ON L5G 1G8
(905) 278-7237
Toll-free: 1-800-268-5229

Falls Pharmacy
6635 Drummond Road
Niagara Falls, ON L2G 4N4
(905) 354-3883
www.fallspharmacy.com

Clinic Pharmacy
117 King Street East
Oshawa, ON L1H 1B9
(905) 576-9090

Glebe Apothecary
778 Bank Street
Ottawa, ON KIS 3V6
(613) 234-4643
www.feelbest.com

Nutri-Chem Compounding Pharmacy
1303 Richmond Road
Ottawa, ON K2B 7Y4
(613) 820-4200
Toll-free: 1-888-384-7855
www.nutrichem.com

Courtesy Compounding Laboratory
1603 Clarkson Road North
Port Credit, ON L5J 2X1
(905) 823-4664
www.courtesylab.com

Habers Pharmacy
1584 Bathurst Street
Toronto, ON MSP 3H3
(416) 656-9800
Toll-free: 1-877-262-1084
www.haberspharmacy.com

Smith's Pharmacy
3463 Yonge Street
Toronto, ON M4N 2N3
(416) 488-2600
Toll-free: 1-800-361-6624
www.smithspharmacy.com

The Medicine Shoppe
Kingsway Medical Building
2917 Bloor Street West
Toronto, ON M8X 1B4
(416) 239-3566
www.themedicineshoppe.on.ca

Toronto Compounding Shoppe
3537 Bathurst Street
Toronto, ON M6A 2C7
(416) 789-1800
Toll-free: 1-800-201-8590

York Downs Pharmacy
3910 Bathurst Street
Toronto, ON M3H 3Z8
(416) 633-2244
Toll-free: 1-800-564-5020
www.yorkdownsrx.com

QUEBEC

Pharmacie Perreault
1435 boulevard Saint-Martin Ouest
Chomedey, QC H7S 1N1
(450) 667-3202

Westmount Medical
5025 Sherbrooke West
Montreal, QC H4A 1S9
(514) 484-2222
Toll-free: 1-800-650-5025
www.montrealpharmacy.com

Yetvart PaylanPharmacie paylan
8897 rue Lajeunesse
Montreal, QC H2M 1R8
(514) 382-5921

ATLANTIC PROVINCES

Parkdale Pharmacy
24 Peter's Road
Charlottetown, PEI C1A 8T4
(902) 894-8553

Central Pharmacy
PO Box 496
Union Street
Grand Falls–Windsor, NF A2A 2J9
(709) 489-5411
www.centralpharmacy.nf.ca

Ford Apothecary
544 St. George Boulevard
Moncton, NB E1E 2B5
(506) 853-0830
Toll-free: 1-888-644-3673

Bio-identical hormone replacement therapy prescriptions may be filled at a compounding service pharmacy. To find out if there is a compounding pharmacy in your area, contact:

International Academy of
Compounding Pharmacists
Toll-free: 1-800-927-4227
www.iacprx.org

Wiler Professional Compounding
Centers of America (PCCA)
744 Third Street
London, ON N5V 5J2
Toll-free: 1-800-668-9453
www.pccacanada.com

All that's required is your postal code, and the referral service will do the searching for you!

Appendix 6

Resources

ASSOCIATIONS

American Menopause Foundation
350 Fifth Avenue, Suite 2822
New York, NY, USA 10119
Tel: 212-714-2398
Fax: 212-714-1252
www.americanmenopause.org

Founded in 1993, the American Menopause Foundation is an independent, nonprofit health organization dedicated to providing support and assistance on all issues concerning menopause. Through a newsletter, literature, and educational programs, the foundation provides the latest information on scientific research and other pertinent facts about menopause.

Canadian Cancer Society
National Office
10 Alcorn Avenue, Suite 200
Toronto, Ontario, Canada M4V 3B1
Tel: 416-961-7223
Fax: 416-961-4189
Cancer Information Service: (Toll-free) 1-888-939-3333
www.cancer.ca

Canadian College of Naturopathic Medicine
1255 Sheppard Avenue East
North York, Ontario, Canada M2K 1E2
Tel: 416-498-1255
Fax: 416-498-1576
www.ccnm.edu

Dietitians of Canada
480 University Avenue, Suite 604
Toronto, Ontario, Canada M5G 1V2
Tel: 416-596-0857
Fax: 416-596-0603
www.dietitians.ca

The Dietitians of Canada is an association of food and nutrition professionals committed to the health and well-being of Canadians. Visit the website to learn about nutrition resources or to find a dietitian in your community.

Heart and Stroke Foundation of Canada
222 Queen Street, Suite 1402
Ottawa, Ontario, Canada K1P 5V9
Tel: 613-569-4361
Fax: 613-569-3278
www.heartandstroke.ca

To contact your nearest Heart and Stroke Foundation office, call toll free: 1-888-HSF-INFO (473-4636)

National Institute of Nutrition
265 Carling Avenue, Suite 302
Ottawa, Ontario, Canada K1S 2E1
Tel: 613-235-3355
Fax: 613-235-7032
www.nin.ca

This private, nonprofit organization is dedicated to providing leadership in promoting nutrition for the benefit of all Canadians. The institute serves as a credible source and objective authority on issues related to nutrition, fosters nutrition research and education in Canada, and informs nutrition-related public policy deliberations. At the website, you can read about Canadian nutrition news and publications prepared by the institute.

North American Menopause Society
P.O. Box 94527
Cleveland, Ohio, USA 44101-4527
Tel: 440-442-7550
www.menopause.org

This is a nonprofit scientific organization devoted to promoting understanding of menopause and improving the health of women through midlife and beyond. You'll find a list of recommended books, newsletters, and web resources, as well as referral lists of menopause clinicians in Canada and the United States.

Osteoporosis Society of Canada
33 Laird Drive
Toronto, Ontario, Canada M4G 3S9
Tel: 416-696-2663
Toll-free: 1-800-463-6842
Fax: 416-696-2673
www.osteoporosis.ca

BOOKS

The Wisdom of Menopause
Christiane Northrup, MD
New York, NY: Bantam Books, 2001

The Change Before the Change
Laura E. Corio, MD
New York, NY: Bantam Books, 2000

A Woman's Guide to Natural Hormones
Christine Conrad
New York, NY: Berkley Publishing Group, 2000

The Menopause Manager
Mary Ann Mayo and Joseph L. Mayo, MD
Grand Rapids, MI: Fleming H. Revell, 1998

Before the Change: Taking Charge of Your Perimenopause
Ann Louise Gittleman
New York, NY: HarperCollins Publishers, 1998

CalciYum! Calcium-Rich, Dairy-Free Vegetarian Recipes
David and Rachelle Bronfman
Toronto, ON: Bromedia, 1998

Dr. Susan Love's Hormone Book
Susan M. Love, MD, and Karen Lindsey
New York, NY: Random House, 1997

Dr. Susan Love's Breast Book
Susan M. Love, MD, and Karen Lindsey
New York, NY: Addison-Wesley, 1995 (2nd ed.)

Eat for a Healthy Menopause
Elaine Magee
New York, NY: John Wiley and Sons, 1996

Estrogen: The Natural Way
Nina Shandler
New York, NY: Villard Books, 1997

Good Nutrition for a Healthy Menopause
Louise Lambert-Lagacé, DTP
Stoddart Publishing, 1999

Menopause
Isaac Schiff, MD, with Ann B. Parson
Toronto, ON: Random House of Canada, 1996

Menopausal Years: The Wise Woman Way
Susun S. Weed
Woodstock, NY: Ash Tree Publishing, 1992

Super Nutrition for Menopause
Ann Louise Gittleman
Garden City Park, NY: Avery Publishing Group, 1998

The Osteoporosis Handbook
Sidney Lou Bonnick, MD, FACP
Dallas, TX: Taylor, 1997

Trouble-Free Menopause: Manage Your Symptoms and Your Weight
Judy Marchel, RD, and Linda Konner
New York, NY: Avon Books, 1995

BOOKLETS AND NEWSLETTERS

Menopause Guidebook: Helping Women Make Informed Healthcare Decisions through Perimenopause and Beyond
   The North American Menopause Society
   Available at: www.menopause.org/edumaterials/guidebook/guidebook.html
Published in 2001, this 60-page booklet contains information on perimenopause, early menopause, menopause symptoms, and long-term effects of estrogen loss, as well as a wide variety of therapies to enhance health.

A Friend Indeed
Initiatives for Women's Health Inc.
Main Floor, 419 Graham Avenue
Winnipeg, MB, Canada R3C 0M3
Tel: 204-989-8028
Fax: 204-989-8029
www.afriendindeed.ca
Published since 1984, this is considered the "grandmother of all menopause newsletters" and is a recommended resource in many books about menopause. Written for women approaching or experiencing menopause, each issue comprises a feature article,

letters, research findings, and other health news. A yearly subscription for six issues costs $35 CDN; back issues are also available for a nominal fee.

Harvard Women's Health Watch
P.O. Box 420068
Palm Coast, FL, USA 32142-0068
Toll-free: 1-800-829-5921

This comprehensive newsletter addresses issues relating not only to menopause but also to myriad health concerns that arise through all stages of a woman's life. An annual subscription of 12 issues costs $32 USD.

SOY COOKBOOKS

Tofu and Soyfoods Cookery
Peter Golbitz
Summertown, TN: Book Publishing Company, 1998

Tofu Mania: Add Tofu to Your Favorite Dishes for Optimum Health
Brita Housez
Regina, SK: Centax Books, 1999

The New Soy Cookbook: Tempting Recipes for Tofu, Tempeh, Soybeans, and Soymilk
Lorna Sass and Jonelle Weaver
San Francisco, CA: Chronicle Books, 1998

The TVP Cookbook
Dorothy R. Bates
Summertown, TN: Book Publishing Company, 1991

The Whole Soy Cookbook: 175 Delicious, Nutritious, Easy-To-Prepare Recipes Featuring Tofu, Tempeh, and Various Forms of Nature's Healthiest Bean
Patricia Greenberg and Helen Newton Hartung
New York, NY: Three Rivers Press, 1998

Virtues of Soy: A Practical Health Guide and Cookbook
Monique Gilbert
Universal Publishers, 2000

Notes

I What is Menopause?

1. Schneider HPG et al. 2000. The Menopause Rating Scale (MRS): reliability of scores of menopausal complaints. *Climacteric* 3:59–64.

2. Pottoff R et al. 2000. Menopause-Rating Skala (MRS II): Methodische Standardisierung in der deutschen Bevolkerung. *Zentralbl Gynakol* 122(5):280–286.

2 The Hormone Replacement Therapy (HRT) Dilemma

1. Writing Group for the Women's Health Initiative Investigators. 2002. Risks and benefits of estrogen plus progestin in healthy postmenopausal women: principal results from the Women's Health Initiative randomized controlled trial. *JAMA* 288(3):321–333.

2. Hulley S et al. for the Heart and Estrogen/progestin Replacement Study (HERS) Research Group. 1998. Randomized trial of estrogen plus progestin for secondary prevention of coronary heart disease in postmenopausal women. *JAMA* 280(7):605–613.

   Grady D et al. 2002. Cardiovascular disease outcomes during 6.8 years of hormone therapy: Heart and Estrogen/Progestin Replacement Study follow-up (HERS II). *JAMA* 288(1):49–57.

4 Hot Flashes and Night Sweats

1. Tang GWK. 1994. The climacteric of Chinese factory workers. *Maturitas* 19:177–182.

2. Albertazzi P et al. 1998. The effect of dietary soy supplementation on hot flushes. *Obstetrics and Gynecology* 91(1):6–11.

3. Washburn S et al. 1999. Effect of soy protein supplementation on serum lipoproteins, blood pressure, and menopausal symptoms in perimenopausal women. *Menopause* 6(1):7–13.

4. Hochanadel G et al. 1999. Soy isoflavone extract ineffective for alleviation of postmenopausal symptoms. Clinical Research Center, MIT. Unpublished.

   Upmalis DH et al. 1999. Effect of biochemical parameters of an oral soy extract used in the treatment of vasomotor symptoms in menopausal women. Abstract report presented at the North American Menopause Society 1999 Meeting. Personal Products Company, North Brunswick, New Jersey.

5. Han KK et al. 2002. Benefit of soy isoflavone therapeutic regimen on menopausal symptoms. *Obstetrics and Gynecology* 99(3):389–394.

   Faure ED et al. 2002. Effects of a standardized soy extract on hot flushes: a multicenter, double-blind, randomized, placebo-controlled study. *Menopause* 9(5):329–334.

6. Barton DL et al. 1998. Prospective evaluation of vitamin E for hot flashes in breast cancer survivors. *Journal of Clinical Oncology* 16(2):495–500.

   Kronenberg F. 1994. Hot flashes: phenomenology, quality of life, and search for treatment options. *Experimental Gerontology* 29(3–4):319–336.

7. Foster S. 1999. Black cohosh: a literature review. *Herbalgram* 45:35–49.

   Einer-Jensen N et al. 1996. Cimicifuga and Melbrosia lack estrogenic effects in mice and rats. *Maturitas* 25:149–153.

   Freudenstein J et al. 1999. Influence of an isopropanolic aqueous extract of Cimicifugae racemosa rhizoma on the proliferation of MCF-7 cells. Abstracts of the 23rd International

LOF-Symposium on Phyto-Estrogens. University of Gent, Belgium.

8. Liske E et al. 2002. Physiological investigation of a unique extract of black cohosh (*Cimicifugae racemosae rhizoma*): a 6-month clinical study demonstrates no systemic estrogenic effect. *J Womens Health Gend Based Med* 11(2):163–174.

Düker E-M et al. 1991. Effects of extracts from *Cimicifuga racemosa* on gonadotropin release in menopausal women and ovariectomized rats. *Planta Med* 57:420–424.

Lehmann-Willenbrock E and Riedel HH. 1988. Clinical and endocrinological examinations concerning therapy of climacteric symptoms following hysterectomy with remaining ovaries. *Zentrallblatt für Gynäkologie* 110(10):611–618.

Stoll W. 1987. Phytopharmacon influences atrophic vaginal epithelium: double-blind study— *Cimicifuga* vs. estrogenic substances. *Therapeuticum* 1:23–31.

9. Bodinet C and J Freudenstein. 2002. Influence of *Cimicifuga racemosa* on the proliferation of estrogen receptor-positive human breast cancer cells. *Breast Cancer Res Treat* 76(1):1–10.

Zierau O et al. 2002. Antiestrogenic activities of *Cimicifuga racemosa* extracts. *J Steroid Biochem Mol Biol* 80(1):125–130.

Dixon-Shanies D and N Shaikh. 1999. Growth inhibition of human breast cancer cells by herbs and phytoestrogens. *Oncol Rep* 6(6):1383–1387.

10. Jacobson JS et al. 2001. Randomized trial of black cohosh for the treatment of hot flashes among women with a history of breast cancer. *J Clin Oncol* 19(10):2739–2745.

11. Knight DC et al. 1999. The effect of Promensil, an isoflavone extract, on menopausal symptoms. *Climacteric* 2:79–84.

Baber RJ et al. 1999. Randomized placebo-controlled trial of an isoflavone supplement and menopausal symptoms in women. *Climacteric* 2:85–92.

12. Nachtigall LB et al. 1999. The effects of isoflavone derived from red clover on vasomotor symptoms, endometrial thickness, and reproductive hormone concentrations in menopausal women (abstract). Presented at the 81st Annual Meeting of the Endocrine Society, San Diego, CA, June 12–15, 1999.

Van de Weijer P and Barentsend R. 2002. Isoflavones from red clover (Promensil) significantly reduce menopausal hot flush symptoms compared with placebo. *Maturitus* 42(3):187.

13. Atkinson C et al. 2002. The effects of isoflavone phystoestrogens on bone: preliminary results from a large randomised controlled study. ENDO 2000—The Endocrine Society 82nd Annual Meeting 2000.

Clifton-Bligh PB et al. 2001. The effect of isoflavones extracted from red clover (Rimostil) on lipid and bone metabolism. *Menopause* 8(4):259–265.

5 Restless Nights and Insomnia

1. Minister of National Health and Welfare. 1990. Nutrition Recommendations: the Report of the Scientific Review Committee.

2. Landolt HP et al. 1995. Caffeine intake (200 mg) in the morning affects human sleep and EEG power spectra at night. *Brain Research* 675(1–2):67–74.

———. 1995. Caffeine reduces low-frequency delta activity in the human sleep EEG. *Neuropsychopharmacology* 12(3):229–238.

3. ———. 1996. Late-afternoon ethanol intake affects nocturnal sleep and the sleep EEG in middle-aged men. *Journal of Clinical Psychopharmacology* 16(6):428–436.

4. Okawa M et al. 1990. Vitamin B12 treatment for sleep-wake rhythm disorders. *Sleep* 13(1):15–23.

Mayer G et al. 1996. Effects of vitamin B12 on performance and circadian rhythm in normal subjects. *Neuropsychopharmacology* 15(5):456–464.

5. Mennini T et al. 1993. In vitro study on the interaction of extracts and pure compounds from Valerian officinalis root with GABA, benzodiazepine and barbiturate receptors. *Fitoterapia* 64:291–300.

6. Lindahl O et al. 1989. Double-blind study of a valerian preparation. *Pharmacology Biochemistry and Behaviour* 32:1065–1066.

Leathwood PD et al. 1982. Aqueous extract of valerian root improves sleep quality in man. *Pharmacology Biochemistry and Behaviour* 17:65–71.

———. 1985. Aqueous extract of valerian root reduces latency to fall asleep in man. *Planta Med* 51:144–148.

7. Vorbach EU et al. 1996. Therapie von Insomnien: Wirksamkeit und vertaglichkeit eines Baldrian-Praparates. *Psychopharmakotherapie* 3:109–115.

6 Mood Swings

1. Carranza-Lira S et al. 1997. Changes in sympto-matology, hormones, lipids and bone density after hysterectomy. *International Journal of Fertility and Women's Medicine* 42(1):43–47.

    Crosognani PG et al. 1997. Endometrial resection versus vaginal hysterectomy for menorrhagia: long-term clinical and quality of life outcomes. *American Journal of Obstetrics and Gynecology* 177(1):95–101.

2. Wurtman RJ and Wurtman JJ. 1996. Brain sero-tonin, carbohydrate craving, obesity and depres-sion. *Advances in Experimental Medicine and Biology* 398:35–41.

    Wurtman JJ. 1993. Depression and weight gain: the serotonin connection. *Journal of Affective Disorders* 29(2–3):183–192.

    Christensen L. 1993. Effects of eating behaviour on mood: a review of the literature. *International Journal of Eating Disorders* 14(2):171–183.

    Blum I et al. 1992. The influence of meal compo-sition on plasma serotonin and norepinephrine concentrations. *Metabolism* 41(2):137–140.

    Sayegh R et al. 1995. The effect of a carbohydrate-rich beverage on mood, appetite, and cognitive function in women with premenstrual syndrome. *Obstetrics and Gynecology* 86(4 pt 1):520–528.

3. Macdiarmid JI and MM Hetherington. 1995. Mood modulation by food: an exploration of affect and cravings in 'chocolate addicts.' *British Journal of Clinical Psychology* 34(pt 1):129–138.

4. Di Tomaso E at al. 1996. Brain cannibinoids in chocolate. *Nature* 382:677–678.

5. Edwards R et al. 1998. Omega-3 polyunsaturated fatty acid levels in the diet and red blood cell membranes of depressed patients. *Journal of Affective Disorders* 48(2–3):149–155.

6. Stoll AL et al. 1999. Omega 3 fatty acids in bipolar disorder: a preliminary double-blind, placebo controlled trial. *Archives of General Psychiatry* 56(5):407–412.

7. McCullough A et al. 1990. Vitamin B6 status of Egyptian mothers: relation to infant behaviour and maternal-infant interactions. *Am J Clin Nutr* 51:1067–1074.

    Wyatt KM et al. 1999. Efficacy of vitamin B6 in the treatment of premenstrual syndrome: systematic review. *British Medical Journal* 318(7195):1375–1381.

8. Linde K et al. 1996. St. John's Wort for depres-sion—an overview and meta-analysis of random-ized clinical trials. *British Medical Journal* 313:253–258.

    Laakmann G et al. 1998. St. John's Wort in mild to moderate depression: the relevance of hyperforin for the clinical efficacy. *Pharmacopsychiatry* 31(suppl.):54S–59S.

    Schellenberg R et al. 1998. Pharmacodynamic effects of two different hypericum extracts in healthy volunteers measured by quantitative EEG. *Pharmacopsychiatry* 31(suppl.):44S–53S.

9. Kinzler et al. 1991. Wirksamkeit eines Kava-Spezial-Extraktes bei Patienten mit Angst-, Spannungs- and Erregungszuständen nicht-psychotischer Genese. *Arzneim Forsch/Drug Research* 41:584–588.

    Warnecke G et al. 1990. Wirksamkeit von Kawa-Kawa-Extrakt beim klimakterischen Syndrom. *Phytotherapie* 11:81–86.

7 Forgetfulness and Fuzzy Thinking

1. Polo-Kantola P et al. 1998. The effect of short-term estrogen replacement therapy on cognition: a randomized, double-blind, cross-over trial in post-menopausal women. *Obstetrics and Gynecology* 91(3):459–466.

2. Sherwin BB. 1998. Estrogen and cognitive functioning in women. *Proc Soc Exp Biol Med* 217(1):17–22.

    Yaffe K et al. 1998. Estrogen therapy in post-menopausal women: effects on cognitive function and dementia. *Journal of the American Medical Association* 279(9):688–695.

    Waring SC et al. 1999. Postmenopausal estrogen replacement therapy and the risk of AD: a population-based study. *Neurology* 52(5):965–970.

    Baldereschi M et al. 1998. Estrogen-replacement therapy and Alzheimer's disease in the Italian Longitudinal Study on Aging. *Neurology* 50(4):996–1002.

    Asthana S et al. 1999. Cognitive and neuro-endocrine response to a transdermal estrogen in postmenopausal women with Alzheimer's disease: results of a placebo-controlled, double-blind, pilot study. *Psychoneuroendocrinology* 24(6):657–677.

3. Smith A et al. 1994. Effects of breakfast and caf-feine on cognitive performance, mood and cardiovascular functioning. *Appetite* 22(1):39–55.

4. Lombard CB. 2000. What is the role of food in preventing depression and improving mood, performance and cognitive function? *Med J Aust* 173(suppl):104S–105S.

Benton D and Parker PY. 1998. Breakfast, blood glucose, and cognition. *Am J Clin Nutr* 67(suppl):772S–778S.

5. Le Bars PL et al. 1997. A placebo-controlled, double-blind, randomized trial of an extract of Ginkgo biloba for dementia. North American EGb Study Group. *JAMA* 278(16):1327–1332.

6. Wesnes KA et al. 2000. The memory-enhancing effects of a Ginkgo biloba/Panax ginseng combination in healthy middle-aged volunteers. *Psychopharmacology* (Berl). 152(4):353–361.

    Stough C et al. 2001. Neuropsychological changes after 30-day Ginkgo biloba administration in healthy participants. *Int J Neuropsychopharmacol* 4(2):131–134.

    Mix JA et al. 2002. A double-blind, placebo-controlled, randomized trial of Ginkgo biloba extract EGb 761(R) in a sample of cognitively intact older adults: neuropsychological findings. *Hum Psychopharmacol* 17(6):267–277.

    Solomon PR et al. 2002. Ginkgo for memory enhancement: a randomized controlled trial. *JAMA* 288(7):835–840.

7. ——. 1988. *Ginkoglides: Chemistry, Biology, Pharmacology and Clinical Perspectives.* Volume I. Barcelona: JR Prous Science.

    Braquet P (ed). 1989. *Ginkoglides: Chemistry, Biology, Pharmacology and Clinical Perspectives.* Volume II. Barcelona: JR Prous Science.

    Itil TM et al. 1996. Central nervous system effects of Gingko biloba, a plant extract. *American Journal of Therapeutics* 3:63–73.

8 Vaginal and Bladder Changes

1. Sarrel P et al. 1998. Estrogen and estrogen-androgen replacement in postmenopausal women dissatisfied with estrogen therapy. Sexual behaviour and neuroendocrine responses. *Journal of Reproductive Medicine* 43(10):847–856.

    Warnock JK et al. 1999. Female hypoactive sexual disorder: case studies of physiologic androgen replacement. *Journal of Sex and Marital Therapy* 25(3):175–182.

    Simon J et al. 1999. Differential effects of estrogen-androgen and estrogen-only therapy on vasomotor symptoms, gonadotropin secretion, and endogenous androgen bioavailability in post-menopausal women. *Menopause* 6(2):138–146.

2. Brzezinski A et al. 1997. Short-term effects of phytoestrogen-rich diet on postmenopausal women. *Journal of the North American Menopause Society* 4(2):89–94.

    Washburn S et al. 1999. Effect of soy protein supplementation on serum lipoproteins, blood pressure, and menopausal symptoms in perimenopausal women. *Menopause* 6(1):7–13.

    Baird DD et al. 1995. Dietary intervention study to assess estrogenicity of dietary soy among postmenopausal women. *Journal of Clinical Endocrinology and Metabolism* 80(5):1685–1690.

3. Avron J et al. 1994. Reduction of bacteriuria and pyuria after ingestion of cranberry juice. *JAMA* 271:751–754.

4. Punnonen R and Lukola A. 1980. Oestrogen-like effect of ginseng. *British Medical Journal* 281(6248):1110.

5. Hirata JD et al. 1997. Does dong quai have estrogenic effects in postmenopausal women? A double-blind, placebo-controlled trial. *Fertility and Sterility* 68(6):981–986.

6. Balon R. 1999. Ginkgo biloba for antidepressant-induced sexual dysfunction? *Journal of Sex and Marital Therapy* 25(1):1–2.

10 Preventing Weight Gain

1. Reubinoff BE et al. 1995. Effects of hormone replacement therapy on weight, body composition, fat distribution and food intake in early post-menopausal women. *Fertility and Sterility* 64(5):963–968.

2. Ferrara CM et al. 2002. Differences in adipose tissue metabolism between postmenopausal and peri-menopausal women. *J Clin Endocrinol Metab* 87(9):4166–4170.

3. Field AE et al. 2001. Impact of overweight on the risk of developing common chronic diseases during a 10-year period. *Arch Intern Med* 161(13):1581–1586.

4. Holt SH et al. 1995. A satiety index of common foods. *European Journal of Clinical Nutrition* 49(9):675–690.

5. Ludwig DS et al. 1999. High-glycemic index foods, overeating, and obesity. *Pediatrics* 103(3):E26.

6. Klem ML et al. 2000. Does weight loss maintenance become easier over time? *Obes Research* 8(6):438–444.

    McGuire MT et al. 1999. Behavioural strategies of individuals who have maintained long-term weight losses. *Obes Research* 7(4):334–341.

7. Walker LS et al. 1998. Chromium picolinate effects on body composition and muscular performance in wrestlers. *Medicine Science and Sports Exercise* 39(12):1730–1737.

   Trent LK and Thieding-Cancel D. 1995. Effects of chromium picolinate on body composition. *Journal of Medicine and Physical Fitness* 35(4):273–180.

8. Hoeger WW et al. 1998. Four-week supplementation with a natural dietary compound produces favorable changes in body composition. *Advances in Therapeutics* 15(5):305–314.

   Grant KE et al. 1997. Chromium and exercise training: effects on obese women. *Medicine Science in Sports and Exercise* 29(8):992–998.

9. Colker CM et al. 1999. Effects of Citrus aurantium extract, caffeine, and St. John's wort on body fat loss, lipid levels, and mood states in overweight healthy adults. *Current Therapeutic Research* 60(3):145–153.

10. Blankson H et al. Effects of conjugated linoleic acid (CLA) on body fat mass in overweight or obese human volunteers: a double-blind randomized placebo controlled study. American Chemical Society 220th National Meeting, Washington, DC; August 20–24, 2000. [Abstract 23]

    Anon. Linoleic Acid Supplements May Help Dieting Adults Keep Weight off. Reuters Health. URL: www.medscape.com/reuters/prof/2000/08/08.22/20000822drgd003.html (August 22, 2000).

11. Heymsfield SB et al. 1998. Garcinia cambogia (hydroxycitric acid) as a potential antiobesity agent: a randomized controlled trial. *JAMA* 280(18):1596–1600.

11 Reducing Your Risk of Osteoporosis

1. Cornuz J et al. 1999. Smoking, smoking cessation, and risk of hip fracture in women. *American Journal of Medicine* 106(3):311–314.

   Hollenbach KA et al. 1993. Cigarette smoking and bone mineral density in older men and women. *American Journal of Public Health* 83(9):1265–1270.

   Egger P et al. 1996. Cigarette smoking and bone mineral density in the elderly. *Journal of Epidemiology and Community Health* 50(1):47–50.

2. Brown JP et al. 2002. 2002 Clinical practice guidelines for the diagnosis and management of osteoporosis in Canada. *CMAJ* 167(10 suppl): 1S–34S.

3. Kiel DP et al. 1987. Hip fracture and the use of estrogens in postmenopausal women. The Framingham Study. *New England Journal of Medicine* 317(19):1169–1174.

4. Writing Group for the Women's Health Initiative Investigators. 2002. Risks and benefits of estrogen plus progestin in healthy postmenopausal women: principal results from the Women's Health Initiative randomized controlled trial. *JAMA* 288(3):321–333.

5. Recker RR et al. 1999. The effect of low-dose continuous estrogen and progesterone therapy with calcium and vitamin D in elderly women. A randomized, controlled trial. *Annals of Internal Medicine* 130(11):897–904.

6. van Staa TP et al. 1998. Use of cyclical etidronate and prevention of non-vertebral fractures. *British Journal of Rheumatology* 37(1):87–94.

   Lyritis GP et al. 1997. The effect of a modified etidronate cyclical regimen on postmenopausal osteoporosis: a four-year study. *Clinical Rheumatology* 16(4):354–360.

7. Hosking D et al. 1998. Prevention of bone loss with Alendronate in postmenopausal women under 60 years of age. *New England Journal of Medicine* 338(8):485–492.

8. Black DM et al. 1996. Randomised trial of effect of alendronate on risk of fracture in women with existing vertebral fractures. Fracture Intervention Trial Research Group. *Lancet* 348:1535–1541.

9. Lufkin EG et al. 1998. Treatment of established postmenopausal osteoporosis with raloxifene: a randomized trial. *Journal of Bone Mineral Research* 13(11):1747–1754.

10. Ettinger B et al. 1999. Reduction of vertebral fracture risk in postmenopausal women with osteoporosis treated with raloxifene: Results from a 3-year randomized clinical trial. *JAMA* 282:637–645.

11. Potter SM et al. 1998. Soy protein and isoflavones: their effects on blood lipids and bone density in postmenopausal women. *Am J Clin Nutr* 68(suppl):1375S–1379S.

    Schieber MD et al. 1999. Dietary soy isoflavones favorably influence lipids and bone turnover in healthy postmenopausal women. Abstract. Third International Symposium on the Role of Soy in Preventing and Treating Chronic Disease.

12. Munger RG et al. 1999. Prospective study of dietary protein intake and risk of hip fracture in

menopausal women. *Am J Clin Nutr* 69(1):147–152.

Schurch MA et al. 1998. Protein supplements increase serum insulin-like growth factor-I levels and attenuate proximal femur bone loss in patients with recent hip fracture. A randomized, double-blind, placebo-controlled trial. *Annals of Internal Medicine* 128(10):801–809.

13. Position of the American Dietetic Association, Dietitians of Canada, and the American College of Sports Medicine: Nutrition and athletic performance. 2000. *J Am Diet Assoc* 100(12):1543–1556.

Manual of Clinical Dietetics. Sixth edition. The American Dietetic Association. Chicago, Illinois, 2000.

14. Feskanich D et al. 1999. Moderate alcohol consumption and bone density among postmenopausal women. *Journal of Women's Health* 8(1):65–73.

15. Lloyd T et al. 1997. Dietary caffeine intake and bone status of postmenopausal women. *Am J Clin Nutr* 65(6):1826–1830.

Harris SS and Dawson-Hughes B. 1994. Caffeine and bone loss in healthy menopausal women. *Am J Clin Nutr* 60(4):573–578.

16. Devine A et al. 1995. A longitudinal study of the effect of sodium and calcium intakes on regional bone density in postmenopausal women. *Am J Clin Nutr* 62(4):740–745.

17. Baran D et al. 1990. Dietary modification with dairy products for preventing vertebral bone loss in premenopausal women: a three-year prospective study. *Journal of Clinical Endocrinology and Metabolism* 70(1):264–270.

18. Sakhaee K et al. 1998. The effect of calcium citrate on bone density in the early and mid–postmenopausal period: a randomized, placebo-controlled study. Abstract. The Second Joint Meeting of the American Society for Bone and Mineral Research and the International Bone and Mineral Society. Mission Pharmacal Company.

Baran DT et al. 1999. A placebo-controlled study of pre-menopausal women: calcium supplementation and bone density. Abstract. Annual Meeting of the American Society for Bone and Mineral Research.

Storm D et al. 1998. Calcium supplementation prevents seasonal bone loss and changes in biochemical markers of bone turnover in elderly New England women: a randomized placebo-controlled trial. *Journal of Clinical Endocrinology and Metabolism* 83(11):3817–3825.

Ricci TA et al. 1998. Calcium supplementation suppresses bone turnover during weight reduction in postmenopausal women. *Journal of Bone Mineral Research* 13(6):1045–1050.

19. Harris SS and Dawson-Hughes B. 1998. Seasonal changes in plasma 25-hydroxyvitamin D concentrations of young American black and white women. *Am J Clin Nutr* 67(6):1232–1236.

20. Brown JP et al. 2002. 2002 Clinical practice guidelines for the diagnosis and management of osteoporosis in Canada. *CMAJ 67* (10 suppl):1S–34S.

21. Feskanich D et al. 2002. High vitamin A intakes can increase hip fracture risk in postmenopausal women. *JAMA* 287(2):47–54.

22. Michaelsson K et al. 2003. Serum retinol levels and the risk of fracture. *N Eng J Med* 348(4):287–349

23. Promislow JH et al. 2002. Retinol intake and bone mineral density in the elderly; the Rancho Bernardo Study. *J Bone Miner Res* 17(8):1349–58.

24. Feskanich D et al. 1999. Vitamin K intake and hip fractures in women: a prospective study. *Am J Clin Nutr* 69(1):74–79.

25. Strause L et al. 1994. Spinal bone loss in postmenopausal women supplemented with calcium and trace minerals. *Journal of Nutrition* 124(7):1060–1064.

26. Wolff I et al. 1999. The effect of exercise training programs on bone mass: a meta-analysis of published controlled trials in pre- and postmenopausal women. *Osteoporosis International* 9(1):1–12.

Dalsky GP et al. 1988. Weight-bearing exercise training and lumbar bone mineral content in postmenopausal women. *Annals of Internal Medicine* 108(6):824–828.

Pruitt LA et al. 1992. Weight-training effects on bone mineral density in early postmenopausal women. *Journal of Bone Mineral Research* 7(2):179–185.

12 Reducing Your Risk of Heart Disease

1. Heart and Stroke Foundation of Canada. 1995. *Heart Disease and Stroke in Canada, 1995.* Ottawa.

Smurawska LT et al. 1994. Cost of acute stroke care in Toronto, Canada. Stroke 25(8):1628–1631.

Wingate S. 1995. Quality of life for women after a myocardial infarction. *Heart and Lung* 24(6):467–473.

2. Connelly PW et al. 1992. Canadian Heart Health Surveys Research Group. Plasma lipids and lipoproteins and the prevalence of risk for coronary heart disease in Canadian adults. *Canadian Medical Association Journal* 146(11):1977–1987.

Health Canada. 1995. *Canadians and Heart Health: Reducing the Risk*. Ottawa.

La Rosa JC. 1992. Lipids and cardiovascular disease: do the findings and therapy apply equally to men and women? *Women's Health Issues* 2(2):102–111.

Austin MA. 1989. Plasma triglyceride as a risk factor for coronary heart disease: the epidemiologic evidence and beyond. *American Journal of Epidemiology* 129:249–259.

3. Kinosian B et al. 1994. Cholesterol and coronary heart disease predicting risks by ratios and levels. *Annals of Internal Medicine* 121:641–647.

4. Kawachi I et al. 1994. Smoking cessation and time course of decreased risks of coronary heart disease in middle-aged women. *Archives of Internal Medicine* 154(2):169–175.

Kawachi I et al. 1993. Smoking cessation in relation to total mortality rates in women. A prospective cohort study. *Annals of Internal Medicine* 119(10):992–1000.

5. Kannel WB and McGee DL. 1979. Diabetes and cardiovascular disease. The Framingham Study. *JAMA* 241:2035–2038.

6. Health Canada. 1995. *Canadians and Heart Health: Reducing the Risk*. Ottawa.

7. Rexrode KM et al. 1998. Abdominal adiposity and coronary heart disease in women. *Journal of the American Heart Association* 280(21):1843–1848.

8. Boers GH et al. 1985. Heterozygosity for homocystinuria in premature peripheral and cerebral occlusive arterial disease. *New England Journal of Medicine* 313(12):709–715.

Whincup PH et al. 1999. Serum total homocysteine and coronary heart disease: prospective study in middle aged men. *Heart* 82(4):448–454.

Bots ML et al. 1999. Homocysteine and short-term risk of myocardial infarction and stroke in the elderly: the Rotterdam Study. *Arch Intern Medicine* 159(1):38–44.

Arnesen E et al. 1995. Serum total homocysteine and coronary heart disease. *International Journal of Epidemiology* 24(4):704–709.

Ridker PM et al. 1999. Homocysteine and risk of cardiovascular disease among postmenopausal women. *JAMA* 281(19):1817–1821.

9. Heart and Stoke Foundation. 1999. Annual Report Card on Canadians' Health. Toronto.

10. Stallones RA. 1983. Ischemic heart disease and lipids in the blood and diet. *Annual Reviews of Nutrition* 3:155–185.

Stamler J. 1979. Population studies pp. 25–88 in Levy RJ et al., eds. Nutrition, Lipids and Coronary Heart Disease: A Global View. *Nutrition in Health and Disease*, Vol. 1. New York: Raven Press.

11. Hu FB et al. 1997. Dietary fat intake and the risk of coronary heart disease in women. *New England Journal of Medicine* 337(21):1491–1499.

Willett WC et al. 1993. Intake of trans fatty acids and risk of coronary heart disease among women. *Lancet* 341(8845):581–585.

Tavani A et al. 1997. Margarine intake and risk of nonfatal acute myocardial infarction in Italian women. *European Journal of Clinical Nutrition* 51(1):30–32.

12. Rogers AE et al. 1986. Chemically induced mammary gland tumors in rats: modulation by dietary fat. *Progress in Clinical Biology Research* 222:255–282.

13. Albert CM et al. 1998. Fish consumption and the risk of sudden cardiac death. *JAMA* 279(1):23–28.

Daviglus ML et al. 1997. Fish consumption and the 30-year risk of fatal myocardial infarction. *New England Journal of Medicine* 336(15):1046–1053.

Menotti A et al. 1999. Food intake patterns and 25-year mortality from coronary heart disease: cross-cultural correlations in the Seven Countries Study. The Seven Countries Study Research Group. *European Journal of Epidemiology* 15(6):507–515.

14. Hu FB et al. 1999. Dietary intake of alpha-linolenic acid and risk of fatal ischemic heart disease among women. *Am J Clin Nutr* 69(5):890–897.

15. Larsen LF et al. 1999. Are olive oil diets antithrombotic? Diets enriched with olive, rapeseed, or sunflower oil affect postprandial factor VII differently. *Am J Clin Nutr* 70(6):976–982.

Lindholm LH et al. 1992. Risk factors for ischemic heart disease in a Greek population. A cross-sectional study of men and women living in the village of Spili in Crete. *European Heart Journal* 13(3):291–298.

16. De Lorgeril M et al. 1999. Mediterranean diet, traditional risk factors, and the rate of cardiovascular complications after myocardial infarction: final report of the Lyon Diet Heart Study. *Circulation* 99(6):779–785.

17. Hu FB et al. 1999. A prospective study of egg consumption and risk of cardiovascular disease in men and women. *JAMA* 281(15):1387–1394.

18. Anderson JW et al. 1995. Meta-analysis of the effects of soy protein intake on serum lipids. *New England Journal of Medicine* 333(5):276–282.

    Washburn S et al. 1999. Effect of soy protein supplementation on serum lipoproteins, blood pressure, and menopausal symptoms in perimenopausal women. *Menopause* 6(1):7–13.

    Crouse JR et al. 1999. A randomized trial comparing the effect of casein with that of soy protein containing varying amounts of isoflavones on plasma concentrations of lipids and lipoproteins. *Archives of Internal Medicine* 159(17):2070–2076.

    Schieber MD et al. 1999. Dietary soy isoflavones favorably influence lipids and bone turnover in healthy postmenopausal women. Abstract. Third International Symposium on the Role of Soy in Preventing and Treating Chronic Disease.

    Han KK et al. 2002. Benefits of soy isoflavone therapeutic regimen on menopausal symptoms. *Obstet Gynecol* 99(3):389–394.

    Wilcox JN and Blumenthal BF. 1995. Thrombotic mechanism in atherosclerosis: potential impact of soy proteins. *Journal of Nutrition* 125(3 suppl):631S–638S.

19. Jenkins DJ et al. 2000. The effect on serum lipids and oxidized low-density lipoprotein of supplementing self-selected low-fat diets with soluble-fiber, soy, and vegetable protein foods. *Metabolism* 49(1):67–72.

20. MacKay S and MJ Ball. 1992. Do beans and oat bran add to the effectiveness of a low fat diet? *European Journal of Clinical Nutrition* 46(9):641–648.

    Braaten JT et al. 1994. Oat beta-glucan reduces blood cholesterol concentration in hypercholesterolemic subjects. *European Journal of Clinical Nutrition* 48(7):465–474.

    Uusitupa MI et al. 1992. A controlled study of the effect of beta-glucan rich oat bran on serum lipids in hyercholesterolemic subjects: relation to

apolipoprotein E phenotype. *Journal of American Coll Nutrition* 11(6):651–659.

Whyte JL et al. 1992. Oat bran lowers plasma cholesterol levels in mildly hypercholesterolemic men. *Journal of the American Dietetic Association* 92(4):446–449.

Davidson MH et al. 1991. The hypocholesterolemic effects of beta-glucan in oatmeal and oat bran. A dose-controlled study. *Journal of the American Dietetic Association* 265(14):1833–1939.

Olson BH et al. 1997. Psyllium-enriched cereals lower blood total cholesterol and LDL cholesterol, but not HDL cholesterol, in hypercholesterolemic adults: results of a meta-analysis. *Journal of Nutrition* 127(10):1973–1980.

21. Liu S et al. 1999. Whole-grain consumption and risk of coronary heart disease: results from the Nurses' Health Study. *Am J Clin Nutr* 70(3):412–419.

    Jacobs DR Jr. et al. 1998. Whole-grain intake may reduce the risk of ischemic heart disease death in postmenopausal women: the Iowa Women's Health Study. *Am J Clin Nutr* 68(2):248–257.

22. Hu FB et al. 1998. Frequent nut consumption and risk of coronary heart disease in women: prospective cohort study. *British Medical Journal* 317(7169):1341–1345.

    Jenkins DJ et al. 2002. Dose response of almonds on coronary heart disease risk factors: blood lipids, oxidized low-density lipoproteins, lipoprotein(a), homocysteine, and pulmonary nitric oxide: a randomized, controlled, crossover trial. *Circulation* 106(11):1327–1332.

    Lavedrine F et al. 1999. Blood cholesterol and walnut consumption: a cross–sectional survey in France. *Preventative Medicine* 28(4):333–339.

23. Sesso HD et al. 1999. Coffee and tea intake and the risk of myocardial infarction. *American Journal of Epidemiology* 149(2):162–167.

    Yochum L et al. 1999. Dietary flavonoids and risk of cardiovascular disease in postmenopausal women. *American Journal of Epidemiology* 149(10):943–949.

24. Geleijnse JM et al. 1999. Tea flavonoids may protect against atherosclerosis: the Rotterdam Study. *Archives of Internal Medicine* 159(18):2170–2174.

    Hertog MG et al. 1993. Dietary antioxidant flavonoids and risk of coronary heart disease: the Zutphen Elderly Study. *Lancet* 342(8878):1007–1011.

25. Hankinson SE et al. 1995. Alcohol consumption and mortality among women. *New England Journal of Medicine* 332(19):1245–1250.

    Gaziano JM et al. 1993. Moderate alcohol intake, increased levels of high-density lipoprotein and its subfractions, and decreased risk of myocardial infarction. *New England Journal of Medicine* 329(25):1829–1834.

    Muntwyler J et al. 1998. Mortality and light to moderate alcohol consumption after myocardial infarction. *Lancet* 352(9144):1882–1885.

26. Appel LJ et al. 1997. A clinical trial of the effects of dietary patterns on blood pressure. *New England Journal of Medicine* 65(suppl):643S–651S.

27. Rimm EB et al. 1998. Folate and vitamin B6 from diet and supplements in relation to risk of coronary heart disease among women. *JAMA* 279(5):359–364.

28. Nyyssonen K et al. 1997. Vitamin C deficiency and risk of myocardial infarction: prospective study in men from eastern Finland. *British Journal of Medicine* 314(7081):634–638.

    Lopes C et al. 1998. Diet and risk of myocardial infarction. A case-control community-based study. *Acta Med Port* 11(4):311–317.

    Simon JA et al. 1998. Serum ascorbic acid and cardiovascular disease prevalence. *Epidemiology* 9(3):316–321.

29. Gatto LM et al. 1996. Ascorbic acid induces favorable lipid profiles in women. *Journal of the American College of Nutrition* 15:154–158.

    Ness AR et al. 1996. Vitamin C status and serum lipids. *European Journal of Clinical Nutrition* 50:724–729.

    Bordia A et al. 1980. The effect of vitamin C on blood lipids, fibrinolytic activity and platelet adhesiveness in patients with coronary heart disease. *Atherosclerosis* 35:1810–1817.

    Calzada C et al. 1997. The influence of antioxidant nutrients on platelet function in healthy volunteers. *Atherosclerosis* 128:97–105.

30. Stampfer MJ et al. 1993. Vitamin E consumption and the risk of coronary disease in women. *New England Journal of Medicine* 328(20):1444–1449.

    Rimm EB et al. 1993. Vitamin E consumption and the risk of coronary heart disease in men. *New England Journal of Medicine* 328(20):1450–1456.

    Meyer F et al. 1996. Lower ischemic heart disease incidence and mortality among vitamin supplement users. *Canadian Journal of Cardiology* 12(10):930–934.

    Stephens NG et al. 1996. Randomised controlled trial of vitamin E in patients with coronary heart disease. *Cambridge Heart Antioxidant Study* 347(9004):781–786.

31. Waters DD et al. 2002. Effects of hormone replacement therapy and antioxidant vitamin supplements on coronary atherosclerosis in post-menopausal women: a randomized controlled trial. *JAMA* 288(19):2432–2440.

32. Kohlmeier L et al. 1997. Lycopene and myocardial infarction risk in the EURAMIC Study. *American Journal of Epidemiology* 146(8):618–626.

    Street DA et al. 1994. Serum antioxidants and myocardial infarction. Are low levels of carotenoids and alpha-tocopherol risk factors for myocardial infarction? *Circulation* 90(3):1154–1161.

    Su LC et al. 1998. Differences between plasma and adipose tissue biomarkers of carotenoids and tocopherols. *Cancer Epidemiol Biomarkers Prev* 7(11):1043–1048.

    Agarwal S and Rao AV. 1998. Tomato lycopene and low density lipoprotein oxidation: a human dietary intervention study. *Lipids* 33 (10):981–984.

33. Fuhrman B et al. 1997. Hypocholesterolemic effect of lycopene and beta–carotene is related to suppression of cholesterol synthesis and augmentation of LDL receptor activity in macrophages. *Biochemistry and Biophysiology Research Communications* 233:658–662.

34. Kontush A et al. 1997. Plasma ubiquinol-10 is decreased in patients with hyperlipidemia. *Atherosclerosis* 129(1):119–126.

35. Mortensen SA et al. 1997. Dose-related decrease of serum coenzyme Q10 during treatment with HMG-CoA reductase inhibitors. *Molecular Aspects of Medicine* 18(suppl):137S–144S.

36. Sing RB et al. 1999. Serum concentration of lipoprotein(a) decreases on treatment with hydrosoluble coenzyme Q10 in patients with coronary artery disease: discovery of a new role. *International Journal of Cardiology* 68(1):23–29.

    Singh RB et al. 1998. Randomized, double-blind placebo-controlled trial of coenzyme Q10 in patients with acute myocardial infarction. *Cardiovascular Drug Therapy* 12(4):347–353.

37. Steiner M et al. 1996. A double-blind crossover study in moderately hypercholesterolemic men that compared the effect of aged garlic extract and placebo administration on blood lipids. *Am J Clin Nutr* 64(6):866–870.

Holzgartner H et al. 1992. Comparison of the efficacy and tolerance of a garlic preparation vs. bezafibrate. *Arzeimittelforschung* 42(12):1473–1477.

Bordia A. 1981. Effects of garlic on blood lipids in patients with coronary heart disease. *Am J Clin Nutr* 34(10):2100–2103.

Bordia A et al. 1998. Effect of garlic (Allium sativum) on blood lipids, blood sugar, fibrinogen and fibrinolytic activity in patients with coronary artery disease. *Prostaglandins Leukotrienes and Essential Fatty Acids* 58(4):257–263.

Ide N and Lau BH. 1999. Aged garlic extract attenuates intracellular oxidative stress. *Phytomedicine* 6(2):125–131.

Ide N and Lau BH. 1997. Garlic compounds protect vascular endothelial cells from oxidized low-density lipoprotein-induced injury. *Journal of Pharmacy and Pharmacology* 49(9):908–911.

38. Song K and Milner J. 1999. Heating garlic inhibits its ability to suppress 7,12-dimethylbenz(a) anthracene-induced DNA adduct formation in rat mammary tissue. *Journal of Nutrition* 129(3):657–661.

39. Singh RB et al. 1994. Hypolipidemic and antioxidant effects of Commiphora mukul as an adjunct to dietary therapy in patients with hypercholesterolemia. *Cardiovascular Drug Therapy* 8(4):659–664.

13 Reducing Your Risk of Breast Cancer

1. Writing Group for the Women's Health Initiative Investigators. 2002. Risks and benefits of estrogen plus progestin in healthy postmenopausal women: principal results from the Women's Health Initiative randomized controlled trial. *JAMA* 288(3):321–333.

2. Miller AB et al. 1997. The Canadian National Breast Screening Study: update on breast cancer mortality. *Journal of National Cancer Institute Monograms* 22:37–41.

3. World Cancer Research Fund/American Institute for Cancer Research. 1997. *Food, Nutrition and the Prevention of Cancer: A Global Perspective.* Washington DC: American Institute for Cancer Research.

4. Hursting SD et al. 1990. Types of dietary fat and the incidence of cancer at 5 sites. *Preventative Medicine* 19:242–253.

    Rose DP et al. 1986. International comparisons of mortality rates for cancer of the breast, ovary, prostate and colon and per capita food consumption. *Cancer* 58:2263–2271.

    Woods MN et al. 1989. Low fat, high fibre diet and serum estrone sulfate in premenopausal women. *Am J Clin Nutr* 49:1179–1193.

    Prentice RL et al. 1988. Aspects of the rationale for the Women's Health Trial. *Journal of the National Cancer Institute* 80:802–814.

5. Boyd NF et al. 1993. A meta-analysis of studies of dietary-fat and breast cancer risk. *British Journal of Cancer* 68:627–636.

    Holmes MD et al. 1999. Association of dietary fat and fatty acids with risk of breast cancer. *JAMA* 281(10):914–920.

    Wu AH et al. 1999. Meta-analysis: dietary fat intake, serum estrogen levels, and the risk of breast cancer. *Journal of the National Cancer Institute.* 91(6):520–534.

6. Boyd NF et al. 1997. Effects at two years of a low fat, high carbohydrate diet on radiologic features of the breast: results from a randomized trial. Canadian Diet and Breast Cancer Prevention Study Group. *Journal of the National Cancer Institute* 89(7):488–496.

    Boyd NF et al. 1997. Effects of a low fat, high carbohydrate diet on plasma sex hormones in premenopausal women: results from a randomized trial. Canadian Diet and Breast Cancer Prevention Study Group. *British Journal of Cancer* 76(1):127–135.

7. Zheng W et al. 1998. Well-done meat intake and the risk of breast cancer. *Journal of the National Cancer Institute* 90(22):1724–1729.

8. Knekt P et al. 1996. Intake of dairy products and the risk of breast cancer. *British Journal of Cancer* 73(5):687–691.

    Ip MM et al. 1999. Conjugated linoleic acid inhibits proliferation and induces apoptosis of normal rat mammary epithelial cells in primary culture. *Experimental Cellular Research* 250(1):22–34.

    Thompson H et al. 1997. Morphological and biochemical status of the mammary glands as influenced by conjugated linoleic acid: implication for a reduction in mammary cancer risk. *Cancer Research* 57(22):5067–5072.

9. Rose DP et al. 1996. Effect of omega-3 fatty acids on the progression of metastases after surgical excision of human breast cancer cell solid tumors growing in nude mice. *Clinical Cancer Research* 2(10):1751–1756.

10. La Vecchia C et al. 1995. Olive oil, other dietary fats, and the risk of breast cancer (Italy). *Cancer Causes and Control* 6(6):545–550.

11. Lu LJ et al. 1996. Effects of soya consumption for one month on steroid hormones in premenopausal women: implications for breast cancer risk. *Cancer Epidemiol Biomarkers Prev* 5(1):63–70.

    Woods, M, 1999. Dietary soy supplement and menopausal hormones and hot flashes. Tufts University, Boston, Massachusetts. Abstract. Third International Symposium on Soy Foods in Treating and Preventing Chronic Disease.

    Cassidy A et al. 1993. Biological effects of plant oestrogens in premenopausal women. *FASEB Journal* 7:A866.

12. Wu AH et al. 2002. Adolescent and adult soy intake and risk of breast cancer in Asian-Americans. *Carcinogenesis* 23(9):1491–1496.

    Shu XO et al. 2001. Soyfood intake during adolescence and subsequent risk of breast cancer among Chinese women. *Cancer Epidemiol Biomarkers Prev* 10(5):483–488.

13. Li D et al. 1999. Soybean isoflavones reduce experimental metastasis in mice. *Journal of Nutrition* 129(5):1075–1078.

    Shao ZM et al. 1998. Genistein exerts multiple suppressive effects on human breast carcinoma cells. *Cancer Research* 58(21):4851–4857.

    Barnes S. 1997. The chemopreventative properties of soy isoflavonoids in animal models of breast cancer. *Breast Cancer Research and Treatment* 46(2–3):169–179.

    Hsieh CY et al. 1998. Estrogenic effects of genistein on the growth of estrogen receptor-positive human breast cancer (MCF-7) cells in vitro and in vivo. *Cancer Research* 58(17):3833–3838.

14. McMichal-Phillips DF et al. 1998. Effects of soy-protein supplementation on epithelial proliferation in the histologically normal human breast. *Am J Clin Nutr* 68(6 suppl):1431S–1435S.

15. Thompson LU et al. 1996. Flaxseed and its lignan and oil components reduce mammary tumor growth at a late stage of carcinogenesis. *Carcinogenesis* 17(6):1373–1376.

    Thompson LU et al. 1996. Antitumorigenic effect of a mammalian lignan precurser from flaxseed. *Nutrition and Cancer* 26(2):159–165.

16. Hunter DJ et al. 1993. A prospective study of intake of vitamin C, E and A and the risk of breast cancer. *New England Journal of Medicine* 329:234–240.

    Freudenheim JL et al. 1996. Premenopausal breast cancer risk and intake of vegetables, fruits and related nutrients. *Journal of the National Cancer Institute* 88(6):340–348.

17. Howe GR et al. 1990. Dietary factors and risk of breast cancer: combined analysis of 12 case-control studies. *Journal of the National Cancer Institute* 82:561–569.

    Bagga D et al. 1995. Effects of a very low fat, high fibre diet in serum hormones and menstrual function. Implications for breast cancer prevention. *Cancer* 76(12):2491–2496.

    Rose DP et al. 1997. Effects of diet supplementation with wheat bran on serum estrogen levels in the follicular and luteal phases of the menstrual cycle. *Nutrition* 13(6):535–539.

18. Van't Veer P et al. 1989. Consumption of fermented milk products and breast cancer: a case-control study in The Netherlands. *Cancer Research* 49(14):4020–4023.

    Biffi A et al. 1997. Antiproliferative effect of fermented milk on the growth of a human breast cancer cell line. *Nutrition and Cancer* 28(1):93–99.

19. Hunter DJ et al. 1992. A prospective study of caffeine, coffee, tea and breast cancer. *American Journal of Epidemiology* 136:1000–1001 (Abstract).

    Rogers AE et al. 1998. Black tea and mammary gland carcinogenesis by 7,12–dimethylbenz[a]anthracene in rats fed control or high fat diets. *Carcinogenesis* 19(7):1269–1273.

    Weisburger JH et al. 1997. Tea, or tea and milk, inhibit mammary gland and colon carcinogenesis in rats. *Cancer Letter* 114(1–2):323–327.

    Nakachi K et al. 1998. Influence of drinking green tea on breast cancer malignancy among Japanese patients. *Japanese Journal of Cancer Research* 89(3):254–261.

20. Cao G et al. 1997. Antioxidant capacity of tea and common vegetables. *Journal of Agriculture and Food Chemistry* 44(11):3426–3431.

21. Longnecker MP et al. 1994. Alcoholic beverage consumption in relation to risk of breast cancer: meta analysis and review. *Cancer Causes and Control* 5:73–82.

    Hankinson SE et al. 1995. Alcohol, height, and adiposity in relation to estrogen and prolactin levels in postmenopausal women. *Journal of the National Cancer Institute* 87(17):1297–1302.

22. Hirose K et al. 1999. Effect of body size on breast cancer risk among Japanese women. *International Journal of Cancer* 80(3):349–355.

Huang Z et al. 1997. Dual effects of weight and weight gain on breast cancer risk. *JAMA* 278(17):1407–1411.

La Vecchia C et al. 1997. Body mass index and post-menopausal breast cancer: an age-specific analysis. *British Journal of Cancer* 75(3):441–444.

23. Rohan TE et al. 1993. Dietary fibre, vitamins A, C, and E and the risk of breast cancer: a cohort study. *Cancer Causes and Control* 4:29–37.

Jain M and AB Miller. 1994. Premorbid diet and the prognosis of women with breast cancer. *Journal of the National Cancer Institute* 86(18):1390–1397.

Zhang S et al. 1999. Dietary carotenoids and vitamins A, C, and E and risk of breast cancer. *Journal of the National Cancer Institute* 91(6):547–556.

Rock CL et al. 1996. Carotenoids, vitamin A, and estrogen receptor status in breast cancer. *Nutrition and Cancer* 25(3):281–296.

24. Howe GR et al. 1990. Dietary factors and risk of breast cancer: combined analysis of 12 case-control studies. *Journal of the National Cancer Institute* 82:561–569.

25. Wu K et al. 1999. A prospective study on folate, B12, and pyridoxal-5'-phosphate (B6) and breast cancer. *Cancer Epidemiol Biomarkers Prev* 8(3):209–217.

26. Zhang S et al. 1999. A prospective study of folate intake and the risk of breast cancer. *JAMA* 281(17):1632–1637.

Index

body weight and, 181–82
cholesterol and (*see* cholesterol)
defined, 172
diabetes and, 181
diet and, 183–200
exercise and, 182–83
family history and, 175
heart attack and (*see* heart attacks)
herbal remedies and, 209–11
homocysteine levels and, 182
HRT and, 12–14
kinds of, 172
menopause, onset of, and, 175
postmenopause and, 3
process of, 172
recommendations for risk reduction, 211–13
reducing risk of, 170–213
risk factors, 170, 173–83
smoking and, 180–81
triglycerides and, 176–77
vitamins, minerals and, 200–9
herbal remedies
forgetfulness and, 73–75
garlic, 209–10
guggul, 210–11
heart disease and, 209–11
hot flashes and, 37–41
insomnia and, 49–50
menstrual cycle changes and, 91–92
mood swings and, 61–63
vaginal and bladder changes and, 82–85
weight gain and, 124–29
HERS, 13–14
high density lipoproteins. *See* HDL
homocysteine levels, 182
hormone replacement therapy. *See* HRT
hormones. *See also* estrogen; progesterone
bio-identical, 16, 17–18
blood tests for, 6–7
bone health and, 131–33
defined, 3
follicle stimulating (*see* FSH)
hot flashes and, 25–27
lutenizing (*see* LH)
menstrual cycle and, 4–6

synthetic (*see* Premarin; Provera)
hot flashes, 2, 24–29
alcohol and, 46
anatomy of, 24–25
causes of, 26–27
diet and, 28–35
ERT and, 11
estrogen and, 25, 29
guide to coping with, 27–28
herbal remedies, 37–41
hormones and, 25–27
recommendations for relieving, 42
HRT
bio-identical, 16, 17–18
breast cancer and, 220
compounded, 19
discontinuing, 15
estrogen, progestin and, 12
guidelines, 14–15
"natural," 16, 17, 18
osteoporosis and, 138–39
risk vs. benefits, 12–15
vitamins C and E and, 205
weight gains and, 96
Women's Health Initiative Hormone Study and, xi, 12–14
hydroxycitric acid, 126–27
hypothalamus, 26–27
hysterectomy
depression and, 53
hot flashes and, 24
premature menopause and, 3

induced menopause, 3
insomnia, 43–52
alcohol and, 45–47
caffeine and, 44–45
carbohydrates and, 47
chronic, 43, 44
diet and, 44–47
guide to coping with, 52
herbal remedies and, 49–50
vitamin B12 and, 47–49
insulin, body fat and, 102
iron, 70–73, 121–22